9.25

Mental handicap and community care

International Library of Social Policy

General Editor   Kathleen Jones
Professor of Social Administration
University of York

Arbor Scientiæ
Arbor Vitæ

Mental handicap and community care

A study of mentally handicapped people in Sheffield

Michael Bayley

Department of Sociological Studies
University of Sheffield

Routledge & Kegan Paul

London and Boston

First published in 1973
by Routledge & Kegan Paul Ltd
Broadway House, 68-74 Carter Lane,
London EC4V 5EL and
9 Park Street,
Boston, Mass. 02108, U.S.A.
Printed in Great Britain by
Western Printing Services Ltd, Bristol
© Michael Bayley 1973

ISBN 0 7100 7662 2

Library of Congress Catalog Card No. 73–81595

To Fleur

Contents

Preface   xix

1 Introduction   1
   Historical   1
   The ambiguity of 'community'   10
   *The face-to-face level of community is the basis on
   which all welfare services rest*   12
   *A consideration of the face-to-face level of
   community*   13
   A comprehensive basis for community care   19
   General method   20

Part I The files

2 The scope of the survey   27

3 A profile of the survey population   35
   Some basic definitions   35
   The mildly subnormal at home   37
   The mildly subnormal in hospital   40
   The severely subnormal at home   43
   The severely subnormal in hospital   44
   Prevalence   46

4 How the subnormal were reported   50
   The mildly subnormal   50
   The severely subnormal   54

5 Factors which precipitated admission to hospital   57
   Introduction   57
   Behaviour or management   58
   Death or illness of parent or parent figure   62
   Social reasons   64

Nursing problem   66
Other   67
The mildly and severely subnormal compared   67
*The factors precipitating admission of the mildly
subnormal and the age admitted*   67
*The factors precipitating admission of the severely
subnormal and the age admitted*   68
The definition of 'children'   70

6   Social class   71

Introduction   71
Some difficulties considered   71
*A consideration of the class distribution of the
subnormal*   74
Is social class related to admission to hospital?   80

7   Housing and money   82

Type of housing   82
Standard of housing   84
Money   87
Conclusions   90

8   The family background   91

Whom the subnormal was living with   91
Size of the household   97
Size of the subnormal's family   99
A look at the members of the subnormal's family   101
Some further details about the subnormal's family   110
Conclusions   113

9   The subnormals themselves   115

IQ and mongolism   115
The subnormals' physical abilities and disabilities   116
Dressing and feeding   122
Behaviour   123
Contact with the law   130
Supervision needed   132
The relative importance of the different factors   138
*The disabilities used as a basis for deciding whom
to visit*   143

10 The help and services the subnormals and their families received   145

Education   146
The careers of the mildly subnormal after school leaving age   150
The careers of the severely subnormal after school leaving age   154
Short-term care   160
Support from social workers   161
Other help   165
Conclusions   166

11 Findings from the files—some conclusions   167

The pattern of admission to hospital   167
Some general points   168

Part II   The visits

12 Introduction to the visits   175

13 The subnormal people who were visited   180

14 The attitude of the parents   186

Different attitudes   186
Whom the subnormal was living with   194
The importance of the subnormal's ability to communicate   195
The place of the subnormal in the family and the attitude of the parents   200
The long-term effect on the family   206

15 The daily grind   208

The daily routine   208
A structure for coping   228
The cost of keeping the structure intact   230
The break-up of the structure   234
Conclusion   235

16   The quality of life   236

    The restrictions on the parents   236
    Other factors affecting parents' outside activities   240
    Evenings and weekends   242
    A structure of living   248
    Holidays   252
    Short-term care   255
    The future   257
    Conclusion   261

17   Family, friends and neighbours   262

    The tolerance and intolerance of society   262
    Help and support from various sources   265
    Help and support from all sources   280
    The various levels of help and support   283
    Two factors affecting the acceptability of help   292
    Conclusion   297

18   The professional helpers   299

    What the mothers thought of the general practitioners
    and mental welfare officers   299
    Factors influencing the effectiveness of help from
    social workers   303

19   Conclusions   312

    An outline of the pattern of service proposed in the
    White Paper 'Better Services for the Mentally
    Handicapped' and the Sheffield Development Project   312
    A summary of the main findings from the visits   316
    A commentary on the Sheffield Development Project
    and the White Paper   317
    A co-ordinated, integrated, locally based service   328
    Conclusion: community care—the relevant
    preposition?   342

Appendix A: Additional tables   345

Appendix B: Figures 1–13   355

Appendix C: Discussion of strength of association using the
phi test and coefficient of contingency   370

Appendix D: Guided Interview Schedule   372

Appendix E: Summary of the Sheffield Development
Project   382

Appendix F: Potential residents for hostels based on a
population of 20,000   384

Notes   387

Bibliography   393

Index   399

Tables

2.1 Cases excluded from survey   29

2.2 Cases for which only a limited amount of data is available   30

2.3 Cases in main survey   30

3.1 Table of all cases included in survey   35

3.2 Residence as at 1 September 1968 (standard groups only)   36

3.3 Age mildly subnormal at home notified (standard group only)   37

3.4 Age structure of mildly subnormal at home on 1 September 1968 (grouped)   38

3.5 Age group related to period notified   39

3.6 Age on admission to hospital (mildly subnormal)   41

3.7 Age severely subnormal at home reported to Mental Health Service   43

3.8 Prevalence rate of subnormality per 1,000 in each age group   47

3.9 Comparison of prevalence rates of severe subnormality in younger age groups, where all subjects are likely to be known   48

4.1 Age at which mildly subnormal reported   50

4.2 Mildly subnormal reported over age of eighteen by Public Assistance Committee and other agencies   53

4.3 Age at which severely subnormal reported   54

4.4 Agency reporting severely subnormal by age reported   55

5.1 Precipitating factors in admission to hospital   57

5.2 Details of 'Behaviour or management' factor   58

5.3 Details of 'Death or illness of parent or parent figure' factor   62

5.4 Details of 'Social reasons' factor   64

5.5 Details of 'Other' factors   67

5.6 Children and adults—institution only   70

6.1 Socio-economic group of father or father figure   72

6.2 Percentage of non-manual fathers according to adjusted and unadjusted figures   73

6.3 Comparison of socio-economic groupings for Sheffield
C.B. with mildly subnormal and severely subnormal
population 75
6.4 Percentage of non-manual fathers among various groups
of severely subnormal compared with percentage for
Sheffield 77
6.5 Percentage of each socio-economic grouping at home 81
7.1 Type of housing 82
7.2 Mildly subnormal and severely subnormal at home in
different categories of housing 83
7.3 Standard of housing of mildly subnormal 85
7.4 Standard of housing of mildly subnormal. Percentages
of each category at home 85
7.5 Standard of housing of severely subnormal 87
7.6 Standard of housing of severely subnormal. Percentages
of each category at home 87
7.7 Financial circumstances 88
7.8 Financial circumstances. Percentages of each category at
home 89
7.9 Financial circumstances of those in institution divided
by precipitating factor (P.F.) 89
8.1 Whom the subnormal was living with—children 92
8.2 Whom the subnormal was living with—mildly subnormal
adults 93
8.3 Whom the subnormal was living with—severely
subnormal adults 95
8.4 Size of the household—children 98
8.5 Size of the household—adults 99
8.6 Physical health of mother or mother figure—children 102
8.7 Physical health of mother or mother figure—adults 103
8.8 Family relationships—children 108
8.9 Family relationships—adults 109
9.1 Mongols 116
9.2 Walking—children 117
9.3 Walking—adults 118
9.4 Mental illness 121
9.5 Behaviour problems at home—children 127
9.6 Behaviour problems at home—adults 128
9.7 Supervision needed—children 134
9.8 Supervision needed—adults 136
9.9 Relative strength of association with admission to

hospital of physical characteristics and behaviour:
mildly subnormal adults: (a) Younger institution group,
(b) Older institution group   139
10.1 Education—children   147
10.2 Education—adults   149
10.3 Present occupation by education: mildly subnormal
adults: (a) at home, (b) in hospital   151
10.4 Helpfulness at home of mildly subnormal, by sex, not
employed outside the home   153
10.5 Present occupation by education: severely subnormal
adults: (a) at home, (b) in hospital   155
10.6 Helpfulness at home of severely subnormal not
employed outside the home   157
10.7 Number of current and non-current cases among mildly
subnormal and severely subnormal adults at home   162
10.8 Mean age reported, period of surveillance and age last
contact of mildly subnormal and severely subnormal
adults at home, by current and non-current cases   163
14.1 Whom the subnormal was living with   194
14.2 Socio-economic group of the families   195
14.3 Talking or communicating   195
15.1 Getting up   211
15.2 Problems with washing   219
16.1 Parents going out together   242
16.2 Parents going out separately   244
16.3 Holidays   252
16.4 Plans for the future   258
17.1 Father's help   265
17.2 Help of siblings not living in the same household   268
17.3 Help and support from relatives   270
17.4 Help and support of neighbours   275
17.5 Help and support from various sources   281
17.6 Extent of support   282
A1 Agency reporting mildly subnormal   345
A2 Socio-economic group by type of housing, showing   346
redistribution of cases where SEG not known
A3 Socio-economic grouping including those classified by   347
type of housing
A4 How many subnormals who could be living with a sib   348
were doing so? Adults only
A5 Subnormality of mother: adults   349

A6 Age of mother at birth of subnormal: children   350
A7 Age of mother at birth of subnormal: adults   351
A8 Live births by age of mother—England and Wales 1963   352
A9 Type of offence: adults   353
A10 The relative strength of association with admission to   354
hospital of physical characteristics and behaviour:
severely subnormal children and adults

Figures

1 Age structure of mildly subnormal at home on
  1 September 1968   355
2 Age structure of total mildly subnormal hospital
  population at 1 September 1968   356
3 Age mildly subnormal admitted to hospital: (a) Pre
  5.7.48 and post 5.7.48 combined,   357
  (b) Post 5.7.48 only   358
4 Age structure of total mildly subnormal hospital
  population at 1 September 1968 by age admitted and
  period admitted   358
5 Quinquennia in which mildly subnormal admitted to
  hospital (including pre 5.7.48)   359
6 Age of severely subnormal at home on 1 September 1968   360
7 Age structure of total severely subnormal hospital
  population on 1 September 1968   361
8 Age severely subnormal admitted to hospital: (a) Pre
  5.7.48 and post 5.7.48 combined,   362
  (b) Post 5.7.48 only   363
9 Age structure of severely subnormal hospital population
  at 1 September 1968 by age admitted and period admitted 364
10 Quinquennia in which severely subnormal admitted to
  hospital (including pre 5.7.48)   365
11 Factors precipitating admission to hospital of mildly
  subnormal by age admitted   366
12 Factors precipitating admission to hospital of severely
  subnormal by age admitted   367
13 The combination of factors (families visited)   368–9

Preface

The preface offers the author his last chance to qualify what he has written before the book appears in print. There is one particular respect in which I would like to do so. At a stage when it was far too late to do anything about it, I realized that I disliked the term 'subnormal'. The families of the mentally handicapped never used the term themselves and it carries a number of undertones which tend to suggest that the mentally handicapped are in some way sub-human, which is false. The mentally handicapped are people with a particular handicap. Use of the term 'subnormal' tends to obscure this. The mentally handicapped are first and foremost people, not a medical condition. It should be mentioned that the names of all clients and their families are fictitious and details have been altered to preserve the anonymity of the families.

The main point of this preface must be to thank all those who helped in this project. It arose out of an essay written while I was a student on the Diploma in Social Studies course at the University of Sheffield, 1966–7. It would never have started but for the encouragement of Mrs Kathleen Ovens and Mr Eric Sainsbury, tutors on the course. Without their support and advice, the research would never have been completed. The Nuffield Provincial Hospitals Trust financed the last four of the five years the study has taken and for this generous support I would like to express my thanks.

During the course of the research, I received help, advice and assistance from many people. None of the research would have been possible without the kind permission of Dr C. H. Shaw, Medical Officer of Health for Sheffield, and Alderman Mrs P. Sheard, then chairman of the Health Committee. The help and co-operation of the Social Psychiatry Service (the Mental Health Service) could not have been more generous and willing. Much of what I have written is critical of the way the service operated. This is in no way criticism of the individual mental welfare officers. Their concern for their mentally handicapped clients was matched only by their awareness of the difficulty they had in giving them a satisfactory service. I would like to thank all the clerical, administrative and social work staff of the Social Psychiatry Service, in particular Mr W. F. Dunne, the Principal Social Worker, for the friendship, kindness and whole-hearted help they offered throughout the research.

Dr W. H. Parry, Medical Officer of Health for the City of Nottingham, and Mr J. E. Westmoreland and the staff of the Mental Health Service gave invaluable help by making it possible for Mrs Lee and myself to carry out pilot visits in Nottingham.

Thanks are also due to the many hospitals who replied to queries about patients from Sheffield, the Sheffield Regional Hospital Board for help with data processing, Dr D. J. Evans, Mrs Rosemary Ross and Mrs Judy Lay for their assistance with the computing and Dr R. A. Dixon for his help with both the statistical and computing side. Miss Suin Kelleher and Mr Lewis Noble both helped with the coding of the information from the files, and Mrs Hazel Anderson with preparation of the final report.

Dr Jaqueline Grad de Alarcon made valuable suggestions about how to tackle the visiting, as did Dr Sheila Hewett. Dr Albert Kushlick and members of his team in Wessex, especially Mr Paul Williams, gave us the benefit of their wide experience. Professor Kathleen Jones gave the project her support from early on and made many valuable suggestions about the text, especially in the Intro-duction. Mr David Boswell, with his extensive knowledge about hostels for mentally handicapped people, and Mr Walter Jaenig also made comments and suggestions which I would like to acknowledge.

I would like to offer my thanks to my colleagues in the Depart-ment, and in particular to Mr Trevor Noble, especially for his advice on the Introduction and the chapter on social class, Mrs Cissie Goldberg, without whose patient advice I could never have made sense of the statistics, Miss Juliet Berry, especially for her suggestions on the casework side, and Mrs Kathleen Ovens and Mr Eric Sainsbury, who, apart from the help already mentioned, made many detailed comments on the whole of the text.

Thanks for secretarial help are no formality. Miss Beryl Ibbotson, Mrs B. Byart and Mrs J. Dunn all interpreted my appalling hand-writing and tolerated innumerable alterations to the text and redrafts of tables with patience and efficiency.

Mrs Audrey Ward did a mammoth job in preparing the data from the files for the computer. Mrs Jennifer Lee shared in the process of working out the Guided Interview Schedule and in doing the pilot visits and visits in the main survey. The wealth of information gathered during the visits owes much to her.

Throughout almost the entire period of the research I have had the encouragement and help of Mrs Janice Hart, for the first two and a half years in an entirely voluntary capacity. She has been involved in virtually every stage of the research and no task, however daunting, has ever discouraged her. Such success as this research project has enjoyed owes a great deal to her. I can only say that I am profoundly grateful for all she has done.

Finally, I must thank the families who agreed to be visited. It is on their ready co-operation that the second half of the book is based. I hope they will feel that the time they gave to be interviewed was not wasted and that this book may do something to improve the lot of the mentally handicapped and their families.

This book is a slightly shortened version of a Ph.D. thesis submitted to the University of Sheffield.

1   Introduction

Historical

Care IN *the community or care* BY *the community*   Community care has become part of the jargon of our day. It is used to cover a wide range of care and an equally wide variety of understandings of community. The aim of this study is to give more substance to the term. The first consideration is which preposition should come between community and care. There is a large difference between care at home *in* the community and care at home *by* the community.

Consider Frank for instance. He was born in 1920. His backwardness was first noticed in infancy and he was reported to the Mental Deficiency Committee by the Education Department when he was six years old and classified as a very low grade imbecile. He was considered totally ineducable, never attended school, work or any kind of centre. His general behaviour was very trying.

He was the youngest of three boys of patient, loving parents. The father was a capstan operator. The home was a seven-roomed terrace house with a yard and was kept as clean and tidy as possible despite threats, complaints and anonymous letters from the neighbours. As time went on, keeping the home clean became increasingly difficult. Throughout the thirty-five years Frank lived at home he was never able to look after himself in any way. He was totally incontinent, unable to move about without assistance, and had to be put in a bed with high sides.

He became very jealous of other people's ability to speak, and when he was in his twenties he became very jealous of his mother as well. As soon as she spoke to anyone or anyone visited the house he would scream continually and pull and eventually claw at the visitors as well as at his mother. When he was thirty-one an attempt was made to quieten his behaviour with drugs but after a while they had no effect. He screamed and made noises all day and half the night. His parents, although showing great patience, were now nearly seventy and looked very worn.

He was admitted to hospital eventually when he was thirty-five years old to clear up a very bad bed sore, as his parents were unable to stop him tearing and scratching at himself.

Frank is a clear example of care in the community. The family's contact with other people in the neighbourhood was minimal.

Arthur's case presents a marked contrast. He was born at the beginning of the century in a poor working-class district. He was classified low grade feeble minded. He worked at the same steel works as his father, where his father was able to keep an eye on him. When his father had to retire because of ill health, another man in the department where Arthur worked took him under his wing and made sure that he was not exploited.

When his father died he went to live with his married sister, who helped him manage his affairs, which he could not do without help. For instance, the case notes record: 'He knows the value of a two shilling piece and all monies therefore have to be given to him in florins.' He was a life-long attender at the Chapel and attended all the social functions. Periodically he went to stay with relations in Somerset. A few years ago he retired after fifty years' service with the steel works.

Arthur was also cared for at home, but in his case, one can call it care by the community.

This distinction between care in the community and care by the community is important. Until fairly recent times the only distinction to be made was between care at home in the community or by the community. Official care specifically for the mentally handicapped was non-existent until the Idiots Act of 1886, although voluntary bodies began providing accommodation in the second half of the nineteenth century. However, the retrogressive 1890 Lunacy Act ignored completely the distinction between the mentally ill and the mentally handicapped and it was not until the passing of the 1913 Mental Deficiency Act that the foundations of a service which was at all comprehensive began to be laid.

The 1913 Act—care OUT OF *the community*   The 1913 Act became law at a time when opinion was strongly in favour of the permanent segregation of the mentally defective (to use the terminology of the Act), and many of the large institutions or colonies for the mentally handicapped are the legacies of this Act. The emphasis and the concentration of active care for the mentally handicapped was directed to care *out of* the community. This was where the greater part of the public resources were directed. The Board of Control, established by the Act, was concerned primarily with the admission and discharge of patients to and from institutions and their care in them. The centre of concern was out of the community.

Growth of services IN *the community, 1913–48* Despite the emphasis of the 1913 Act on care out of the community, it contained provisions which made possible the growth of services for mentally defective people living at home. Chief among these was the provision for 'supervision' of those cases where neither institutional care nor statutory guardianship appeared necessary. The requirement that each local authority should set up a Mental Deficiency Committee gave the necessary administrative base for this.

Parallel with this the scope and effectiveness of the voluntary organizations increased. This work was co-ordinated by the Central Association for the Care of the Mentally Defective, founded in 1914. In 1923, it became the Central Association for Mental Welfare.

Awareness of the value of care at home came gradually. Kathleen Jones (1960, p. 77) points out that at first the Board of Control thought of community care 'as only a rather unsatisfactory expedient', compared with institutional care. However, during the nineteen-thirties there was an increasing realization of the value of care at home. The voluntary associations had a good deal to do with this. As early as 1918 they were advocating the setting up of occupation centres, and by 1927 there were ninety-nine centres for defectives living at home. Some local authorities delegated their duties of supervision of defectives living at home to local voluntary welfare associations. In this way a considerable body of expertise was built up. This can be seen in the range of special training courses provided by the Central Association for Mental Welfare. By 1927 there were courses in mental deficiency work for social workers, for medical officers, for teachers, and for occupation centre workers.

The Mental Deficiency Act of 1927 and the report of the Wood Committee (1929) both marked an increasing emphasis on care outside institutions. The reorganization made possible by the Local Government Act of 1929 brought many more mentally defective people under the care of the mental deficiency authorities, as the Wood Committee had recommended. This increasing awareness of the value of care at home was matched in the field of mental illness, of which the Mental Treatment Act of 1930 is evidence, and received further impetus from the Feversham Committee. This committee reported to the Minister of Health in 1939 and emphasized strongly the community aspects of the mental health services.

This growth of services brought some help to some of those being cared for at home, but the services were essentially *in* the community.

The National Health Service Act and the move away from care out of the community   The National Health Service Act made the local authorities directly responsible for the supervision, guardianship, training and occupation of those in the community. The supervision of those at home, which had grown up since the 1913 Act, whether carried out by a voluntary association or directly by the Mental Deficiency Committee, meant that these new departments did have at least some social workers with experience in the care and supervision of mental defectives living at home.

After 1948 there was a steady movement of opinion in favour of care outside institutions. Bowlby's findings (1951) on the effects of institutional care on children had considerable influence. The pamphlet *50,000 outside the law*, produced by the National Council for Civil Liberties in 1950, citing 200 cases of alleged wrongful detention of mental defectives, was another indication; so was the decision of the Ministry of Health in 1952 to make it possible for hospitals to give short-term care to defectives living at home. Another significant factor was the increasing range of drugs available for modifying anti-social behaviour and curing, or at least alleviating, some forms of mental illness. The most important of these from the point of view of mental defectives were probably the tranquillizers. These made care at home possible in more cases. But whatever instances one cites, the basic fact is that the tide was turning. Institutional care was no longer generally considered the answer. Care at home was given serious thought.

The 1959 Mental Health Act and care IN *the community*   The setting up of the Royal Commission on Mental Illness and Mental Deficiency in 1954 arose out of and reflected this movement of opinion. The changed emphasis was expressed clearly by the Minister of Health, Mr Derek Walker-Smith, when introducing the 1959 Mental Health Bill, based on the findings of the Royal Commission, in the House of Commons (see Jones, 1960, p. 187). He said:

> One of the main principles we are seeking to pursue is the re-orientation of the mental health services away from institutional care towards care in the community.

It can be seen that this care at home, in the community, was nothing new. But the emphasis on care at home was now backed by the authority of the new Act. It had become official policy enshrined in an Act of Parliament. However, it is one thing to pass an enlightened Act of Parliament, it is another for the will, skill and resources to be available to put that Act into effect. It is true there were people who had much experience of caring for mentally handicapped people at home; but it is also true that in many respects the changed attitude, which led to the passing of the 1959 Mental Health Act, arose not so much out of knowledge about the advantages of caring for mentally handicapped people at home (though this was not totally absent), or out of knowledge about the care the community could give, as out of the increasing knowledge about the disadvantages of care in institutions, out of the community, and the damage that it could do. The lack of local authority social workers and facilities such as training centres and hostels provides ample evidence for the truth of this at the administrative level.

Community care as a positive principle Community care as an explicit, recognizable policy with that name dates from the 1961 Annual Conference of the National Association for Mental Health. At this conference Mr Enoch Powell, then Minister of Health, said (National Association for Mental Health, 1961):

> In fifteen years' time there may well be needed not more than half as many places in hospitals for mental illness as there are today. Expressed in numerical terms, this would represent a redundancy of no fewer than 75,000 hospital beds.

As the association's annual report said: 'These phrases sent a shiver through the Conference audience, this shiver has continued to oscillate in the mental hospitals ever since.'

This is the genesis of the policy as a political fact. It was made an administrative reality by the Hospital Plan of 1962 (revised in 1966) and the complementary Blue Book, *Health and Welfare: The Development of Community Care*, which appeared the following year. Revised editions appeared in 1964 and 1966. This contained the existing and planned local authority services which would be needed if it was going to be possible to care for more people in the community, who otherwise might need care out of the community, generally in hospital. In practice some authorities' plans fell far short of what was needed.

However, in terms of a positive move from care out of the community to care in the community, these plans referred primarily and most specifically to the mentally ill. Beds were to be reduced from 3·3 per 1,000 population to 1·8 per 1,000 population. For the mentally subnormal no reduction of hospital beds was envisaged but it was anticipated that the number needed would remain about the same. It was not until the 1971 White Paper that there came a similar positive move for the mentally subnormal from care out of the community to care in the community. This is considered a little further on.

The need for more services at the local authority level, from more training centres and old people's homes to more home helps, was very real and the plans did something to speed up the expansion of these services. This was valuable, but the Blue Book makes it obvious that at this stage the Government was thinking about community care in administrative terms entirely, in fact in terms of services in the community.

The studies of Tizard and Grad   In 1959, the year the Mental Health Act was passed, a pioneer study of 250 severely mentally handicapped people and their families in London was carried out by Professor Jack Tizard and Dr Jaqueline Grad (1961). One hundred of the handicapped were in hospital and the rest at home. Many of those in institutions were severely handicapped, and problems of management accounted for about half the placements. Possibly more interesting was the way Tizard and Grad showed the heavy price paid by the families who kept their handicapped member at home. They were on average worse off economically, more overcrowded, with poorer housing, and had fewer social contacts than the families with a child in an institution. Two-thirds of the families with their handicapped member at home had at least three severe family problems compared to 45 per cent of those with a similar child in an institution.[1]

These families where the handicapped person was still at home were followed up about seven years later in a study undertaken for Political and Economic Planning by Miss Jean Moncrieff (1966). This showed that the main causes for concern were the shortage of money in an ageing group of parents, the poor quality of the social work help received and the fact that 'although informal community support for the families in this study did exist it was slight in content and sporadic in application' (ibid., p. 79). The impression given by reading these two studies is that what was called community care was, in fact, care by overworked parents, with minimal help from the authorities and an attitude of indifference shown by the neighbours. They evidenced the need for much-improved services in the community and also, though this is not a central theme, began to indicate the need for care by the community.[2]

In 1964 Tizard published a further book, *Community Services for the Mentally Handicapped*. This summarized the findings of his previous study undertaken with Dr Grad, contained a study of the prevalence of mental handicap in London and Middlesex and gave an account of a small experimental children's unit for sixteen children of imbecile grade run for two years (1958–60) at Brooklands, where the children were treated on the principles developed in residential nurseries for children, rather than on medical and nursing lines. Finally he suggested a model pattern of service for the integrated care of the mentally handicapped and their families based on an area of 100,000 population. This line of development has been followed through in Wessex under the direction of Dr Albert Kushlick in collaboration with Professor Tizard.

The main emphasis in these studies and the consequent developments has been on services in the community rather than care by the community.[3]

Conditions in long stay hospitals   The impetus towards care in the community has almost certainly been increased by the series of revelations about conditions in long stay institutions.

Sans Everything (Robb, 1967) was concerned mostly with mentally ill and geriatric patients but it was followed shortly by reports of ill-treatment of subnormal patients at Ely Hospital, Cardiff. The allegations were made by a correspondent of the *News of the World* in July 1967 and they led to an official enquiry whose report was published in March 1969 (the Howe Report). This revealed a drab and sometimes grim life for the inmates, a finding which was substantiated on a wide scale, with extensive documentation, by Pauline Morris in her book *Put Away*, which was published in the same year. The following year three male nurses from Farleigh subnormality hospital were convicted on charges relating to treating patients cruelly, and the committee of enquiry (the Watkins Committee) revealed an appalling administrative situation, and grossly inadequate resources for and supervision of the most difficult and disturbed patients.

The report on Whittingham Hospital, published in February 1972 (the Payne Report), was concerned with the mentally ill but the now all-too-familiar revelations underlined the extreme difficulties under which large, isolated institutions for the chronically ill or handicapped labour.

The cumulative effect of these disturbing reports must have increased public and political pressure for care in the community rather than care out of the community in long stay institutions.

Developments in Wessex   The work in the Wessex Regional Hospital Board has been based on a careful epidemiological study of the area (Kushlick, 1964). This presented the need for residential care and other services by grade, handicaps and age in rates per 100,000 of population. It is on the basis of areas of 100,000 that the Wessex plans are formulated. Dr Kushlick (1967a) has shown, for instance, that it is possible to cater for the residential needs of *all* children in an area of 100,000 population by providing one hostel with twenty places. Two such hostels were opened in 1970, one in Portsmouth, one in Southampton. Their effectiveness is being evaluated by comparison with the other half of the town, which in each case is served by a traditional hospital service. This pattern allows for more effective use of services already available within the community and does not take the child so far from his home. The Wessex experiment is discussed in more detail in the final chapter (p. 335-7).

In many respects the Wessex experiment concentrates on providing services in the community, but such a pattern does make care by the community more of a possibility. When giving a paper to the National Society for Mentally Handicapped Children in 1967, Dr Kushlick (1967b) said: 'Parents will be invited to participate with the staff in the running of the units and to take their children on outings, and where possible for weekends or longer periods. Unit heads will also be encouraged to recruit volunteers from the area to join in the activities of the unit.'

The policy which has been adopted in Wessex shows a move from thinking entirely in terms of care and services in the community towards an approach which takes more account of care by the community.

The Seebohm Report 1968   The Seebohm Report (see Home Office *et al.*, 1968) is in one respect dealing with the creation of an effective family service *in* the community but the authors of the report saw beyond this. The report lays considerable emphasis on care *by* the community, not just *in* the community. However, it is made clear that we are now having to think about care by the community in rather more complex terms. It is more than the simple care at home given by the community in the case of Arthur, who was mentioned earlier. The report sees care by the community in terms of an interweaving between the statutory social services and all manner of mutual aid and informal caring. This marks an important step forward in official thinking. It is not simply a return to care by the community or nothing, but recognizes that 'the whole community "consumes" the social services, directly or indirectly, as well as paying for this through taxation, and consumers have an important contribution to make to the development of an effective family service' (para. 492). This is discussed at greater length in the final chapter (pp. 330 and 342-3). The Seebohm Report can be criticized, not for the terms in which it viewed the role of the community in the provision of an effective family service, but for providing inadequate guidance on how this could become an administrative reality. In a report which was giving guidelines for the future development of the social services, this was a sad omission, even though the difficulty of the task can be appreciated.

The White Paper, Better services for the mentally handicapped, 1971   The White Paper shows the influence of both Professor Jack Tizard and Dr Kushlick. The critical table (table 5) uses a base of 100,000 of population and the small homely unit is commended, even though there is no commitment to close all the large hospitals. It marks a decisive switch from care out of the community to care in the community, halving the number of hospital places for adults and making the number good by a sevenfold increase in local authority residential places.

It shows an awareness of the importance of the community but not in such fundamental terms as does the Seebohm Report. In particular it does not really see the need for an *interweaving* of statutory and informal care. The White Paper is considered in detail in the final chapter.

The implications of care by the community   The effect of the White Paper and the Seebohm Report, and of the consistent official emphasis on care in the community, taken together with the increasing realization of the importance of the insights of community development (of which the Home Office Community Development Projects are only one instance), means that the helping services are being faced increasingly by the question of what care by the community means. They cannot consider this in simple terms, such as is illustrated by the care given to Arthur (see page 2), but they have to consider it in relation to and in conjunction with the service they themselves are seeking to provide.

Care out of the community need not concern itself with the community from which it is removing the client. Even care in the community need not concern itself overmuch with what the community is or the way it functions. But care by the community demands understanding of what it is, sympathy with the way it works and insight into the way the community can help. It demands that some consideration should be given to what is meant when we use the word community.

The ambiguity of 'community'

The Seebohm Report recognized this need and produced a definition of community at the beinning of the chapter on 'The community' (para. 476):

> The term 'community' is usually understood to cover both the physical location and the common activity of a group of people. The definition of a community, however, or even of a neighbourhood, is increasingly difficult as Society becomes more mobile and people belong to 'communities' of common interest, influenced by their work, education or social activities, as well as where they live. Thus, although traditionally the idea of a community has rested upon geographical locality, and this remains an important aspect of many communities, today different members of a family may belong to different communities of interest as well as the same local neighbourhood. The notion of a community implies the existence of a network of reciprocal social relationships, which among other things ensure mutual aid and give those who experience it a sense of well being.

This definition covers what are generally accepted as basic elements which go to make up what is meant by 'community', that is a sense of belonging, locality and the existence of reciprocal social relationships. It is possible to talk about community meaningfully in terms that take little account of place; for instance, one can talk about the community of scholars. Such a community is an example of communities where interest is prior and place is secondary. However, the notion of locality is usually present and once one comes to consider community in more spatial terms, the size of what is considered a community and the number of people in it varies, naturally enough, according to the criteria used.

Three levels may be suggested. If one takes as the main criterion the extent to which it is a complete social system, one would have to agree with MacIver (quoted in Dennis, 1958) that 'the completest type of community is the nation'. Other writers stress socio-cultural aspects and the awareness of a separate identity. It is far from easy in modern urban society to determine the extent to which the people of any area are aware of their separate identity as a group. A community based on this definition could cover areas of vastly differing size. It might be a county, a town or a district within a town. Whatever size of community such a definition would suggest, it would certainly be larger than that suggested by G. P. Murdock and colleagues (quoted in Gould and Kolb, 1964). Theirs is a small-scale understanding of community. 'The term "community" connotes the maximal group of persons who normally reside together in face-to-face association.'

It seems unprofitable to say that any one of these, or any other understanding of community, is right and the others wrong, for man is a complex being and has a complex organization which reflects this. From the point of view of the care of the mentally handicapped it is possible to equate very crudely the three levels of community just outlined with three administrative levels.

First, there is the central government level. Care of the mentally handicapped by the nation means that the central government has to pay for and provide certain services, among them the hospital service. This is not what is generally understood by community care but it does reflect one essential aspect of it.

Second, there is the local authority level. The Sheffield City Council, along with other local authorities, is responsible for providing a variety of services for the mentally handicapped among a host of other groups of people in need of various forms of help and care. This includes such facilities as social work services, hostels and training centres. In one sense it is quite fair to talk about the provision of such services as community care, because it does represent the services offered by the community at a certain level of organization. Such services are indeed essential, but the unjustified assumption is made that the provision of services at this level automatically provides care at the face-to-face level. It is the failure to make a distinction between these different levels of community function that leads to much of the confused thinking about community care.

Third, we need to find an administrative equivalent for the face-to-face level. It might be possible to equate this with the ward or parish level, indeed there is really no administrative alternative, but the attempt to find an administrative equivalent starts to break down at this point because the welfare services are rarely, if ever, organized on a ward or parish basis or, to express the same idea in Elizabeth Bott's terms, in relation to 'the effective social environment of a family [and] its network of friends, neighbours, relatives and particular social institutions' (1971, p. 159). However, the fact that there is no satisfactory administrative equivalent does not mean that this face-to-face level can be ignored, for when one is considering care by the community it is generally this level which is the most relevant.

For this reason the following discussion focuses on community at this small-scale level. First a case is argued for its fundamental importance to the welfare services, and then the face-to-face level of community is examined in more detail.

The lack of effective administrative contact with the community at this level is given further consideration in the final chapter.

The face-to-face level of community is the basis on which all welfare services rest

The three levels of community which have been suggested make it clear that it is not possible to consider any one level in isolation from the others when discussing community care. However, care by the community at the small-scale level of the intimate, face-to-face relationships of the social networks of kin, friends and neighbours can be seen to be the basis on which care at the larger scale levels depends.

This can be illustrated by the National Health Service. It is not based on the general practitioners, vital though they are, but the mothers who nurse their children through the common infectious diseases, the relatives who help during childbirth, the neighbours who lend a hand when a mother is ill at home. If it were not for this the hospitals would be ludicrously inadequate and the general practitioners would be overwhelmed. The National Health Service does not replace care by the community at this level but it builds on it and strengthens it. Indeed, its efficiency depends to a considerable extent on its success in doing this, rather than creating its own empire apart from the caring which is already done by families and friends within the community. The futility of even thinking of creating a service apart from the community (in the microcosmic sense) is shown by the elderly. Over 94 per cent live at home and the vast majority live at home because they want to. Here, as clearly as in any branch of the social services, we can see that the community caring at the small-scale, face-to-face level is and must be the basis on which all services depend.

A consideration of the face-to-face level of community

(a) *Local communities are under pressure*

Communities, as has been said above, are often thought of in local terms. Historically this is certainly justified. The model of such a community in many people's minds is the village community, or the old-established urban working-class area. But as Minar and Greer say (1969, p. xi):

> Change has destroyed the validity of the oldest and in many ways still archetypal form of community, the agricultural village. Created ten thousand years ago during that great creative period we call the Neolithic, it is still the home of most of mankind. But the superior energy sources and power of the urban technological societies everywhere (including nations where a majority still live in the villages), and their expansive tendencies, indicate the obsolescence of the older form.

The pressures against integrated local communities, whether in town or village, are indeed strong. Possibly the most obvious is the physical one of rehousing in new housing estates.

Norman Dennis in an article in *New Society* (Dennis, 1963, pp. 8–11) gives a good overall picture of these pressures. He shows very clearly how some of the factors which undermined communal solidarity and reduced the extent of mutual help, for instance the increased provision of welfare benefits, were commendable in themselves.

From his studies on two housing estates in a large southern city, he came to the conclusion that:

> This suggests that the neighbourhood culture of the urban working class as reported by Young, Horobin, Hoggart and others may be facing difficulties in the housing estate milieu. Some people argue that it is just a matter of time. Places like Hunslet and Bethnal Green in their early days prompted Disraeli's comment in *Sybil*: 'There is no community . . . there is aggregation . . . modern society acknowledges no neighbours'. Time alone, however, does not produce social relationships. Working-class mutual aid, sociability, control of neighbourliness and tolerance of other behaviour were rooted in both the work situation and the urban environment.

He goes on to explore these features of the work situation and the urban environment. He shows how willingness to help neighbours depended on insecurity of income and the inability to meet unexpected calls on the budget. However, since the end of the Second World War, full employment and increased welfare benefits have lifted large segments of the population above the likelihood of real dependence on neighbours, and thus there is not the same scope for *reciprocal* neighbourliness.

The husband tended to be workmate-centred rather than wife-centred and so the woman turned to her neighbours for sociable contact. Wives shared common facilities, such as the wash-house, and the difficulty of travel confined the woman to her own district and also tended to limit men to working in one particular occupation. Finally, lack of competitiveness helped solidarity to grow. People were on the same level now and would remain so.

> The result of these influences was an accumulation of knowledge about and a commitment to fellow residents and the physical neighbourhood. Every connection of kin and neighbours formed a bridge to other people and the pattern was stabilized by a *network* of congeniality and contact and not just by *feelings* of *individual* liking and obligation.

Dennis goes on to point out that all these conditions are altering:

> More wives go out to work themselves, and companionship within marriage becomes more important. On estates the home is well equipped for leisure and the neighbourhood poorly

equipped. Instead of the neighbourhood being 'the railwaymen's district' or 'the fishermen's district' or 'the dockers' area' or nearly all the neighbours steelworkers, many occupations are represented. . . . The possibility of the children bettering themselves through education reduces the sense of fundamental and inescapable equality among neighbours. The location of the estate in relation to the facilities of the rest of the town reduces the number of occasions on which a woman is likely to come across a particular neighbour as she goes to any one of a number of nearby shopping centres, any one of a number of churches, and so forth.

Practice and preference appear to be towards the abrogation of neighbourly duties and interests. . . . Neighbours are regarded as expendable in the search for middle class success. And as the old values are discarded, as the old patina is eroded, the population becomes ever more open to the general cultural media, and their recommendations are out of harmony with the neighbours' traditional role.

The case that Dennis puts forward for the declining importance of neighbours is a strong one. It agrees broadly with the rather depressing picture of social isolation which people who had moved from Bethnal Green to 'Greenleigh' reported (Young and Willmott, 1957). Dennis (1962, p. 86) reiterates his belief in the decline of neighbourly contacts in another article:

In the elaboration of modern social institutions marriage has become the only place in which the individual can demand and expect esteem and love. Adults have no-one on whom they have a right to lean for this sort of support at all comparable to their right to lean on their spouse.

This perception of the way in which society is developing is consistent with much past sociological analysis, such as, for instance, that of Tönnies, who, in *Community and Association* (1955) distinguished *Gemeinschaft* (community) and *Gesellschaft* (association), and saw modern society as abandoning the first kind of grouping in favour of the second.

(b) *The resilience of neighbourly activity*

There are, however, grounds for questioning whether society in this country is developing so remorselessly in this direction. An important work in this respect is Willmott's study of Dagenham after forty years (1963). The Dagenham estate itself epitomizes all that is awful about council building between the wars. It suffers from a number of disadvantages, of which possibly the most serious is that no provision was made for an expanding population, which has often frustrated the wish of children to find a house near their parents. Despite this (ibid., p. 109):

> At the end one is impressed by how similar, not how different they [Dagenham and the East End] are. Local extended families, which hold such a central place in the older districts, have grown up in almost identical form on the estate, so have local networks of neighbours—people living in the same street who help each other, mix together and are on easy going terms. . . . In part Dagenham is the East End reborn.

He says a little later (ibid., p. 111):

> Although working-class life is obviously changing in many ways—people have more possessions, are more home-centred, and, whether they live in the old districts or the new, probably spend more time with their families—there are, apparently, some fundamental regularities in working-class life which, given time, will reassert themselves.

This is a direct contradiction of Dennis's supposition (p. 14). The conclusions Dennis draws also appear to disregard the importance of the family life cycle and the considerable impact this has. The importance of this point has been well made by Peter Mann (1965). Having small children or being old are likely to make the immediate neighbourhood far more important to some families. The same applies to families who have a handicapped member.

R. E. Pahl (1970, p. 109) makes the very basic point, as comment on Dennis's article 'Who needs neighbours?', that:

> The normal business of life creates emergencies and difficulties, which force some kind of relationship with those living in the immediate area. Even if the nearest kin or friend can be at an individual's house within half an hour, this may be too long if someone has had a severe accident or a fire has started in the living room.

The proportion of the population who are at a stage in the life cycle that means that they spend much time in their locality, and

the ordinary contingencies of life to which even the most inter-
nationally mobile spiralist is subject, taken together with such
evidence as the Dagenham study, make it clear that a significant
amount of interaction is likely to take place at a local level. Neither
the locality nor neighbourly actions can be dismissed arbitrarily
from any view of society which seeks to take account of all its
members. It is true that the Dagenham study relates to a working-
class estate, but there is considerable evidence that the middle class,
including those who are geographically mobile, are likely to take
a great deal of interest in what goes on locally.

This is not to suggest that the social pressures which militate
against traditional forms of community are not real. They are clearly
powerful and the structures of society are changing. This is not
disputed, but in considering the decline of the *traditional* community
it is important not to ignore aspects of community which remain and
also new forms of community functioning which are developing.
While on the one hand the breakdown of many aspects of community in its traditional form must be acknowledged, yet, on the
other hand, it is quite evident that mutual aid, social intercourse and
friendly help still happen. Furthermore, in considering the way in
which such community activity does happen, the importance of the
locality cannot be ignored. It is clear that the tide is not turning
inexorably against the formation and cultivation of neighbourly
contacts.

(c) *Social networks*

Little has been said so far of the way in which such interaction might
take place. To discuss it, the concept of the social network, which
owes much to Elizabeth Bott's book *Family and Social Network*
(1957), is most useful. Pahl (1970, pp. 104–5) introduces the concept
with commendable clarity:

> The rich and privileged have always sought to escape from the
> community of common deprivation. Even if physically *in* small
> communities they are not socially *of* them. The so-called 'decay
> of the village community' was not thought of until the increasing
> wealth of the less-privileged enabled them to follow the example
> of the well-to-do. Darcy in Jane Austen's *Pride and Prejudice*
> offended his hosts when he remarked: 'In a country
> neighbourhood you move in a very confined and unvarying
> society.' However, Mr Bingley does not feel inhibited by this:

'When I am in the country . . . I never wish to leave it; and when I am in town it is pretty much the same. They each have their advantages, and I can be equally happy in either.' Later, Mrs Bennett, still smarting from Darcy's remark returns to the attack:

> 'Aye—that is because you have the right disposition, but that gentleman,' looking at Darcy, 'seemed to think the country was nothing at all.'
>
> 'Indeed, Mama, you are mistaken,' said Elizabeth, blushing for her mother. 'You quite mistook Mr Darcy. He only meant that there were not such a variety of people to be met with in the country as in town, which you must acknowledge to be true.'
>
> 'Certainly, my dear, nobody said there were; but as to not meeting with many people in this neighbourhood, I believe there are few neighbourhoods larger, I know we dine with four and twenty families.'

It is clear that the characters in Jane Austen's world lived in *social networks*, not communities. They moved about the country, staying in each other's houses, wintering in London or spending the season in Bath. The so-called 'rural communities' in which their friends' houses were located were rustic prisons only for those without the means to escape from them.

One slightly confusing aspect of Pahl's explanation is that he contrasts social networks with communities, which is in effect comparing a part with the whole. The social network can be taken more usefully as a valuable way of explaining how communal intercourse can take place or how community happens, not as a rival concept. The point that concerns us here is the relationship between social network and locality. When there was little population movement the two would in most cases coincide. The (close-knit) networks of interaction in a mediaeval village would coincide with the village: the same could be said of, for instance, the Welsh village studied by Alwyn Rees (in Frankenberg, 1966).

In a large urban area social network and local area do not coincide so often and we are presented with a very much more complex picture. The basic approach adopted in this study is to consider what geographical area is meaningful in terms of social networks. This implies no lack of concern about nearness: a case has just been argued for its importance and this is stressed in the second half of the book. It is the order that is important: the families' social networks are looked at first; and then, and very important it is, comes the geography of those networks. The geography is considered in terms of the social networks. The consideration of the networks is not subjected to any geographical *limitation* though the geographical *aspect* of the networks is treated as a matter of great importance.

The social networks of the families who were visited in this study were naturally affected very much by the needs of the subnormal. They affected almost every aspect of the family's life. By exploring the framework of care and support within which the subnormal was looked after, and by considering the various sources of help available to the family as a whole, it was possible to gain quite a clear picture of the social networks of the families. The very practical function of these networks served to make them rather clearer than might otherwise have been the case.

The discussion of the geographical implications of these networks is left to the final chapter, because they are closely linked with administrative considerations which arise out of the findings. It is sufficient at this stage to say that the findings in this study agree in large measure with three other studies carried out in Sheffield, that a very small localized area is often the critical one for social inter-action (Mitchell *et al.*, 1954; Skipper: Sheffield Council of Social Service; Hampton, 1970).

A comprehensive basis for community care

The face-to-face level of community which has been discussed is of fundamental importance if one is to gain an understanding of community care which gives meaningful expression to care by the community. But it was also shown in the section on 'the ambiguity of "community"' in this chapter that the community at the central government and local authority levels have a vital role to play as well.

A view of community care which takes account of the complexity of human organization, and the realities of our political and admini-strative system, entails consideration of society at four levels: (a) the client and his family which merges into (b) the social network of the family's kin, friends and neighbours; (c) the social worker and the local authority services which may or may not include (d) some form of residential care. This residential care may, of course, be provided by the Regional Hospital Board. All these four elements need to be considered if one is going to examine community care satisfactorily. A vital aspect of any such consideration is the interaction between these four elements. This involves looking at care by the community, care in the community, care out of the community, and how the three combine. It involves considering whether there is any place for care out of the community, and if not, what measures are needed to make care in the community and by the community a reality.

It is on this fourfold understanding of community care that this book is based, but the emphasis is wholeheartedly and unashamedly on the first two—the client and his family and the social network within which they live. The consideration of the services is based on what the families experienced and needed, not the other way round: it is care by the community that is central to the study. The official services are considered in relation to how they can help and strengthen and interweave with care by the community.

General method

The first aim of this study was to try to establish what factors make for good care at home, and then to explore ways in which what is called community care can be based more realistically on the resources that are available within the community. It was not easy to decide how to tackle this. The distinctive feature of the study was its attempt to make a specific tie-up between the patterns of community interaction on the microcosmic scale that has been indicated, and the way in which the social services operate. But how was this to be done?

One possible approach was to examine a particular locality and then see how the various social work agencies linked in with the various social networks. But what locality would be chosen and why? Which social networks would be chosen and on what basis, and how would they be traced? What characteristics of community would be sought and why, and would this not presume what the study was trying to find out? The sheer complexity of this and the apparent operational impossibility of it led to this approach being abandoned.

The approach that was adopted took account of the fact that the subnormal and his immediate family need a good deal of help and support. It was after all the care of the subnormal with which the study was concerned. This help and support was used as the means by which to examine the network of relationships and contacts within which the family lived. The contacts of the family with the social services were not ignored but these contacts were considered in the light of the family's more immediate relationships.

Before this part of the study was possible, however, the families that were to be visited had to be chosen, and the criteria on which they were to be chosen had to be worked out. Therefore it was decided to take all the subnormals on the books of the Sheffield Mental Health Service, read their files and code the information. The information coded covered the extent of the subnormal's abilities and disabilities, details about his family, his education, training and employment (if any), extent of help from family, friends and neighbours, and local authority services, in addition to basic data about age and sex, etc.

These files produced a great deal of information which had to be analysed to produce not simply a long list of the needs of the subnormal, but a list which highlighted the needs of the subnormal *at home*, that is of the community care needs. The files covered subnormals both at home and in hospital, so the obvious method was to compare the circumstances of those subnormals who were then at home with those then in hospital. In the case of those in hospital the information which was coded was of their *home* circumstances *at the time they were admitted to hospital*. It is the *home* circumstances of both the home group and the hospital group which are compared. The home circumstances are the circumstances of the home from which they were admitted to hospital.

This data from the files made it possible to compare the home group with the hospital group and to pick out those factors which were associated most strongly with admission to hospital. It turned out that it was difficulties with behaviour, some major physical handicaps and gross social incompetence that were related most unambiguously to hospital admission.

This collection of factors associated with admission to hospital having been established, a group which was still at home and in which two or more of these factors were present was picked out. In other words a deviant group was selected which, according to the data from the files, one might have expected to be in hospital. This group, whose families had managed to keep its member at home in spite of the presence of these major handicaps, was visited to see what compensating factors had enabled them to do so. The theory was that this group of extremely handicapped people was one whose care was a considerable burden on the families concerned, and therefore might be expected to produce examples of cases where there was much support from the community, whether from families or neighbours or both. In addition the group visited was limited to subnormals over the age of fifteen, which meant that the families had borne this burden for some years. In the interview much time was devoted to the extent and range of help the families had received, and quite a full picture was built up.

It is the needs of these families which are used as the baseline from which to examine the community caring. Their needs are used as a way of discovering something about the resources available from their family, friends and the area in which they live: their needs are used as an indication of the way a local authority social work service works: their needs are used to indicate ways in which the local authority services interact with the social environment within which the families live. In meeting the needs of the subnormal all the four elements mentioned above meet—that is (a) the client and his family which merges into (b) the social network of the family's kin, friends and neighbours; (c) the social worker and the local authority services which may or may not include (d) some form of residential care, which is more likely to be provided by the Regional Hospital Board.

The second part of the study is purely descriptive. No attempt was made to visit families where the subnormal had gone into hospital, as Tizard and Grad did. The aim of the second part was to search for clues of positive factors about care in the community and by the community among the many years of experience of the fifty-four families visited. As such it is only the beginning of an attempt to define the link between the community as it functions at the level of a family's daily experience and the way the social services operate.

The information from the visits is augmented and put into context by the information from the files. Generally the files said little about the help that neighbours did or did not give but some files gave full accounts of what families had experienced. The files also made it possible to put the results of the visits into context. This is important because it is easy for one particularly harrowing case to distort the total perspective. For instance the files made it clear that many people who at some stage in their life had been labelled subnormal managed extremely well with little or no help. The information gathered from the files is able to show not only where much more help is needed, but also to suggest where scarce resources can be used to best advantage.

Part I (chapters 2–11) deals with the material gathered from the files. These findings are summarized in chapter 11. Part II (chapters 12–19) describes these visits, and in the final two chapters there is a discussion of how community care could become more effectively care by the community.

Part I

The files

2   The scope of the survey

The scope of the survey was very simple. Basically it covered all subnormals on the books of the Sheffield Mental Health Service on 1 September 1968. This was the only source of cases. No cases from any other source were considered. The scope of the survey is therefore an administrative one.

Within this broad definition certain other limits had to be set. First, all the subnormals had to be alive on 1 September 1968. This must appear obvious, but we found three of those listed in the home filing-cabinets and no less than seventy-one of those listed in the hospital filing-cabinets were in fact dead on that date. The large number of those listed as being in hospital who were dead gives some indication of the problems of communication between the hospitals and the local authority services.

It was decided to set an upper IQ limit of 70. Six hospital cases and forty-three home cases were excluded on this basis; one of the hospital cases had a university degree. Most of those at home excluded for the above reason had an IQ that fell in the 70s, but two had an IQ of over 100—one of 101, the other of 109.

Some cases could not be taken into consideration because the information in the file was inadequate. In addition all cases where the subnormal was never visited at all by a mental welfare officer (or before 1960 by an inspector under the Mental Deficiency Acts) were excluded. In practice the information in such files was generally inadequate. This caused the removal of three hospital cases and twenty-four home cases from the survey. Cases where the subnormal had left Sheffield reduced the total at home by a further twenty-seven.

All those cases that came into the Sheffield area when the boundaries were extended on 1 April 1967 were excluded. The sixty-five home cases concerned had been in Sheffield's care for only eighteen months and before that provision for them and the facilities available had been different. Therefore it was considered wisest to exclude them. In addition a further seven cases which were reported between 1 April 1967 and 1 October 1968 who lived in the 'new' Sheffield areas were excluded so that the area covered was defined clearly as

27

the Sheffield boundaries before 1 April 1967, for which the population is known.

Information about patients in hospital was obtained by visiting or writing to the hospital indicated by their files. If they had been transferred to another hospital we wrote to that hospital, and so on, until they were tracked down. In ten cases the patients could not be traced, and so they had to be excluded.

Among the hospital population, or to be more accurate the people listed in the hospital filing-cabinets, fifteen had been discharged or absconded and nothing was known about what had happened to them subsequently. Sixteen had been discharged from hospital and had gone to live outside Sheffield. These thirty-one cases were excluded.

The most important limit set on the survey was the exclusion of all the subnormals living at home with whom there had been no contact since the day that the National Health Service came into operation, that is 5 July 1948. In such cases the information was over twenty years old and conditions before that date were so different that it seemed unwise to consider these cases together with the later ones. Therefore they were all excluded, though they gave some fascinating and horrifying glimpses into a bygone age. There was, for instance, the file which, under the question 'Supposed cause of mental deficiency', said 'Starvation of mother during pregnancy'. The last entry in some of these files was many years ago. There were three imbecile sisters who were last contacted in 1915 and two others where the last contact was 1914. Pressure of time was a factor in this decision. Approximately 800 files were excluded on this basis. They could produce much valuable information for the period from about 1890 to 1948 if someone had the time and resources to look at them carefully. They illustrate very graphically the change in attitudes.

The effect of this limitation is that the cases of those at home cover a period of just over twenty years from 5 July 1948 to 1 September 1968.

Another minor exclusion was designed to cut out those who were likely to be dead. All those who were at home who were born before 1 September 1898 (i.e. aged seventy or more) and with whom there had been no contact for the previous three years were excluded. In the event only two cases were excluded for this reason.

Finally eighty-eight home and thirteen institution cases had to be excluded because their files could not be found before the deadline that had to be set for finishing the coding of the files. An attempt was made to obtain certain basic data from their index cards. However, in many cases it was not even stated whether they were mildly or severely subnormal and the information was so sketchy and uncertain that it was decided to exclude these cases completely. Table 2.1 shows the total numbers excluded.

Table 2.1   Cases excluded from survey

	Home	Institution	Total
IQ 70+	43	6	49
Inadequate information or never visited	24	3	27
Left Sheffield	27	0	27
Came in at Sheffield boundary change	72	0	72
No trace in hospital	0	10	10
Discharged from hospital, nothing subsequent known	0	15	15
Discharged from hospital to an address outside Sheffield	0	16	16
Aged over 70 and no contact for previous three years	2	0	2
File could not be found in time	88	13	101
Total	256	63	319

Note: In addition there were approximately 800 home cases where the last contact was before 5 July 1948, who were all excluded.

In addition to these cases which were excluded totally, there are a number of cases where only a limited amount of data is available.

The most important group of these consisted of the cases which were admitted to hospital before 5 July 1948. As regards the hospital population it was felt that it would be valuable to have some basic information about the total number of inhabitants. It would have been impossible to discover if all the home cases where there had been no contact since 5 July 1948 were alive, but it was far easier to discover what had happened to those who had been admitted to hospital. There were only ten cases which could not be traced, as we have seen already.

Basic data were obtained for those who were admitted to hospital before 5 July 1948. These covered their sex, age, degree of disability, and age and year they were admitted to hospital. From this information it has been possible to see the age structures of the total hospital population of subnormals admitted from Sheffield and to see changing patterns in, for instance, the age at admission. Those who were admitted to hospital before 5 July 1948 will be referred to as the 'early hospital cases'. There were 270 cases in this category.

It happens that the population of Sheffield is approximately 1 per cent of the population of England and Wales and the population of subnormals in hospital is approximately 1 per cent of the total for England and Wales.

The next group for whom there is only a limited amount of data consists of those cases which were first reported in another local authority area, and subsequently moved to Sheffield; in these, the quality of recording and the range of information varied considerably; and, in addition, the facilities, such as training centres, provided by different local health authorities also varied considerably. One aim of the study was to see what impact the provision of facilities, such as training centres, had on admission to hospital. Therefore in these cases just the basic data already mentioned are available. There were sixty-six cases at home and twenty-eight in an institution in this category. Table 2.2 shows the number of cases for whom only this limited amount of data is available.

Table 2.2   *Cases for which only a limited amount of data is available*

	Home	Institution	Total
Cases admitted to hospital before 5.7.48	0	270	270
Cases first reported in another local authority area	66	28	94
Total	66	298	364

When those cases that have been excluded completely and those for which only a limited amount of data is available have been taken away, there remain 1,763 cases for which comparatively full data are available, and it is on these cases that the main part of the survey is based. Table 2.3 shows how this number is made up.

Table 2.3   *Cases in main survey*

	MSN Home	Institution	Total	SSN Home	Institution	Total	Total
Total	746	120	866	674	223	897	1,763

These four groups—the mildly subnormal at home, the mildly subnormal in an institution, the severely subnormal at home and the severely subnormal in an institution—will be referred to as 'the four standard groups'.

The distinction has been made between the mildly subnormal (MSN) and the severely subnormal (SSN). The first criterion for making this distinction is IQ. All those with an IQ below 50 have been classed as severely subnormal. If no IQ was mentioned in the file, the category in which the subnormal was placed on ascertainment or examination was used. If there was no information about this, the subnormal was classed as mildly subnormal if he had been to a school for the educationally subnormal, and severely subnormal if he had been excluded from the educational system. By these means it was possible to classify all the cases included in the survey.

In spite of its arbitrary nature the distinction between the mildly and severely subnormal is basically sound. This distinction is well documented and widely accepted. Dr Albert Kushlick (1966, pp. 73–82) writes:

It has long been known that in industrial societies, parents of severely subnormal children are evenly distributed among all the social strata in the society, while those of mildly subnormal subjects come predominantly from the lower social classes. Recent evidence suggests that mild subnormality, in the absence of abnormal neurological signs, epilepsy, electroencephalographic abnormalities, biochemical abnormalities, chromosomal abnormalities or sensory defects, is virtually confined to people in the lower social categories. Almost no children of higher social class parents have IQ scores of less than eighty, unless they have one of the pathological processes mentioned above.

This has been observed among ESN subjects, subjects referred to school psychological services and those taking the 11 plus examination [Saenger, 1960: Stein and Susser, 1963]. The Scottish Mental Survey of 1947 gave similar results. No child who scored less than an IQ of 86 had a professional father while no fewer than 26 per cent of children whose father had unskilled occupations had IQ equivalents under 86 [Scottish Council for Research in Education, 1953].

One incidental aspect of this study is to confirm this distinction. In general the mildly and severely subnormal are considered separately, and so the many ways in which they differ will be apparent throughout the text. The only point on which the data throw any doubt is whether the severely subnormal are quite as evenly distributed among all social strata as Dr Kushlick suggests in this quotation.

There is another less obvious, more general and unspecific factor which affects the scope of this survey. This is how and why society labels some people as subnormal. How did it happen, for instance, that a man with a university degree was certified as mentally defective? It is clear that criteria other than those simply of intelligence were applied.

But even criteria of intelligence are not simple and this matter must be considered first. The impact of social class was made clear in the above quotation from Dr Kushlick. Professor Townsend, in his foreword to Pauline Morris's book *Put Away* (1969, p. xv), points out the positive advantages that a middle-class child may have when it comes to intelligence testing:

> When eleven-year-olds are given two complete practice tests and a few hours of interspersed coaching the average gain is about nine points. A significant minority of children gain from fifteen to twenty-five or more points [Vernon, 1960]. The implications are important. If this is what can be done by familiarity and concentrated practice for a few hours or weeks, how much more important may be the years of 'coaching' in a privileged social setting?

Townsend goes on to say: 'Any wide-ranging analysis of recent evidence must conclude that human excellence is a social product as well as an individual quality' (pp. xvf). The impact of a person's social background is so pervasive that it is easy to forget its importance and consider him just as an individual, but the immense overall effect must be borne in mind. It will have affected the scope of the survey though not in any way that it is possible to quantify accurately. The social background of those who were included in the survey is considered in chapter 6. Behind the detailed discussion in that chapter lie the intangible but important factors mentioned here. The fact that virtually two-thirds of the mildly subnormal adults at home and one-fifth of the severely subnormal adults at home were either in open employment or were housewives must at least put a question mark against the relevance of the label that was attached to them.

Once that label had been attached it was very difficult for them to get rid of it. The spurious scientific exactness of an IQ score had the most undesirable effect of making people who were not aware of its limitations think that it was a fixed, unalterable and final judgment of that person's ability. Once an IQ score of 57 had been attached to someone, he tended to be considered as feeble-minded for ever more.

But this does not explain how a man with a university degree, and suffering from no intellectual impairment, could be sent to a mental deficiency institution. This particular man had interfered sexually with small children and he had been labelled as mentally defective because his behaviour was socially unacceptable. In the past, mental deficiency was considered to cover social incompetence and emotional immaturity. This was explicit in the classification of 'moral defective'. Indeed, there was even a category 'moral imbecile', which seemed on the evidence of the files to reflect the disgust with which the examining psychiatrist viewed the person's behaviour more than anything to do with the person's intelligence.

Deviant behaviour that evoked moral disapproval was likely to lead to a person being labelled mentally defective. A cruder way of putting it is that mental deficiency was used as a dustbin category. People were not labelled just for the sake of being labelled, but so that they could be dealt with. There were cases where a mental deficiency institution was used simply because nobody else would have those concerned. Labelling people as mentally defective was not just a matter of psychological fashion but of administrative convenience or necessity.

The 1959 Mental Health Act countered this misuse by including subnormality of intelligence within the definition of mental subnormality. Unfortunately the evidence from the Sheffield files lends some support to Professor Townsend's claim that 'a substantial number of people are classified either as "subnormal" or "severely subnormal" when their intelligence test scores considerably exceed the limits normally accepted for purposes of definition by psychologists.' Subnormality remains a dustbin category, just as mental deficiency was, in which some awkward customers, though probably fewer than before the 1959 Act, are dumped wrongly.

The fifty-four subnormals who were visited in this study were all severely subnormal and there was no question about their subnormality. A study in the United States by Edgerton (1967) looked at a very different group. He had extensive interviews with fifty-one ex-patients of Pacific State Hospital in California, choosing people who had a reasonable chance of success in independent city living.

'Thus, members of the research cohort are near the upper limit of the mildly retarded range in intelligence, they have a demonstrated ability for self-support, and they are old enough to have achieved some emotional stability,' he states (p. 11).

Of all the many burdens these people bore in the outside world the most crushing was the stigma of having been labelled as mentally defective: Edgerton writes (p. 205f):

> To find oneself regarded as a mental retardate is to be burdened by a shattering stigma. Indeed, for the former patient, to be labelled as a mental retardate is the ultimate horror. They reject it with all their will.

There was some evidence of this very understandable attitude in the files of some of the mildly subnormal.

However, as was said at the beginning of this chapter, the scope of this survey is an administrative one and in the first part of the book public attitudes are only seen as reflected in administrative procedures. Thus, the impact of education, and who should be treated as educable, will be seen in the age at which the subnormal was notified (chapters 3 and 4). The impact of social conditions can be seen in those notified because their fathers were out of work during the Depression between the two world wars (chapter 4). Changing social attitudes led to the 1959 Mental Health Act. The sharp drop following this legislative change in the number of people reported to the Mental Health Service is illustrated in the next chapter.

The basis for deciding the scope of this survey was primarily administrative, but administrative criteria are ultimately decided by social attitudes. It is worth remembering that the people considered in this survey were born any time between the 1880s and the 1960s. During that period social attitudes changed.

3   A profile of the survey population

Some basic definitions

The scope of the survey has been set out in chapter 2. In chapter 3 we shall be concerned with both the four standard groups, totalling 1,763 cases, and those persons for whom only a limited amount of data is available, totalling 364 cases. These latter cases are divided into two. First, there are 270 patients who were admitted to hospital before 5 July 1948 and, second, there are the ninety-four cases who moved into Sheffield from another local authority area. Five of these were also admitted to hospital before 5 July 1948.

Table 3.1   Table of all cases included in survey

	MSN Home	Institution	SSN Home	Institution	Total
Standard groups	746	120	674	223	1,763
Admitted to institutions before 5.7.48		116		154	270
Moved into Sheffield from elsewhere	25	16	41	12	94
Total	771	252	715	389	2,127

Naturally the early hospital cases appear only in the sections dealing with the mildly and severely subnormal in hospital. The discussion of prevalence in the seventh section includes people who moved into Sheffield from elsewhere.

The distinction between 'home' and 'institution' is generally clear-cut. For the vast majority of the cases this meant living at home or living in hospital, but for a few cases the distinction is not as clearly defined, as table 3.2 shows.

A 'hospital' was almost always a subnormality hospital; occasionally it referred to a subnormality ward in a mental hospital.

The general principle in deciding to which group any individual should belong was that once the subnormal had to leave his home he should be counted among the institution group. The new local authority hostel is an expression of the policy of 'community care' and part of the idea of the hostel is to keep people 'in the community'. However, the people in the hostel have had to leave their homes, whatever the reason, and therefore they, together with those in the hospital hostels and those in old people's homes, were put into the institution group. The two in prison were also put into the institution category for the same reason. They were difficult to categorize but being only two they do not make a great deal of difference.

Table 3.2   Residence as at 1 September 1968 (standard groups only)

Home	MSN	SSN	Institution	MSN	SSN
Home	743	671	Hospital	97	206
Children's home	3	3	Hospital hostel	10	3
			Local authority hostel	7	10
			Old people's home	4	4
			Prison	2	
Total	746	674		120	223

It must be admitted that to include those in a children's home among the home group is a little illogical. The reasons for doing so were of a practical nature. The child was often reported to the Mental Health Service when he was already in a children's home and there was often very little, if any, information about his own home. Furthermore, the criteria for admission to a children's home are likely to be different from those for admission to a subnormality hospital, and to equate the two seemed questionable. Fortunately there were only three mildly subnormal cases and three severely subnormal in a children's home on 1 September 1968, so the difference they make is minute.

The same might be said of an old people's home, but the files in these cases were generally much more informative about the home from which the subnormal came. More important, the reasons for subnormal old people being admitted to an old people's home are not likely to be so very different from the reasons for which subnormal old people are admitted to a subnormality hospital or hostel. In practice none of these categories was large enough to make much difference.

Table 3.1 divided the population surveyed into four groups. In the next four sections each group is considered in turn.

The mildly subnormal at home

If the definition of the mildly subnormal is taken as those whose IQ falls in the range 50–70, the total number of mildly subnormal in Sheffield would be in the region of 10,000. In practice the number of known mildly subnormal is less than a tenth of this. This figure is due to the administrative procedures for defining an ill-defined category. Many people who fall into this range of IQ manage to remain in the normal educational system and of those who do go to an ESN school, only a proportion are reported to the Mental Health Service when they leave.

The number of mildly subnormal on the books of the Mental Health Service is further reduced because the great majority are not reported until they actually leave ESN school. Table 3.3 shows the numbers reported at various ages, and illustrates clearly the high proportion of notifications at the age for leaving ESN school.

Table 3.3 Age mildly subnormal at home notified (standard group only)

Age	No.	%
0–8	23	3·1
9–13	87	11·7
14–16	502	67·5
17–18	36	4·8
19–39	89	12·0
40–55	7	0·9
Sub-total	744	100·0
Not known	2	
Total	746	

There is a steady increase in the numbers notified up to the age of sixteen. Those notified at fourteen, fifteen and sixteen have been grouped because some of the mildly subnormal were allowed to leave the ESN school early in order to start working, and therefore were reported before sixteen. Those who did this were considered to have completed their education. This happened more in the past, especially before the Second World War. Those reported in this age bracket account for two-thirds of the mildly subnormal at home. The thirty-six reported when aged seventeen or eighteen are likely to have encountered some problem in finding work or keeping it. Those who were reported earlier, that is up to the age of thirteen, tended to be on the borderline between mild and severe subnormality.

After eighteen the number reported at any one age never reaches double figures. The number reported after the age of thirty-nine is insignificant. Fifty-five was the highest age at which anyone in this group was reported.

The age at which the mildly subnormal tend to be reported has its effect on the age distribution of the mildly subnormal at home. This can be seen in figure 1 and table 3.4. The conventional quinquennia used in the diagram coincide with the actual dividing points, with two exceptions. There are three children aged fifteen who go most naturally into the age grouping below, and sixteen aged twenty-four who would go most naturally into the age group above. These adjustments give the broader age groupings shown in table 3.4.

Table 3.4　Age structure of mildly subnormal at home on 1 September 1968 (grouped)

Age	No.	%
0–4	0	
5–15	16	2·1
16–23	46	6·2
24–39	341	45·7
40–54	253	33·9
55+	90	12·1
Total	746	100·0

The very small number under sixteen is due to the fact that most mildly subnormal are notified at about sixteen years of age, as we have seen. The IQ was given in the file for thirteen of these sixteen mildly subnormal children. In twelve cases their IQ fell in the 50–54 range. This comes within the limit of fifty-five, which is sometimes set as the upper limit for severe subnormality. The remaining case fell into the 55–59 range.

The small number of mildly subnormal under sixteen is easy to understand; the small number in the next age grouping from sixteen to twenty-three, inclusive, is not. This is particularly puzzling in view of the very marked jump that takes place between those aged twenty-three and twenty-four. As the majority of the mildly subnormal were notified when they were about sixteen years old, the first thing to check was whether there had been a drop in the number of mildly subnormal being reported. Table 3.5 relates the number in selected age groups to the numbers notified in the period in which they are most likely to have been reported (i.e. when they were about sixteen).

Table 3.5 Age group related to period notified

Age group	16–23	24–29	30–34	35–39
No. in age group	46	113	122	106
No. notified	45	108	128	108
In period	1961–8	1955–60	1950–4	1945–9

This shows very clearly that the sharp drop between the number aged twenty-four and above and twenty-three and below is due to the much smaller number being notified. It does not explain in itself why the number notified should drop so sharply in 1960, but the year is significant. In November 1960 the 1959 Mental Health Act came into force and it was no longer necessary for local education authorities to refer cases for supervision after leaving school. In line with this, the policy in Sheffield changed. Up to 1960, when the old system was in operation, roughly half of the ESN school leavers were notified and the majority were ascertained as 'Feeble-minded'. After 1960 only those children whom the head teacher thought to be at risk were reported, and not all of these were taken on by the Mental Health Service.

We have just seen that the big increase in numbers from the age of twenty-four onwards is due to the greater number who were notified before 1961. This leaves unanswered the question of why the numbers of mildly subnormal at home should be so small in the older age groups. The life expectancy of the mildly subnormal is not vastly different from that of the general population. Why, then, should there be fewer in the forty to fifty-four age grouping than there are in the twenty-four to thirty-nine age grouping? Why is there such a sharp fall off over the age of fifty-five? Neither deaths nor hospital admissions can explain this adequately.

The answer lies in the limits imposed on the population surveyed. No one was included in the populations of mildly subnormal or severely subnormal at *home* with whom there had been no contact since before 5 July 1948. This cut-off date is likely to reduce the thirty-five to thirty-nine age group and onwards,[1] which has probably had a considerable effect because in a high proportion of the mildly subnormal cases contact was only maintained for a few years before they were discharged under the Mental Deficiency Acts (which were in operation until 1960, when the 1959 Mental Health Act came into force).

If the age structure of the mildly subnormal at home is compared to that of the mildly subnormal in hospital, which includes *all* patients irrespective of when they were admitted, it is quite clear that the exclusion of those at home with whom there had been no contact since before 5 July 1948 has reduced the numbers in the older age groups very considerably.

There are three additional minor factors which will have played a part in making the twenty-four to thirty-nine age grouping the largest. First, very few will die before the age of thirty-nine. Second, there is a steady trickle of mildly subnormal notified up to the age of thirty-nine, as can be seen from table 3.3. Third, except for those mentioned in chapter 2, none of those with whom there had been contact since 5 July 1948 have been excluded, even if the last contact was on that day.

It can be seen that the number of people who fall into this mildly subnormal group is determined to a considerable extent by administrative decisions and the limits of the survey. They have been affected in this way more than any of the other three groups.

The mildly subnormal in hospital

There are two groups to be considered—those who were admitted after the National Health Service Act came into effect and those who were admitted before. The amount of data available for those admitted before the Act is limited, as explained in chapter 2. Figure 2 (see p. 356) shows the age structure of the total mildly subnormal hospital population, which includes both groups.

One of the points made about the mildly subnormal at home applies with equal force to those now in hospital; they were reported only rarely before sixteen. Figure 2 makes this clear. There were only three mildly subnormal under sixteen in hospital. In both cases where the IQ was known it was in the 50–54 range.

On the other hand the fall off from the thirty-five to thirty-nine age group onwards, which occurs in the mildly subnormal group at home, does not occur in the hospital group. This is because those admitted to hospital before the National Health Service Act came into force have *not* been excluded from the table, but those at home with whom there has been no contact since 5 July 1948 *have* been excluded. What has to be explained here is the steep rise which occurs in the forty-five to forty-nine group onwards.

In the case of those in hospital the key factor was not the age at which they were reported but the age at which they were admitted to hospital. Figure 3 shows this. Figure 3a shows both those admitted before and after 5 July 1948 and figure 3b shows just those admitted after.

In figure 3a the outstanding feature is the very high proportion who went in between the ages of fifteen and nineteen inclusive. It amounts to no less than 28 per cent of the total. It is clear that this is largely due to those who were admitted before 5 July 1948. The forty-four in the early hospital group who were admitted between fifteen and nineteen inclusive are 38 per cent of the total of 116. However, this percentage is inflated because patients admitted before 5 July 1948 who were older when they were admitted are likely to have died.

The probable effect of this can be seen by looking at figure 3b, which shows the age on admission of those admitted to hospital since 5 July 1948. Here, the largest single age group is still the fifteen to nineteen age group, but it does not predominate in the same way. It is only 18 per cent of the total of 120. There is a second peak in the thirty-five to forty-nine age range. This is lacking in the early hospital group, probably because of deaths, though there is a small increase in the forty to forty-four age group.

The pattern of figure 3b suggests four wider age groupings, nought to nineteen, twenty to thirty-four, thirty-five to forty-nine and fifty plus. These take account of the two peaks, the slight dip in between, and the sharp fall off over fifty. Table 3.6 shows the figures for these larger groupings. In this table those admitted after 5 July 1948 have been divided.

Table 3.6   Age on admission to hospital (*mildly subnormal*)

	Years old 0–19		20–34		35–49		50+		Total	
	No.	%	No.	%	No.	%	No.	%	No.	%
Pre 5.7.48	60	51·7	40	34·5	15	12·9	1	0·9	116	100·0
6.7.48–1960	17	25·0	16	23·5	29	42·6	6	8·8	68	99·9
1961–8	12	23·1	14	26·9	16	30·8	10	19·2	52	100·0
Total	89		70		60		17		236	

Within these larger groupings the thirty-five to forty-nine age grouping is the largest in both groups admitted after 5 July 1948, with very little to choose between those admitted before they were twenty and those admitted between twenty and thirty-four. Among early hospital cases the under twenty grouping is by far the largest, as might be expected. It is the largest single category.

Now that the pattern of the age at which the patients were admitted has been considered, it is possible to see its effect on the age structure of the mildly subnormal hospital population. Figure 4 shows how the age on 1 September 1968 and the age at which the patients were admitted are related. It also shows the period in which they were admitted.

This figure indicates the cumulative effect of each of the three largest age brackets within which people were admitted. The result is a plateau from forty-five to sixty-four after which deaths start taking noticeable effect. It is worth drawing attention to the impact of those admitted before they were twenty in the early hospital group. There were sixty of them still in hospital on 1 September 1968 and they comprise just over one quarter of the mildly subnormal admitted to hospital from Sheffield. One reason why so many of them went into hospital in the first place was the total lack of training facilities for subnormals staying at home. The first occupation centre in Sheffield was not opened until 1938. Figure 4 also shows that the jump in the numbers in the forty-five to forty-nine age group onwards is due to the people admitted when they were aged between thirty-five and forty-nine inclusive. As those admitted when they were younger had neither died nor been discharged, generally speaking, the inevitable result is the increase in those aged forty-five to sixty-four.

Mention has been made in passing of the year in which patients were admitted but no attempt has been made to see if there is any discernible pattern. Figure 5 shows the quinquennium in which the total mildly subnormal hospital population was admitted.

The final 'quinquennium' is only three and two-third years because it finished on 1 September 1968. The dotted extension of the 1965–8 column shows the number that might have been expected in a full quinquennium. If we accept this estimate, then the picture is one of a steady rise. The smaller numbers admitted in the earlier part of the century can be accounted for by deaths. What is not so expected is the continued increase in admissions after 1960. In that year the 1959 Mental Health Act came into force and emphasized care at home in preference to care in hospital. These figures underline the point made in the first chapter, that the decisive shift in policy for the residential care of the subnormal did not come until the White Paper, *Better Services for the Mentally Handicapped* (see Department of Health and Social Security, 1971). However, the 1959 policy did have some effect. Out of the twenty-nine patients admitted between 1 January 1965 and 1 September 1968, seven went into the new local authority hostel. If these seven were removed, the estimate for the full quinquennium would be only twenty-nine, compared with thirty-five in the previous one.

The severely subnormal at home

The severely subnormal are a very different group from the mildly subnormal. Much of the data underlines how marked that difference is. Figure 6 shows the age structure of the severely subnormal at home. It is very different from that of the mildly subnormal. There is a steady fall from the five to nine group down to the few who are sixty-five or more. There are probably some who have been excluded because there has been no contact with them since 5 July 1948. The age structure of those in hospital suggests that this is the case (see figure 7). However, this steady fall is probably due for the greater part to the lower life expectancy of the severely subnormal and the increasing proportion in hospital.

There were only four under five years old known to the Mental Health Service on 1 September 1968. Generally, the severely subnormal start being reported when the education authorities find that they are unsuitable for school. As a result, 207 (31 per cent) were reported when they were four or five. They continue being reported in considerable numbers during school age. There is a final bump at sixteen when seventy-two (11 per cent) were reported. Table 3.7 summarizes this.

Table 3.7   Age severely subnormal at home reported to Mental Health Service

Age reported	0–3	4	5	6–10	11–15	16	Over 16	Total
No.	27	84	123	194	155	72	19	674
%	4·0	12·5	18·2	28·8	23·0	10·7	2·8	100·0

The severely subnormal in hospital

Two distinct groups fall into this category, as was the case with the mildly subnormal. There are those who were admitted before the National Health Service Act came into effect, and those who were admitted after. Figure 7 shows the age structure of all the severely subnormal from Sheffield who were in hospital on 1 September 1968. This includes both groups. In this diagram they are not distinguished.

The pattern is quite different from that of the mildly subnormal hospital population. The biggest peak is much earlier, reaching its height in the thirty to thirty-four age group. Then there is rather a puzzling drop, which raises the question of whether the thirty-five to thirty-nine and forty-five to forty-nine age groups are freakishly low or whether the forty to forty-four age group is freakishly high. If the latter is the case, does this mean that it is a bi-modal distribution, and if so, why?

One thing that figure 7 does show clearly is that many of the severely subnormal are not short-lived. This suggests that the age structure of the severely subnormal at home has been affected by the exclusion of those with whom there has been no contact since 5 July 1948.

The answer to some at least of the questions raised by the age structure can be seen in figure 8, which shows the age at which the severely subnormal were admitted to hospital. Figure 8a shows those admitted both before and after 5 July 1948. Figure 8b shows only those admitted after that date.

The lack of early hospital cases admitted in the older age groups can be explained by deaths. There does not appear to be a fundamentally different pattern of age on admission before and after the National Health Service Act. It will be remembered that in the case of the mildly subnormal in hospital there did appear to be a different pattern.

The age at which the severely subnormal tend to be admitted is younger. Twenty-eight per cent were admitted before the age of ten. Less than 4 per cent of the mildly subnormal were admitted to hospital before that age. A further substantial proportion of the severely subnormal were admitted between the ages of ten and nineteen inclusive. This was 38 per cent of the total: seventy-three of these (19 per cent) were in the fifteen to nineteen age group in which the mildly subnormal are so heavily concentrated. It is likely that some of these were on the borderline of mild and severe subnormality.

The big difference between the mildly and severely subnormal comes in the older age groups. There is no second peak in the age on admission among the severely subnormal, as there is with mildly subnormal. There is a steady falling away, with the sole exception of the unusually low figure for the twenty-five to twenty-nine group. There is no obvious reason for this. The twenty to twenty-four age bracket is the last one of any size. Fifty-two patients (14 per cent) were admitted in their twenties, and seventy-seven (20 per cent) were admitted when aged thirty or more.

This gives some clues to the reasons behind the age structure of the severely subnormal in hospital, but not much more. Figure 9 shows how the age structure is made up by the age grouping in which the patient was admitted and the period in which he was admitted. Note that the age groupings are different from those used for the mildly subnormal.

This figure shows some of the reasons underlying the age structure. Those admitted before ten tend to die early, and as a result there is nothing comparable with the jump in the mildly subnormal hospital population in the forty-five to forty-nine age bracket. This early mortality does not appear to affect those admitted between ten and nineteen years old. There are six of them in the seventy to seventy-four age group.

The grouping who were oldest on admission (thirty or older) provide a consistent proportion of each age group from forty to forty-four onwards. It is they who form the second peak in the age structure, in conjunction with a considerable number of those admitted before 5 July 1948, when aged between ten and nineteen years old.

There is no obvious reason for the fluctuation in the thirty-five to forty-nine age groups. The diagram shows that most of the jump in the forty to forty-four age bracket is due to those admitted while in their twenties, between 5 July 1948 and 31 December 1960. It can however provide no explanation for why this should be. The relationship between why patients were admitted and the age at which they were admitted is considered in chapter 5.

Year of admission The length of time that many of these people have been in hospital has been mentioned already. Figure 10 shows just how long. The fluctuations before 1950 are not very marked but there is a sharp increase in the quinquennium 1950–4. Thunder-cliffe Grange, a subnormality hospital for children, was opened in

1950. Not all of its sixty beds were for Sheffield children, but a backlog of urgent cases was admitted when it first opened. This illustrates as clearly as anything the acute shortage of beds in the Sheffield area. The estimated number for the full quinquennium 1965–9 (i.e. allowing for the missing one and one-third years) is sixty-eight, which is shown by the dotted line. However, ten of those admitted between 1 January 1965 and 1 September 1968 went to the new local authority hostel, which opened in April 1968. If these ten are taken away, the estimated figure for 1965–9 is fifty-five, almost exactly the same as the previous three quinquennia.

It seems that figure 10 is merely an indication of beds available. So long as there is a shortage of beds any increase in admissions will relate directly to an increase in the number of beds available, not the need for beds.

Prevalence

The discussion so far has not considered those who came into Sheffield from other local authority areas. As only limited data were available for these cases, it was difficult to include them in the general discussion. To have done so would have meant continually altering the totals being considered. There is one place where they must be included and that is in any discussion of prevalence. Therefore in this section the figures used include the four standard groups, the early hospital cases and the immigrants from other local authority areas. This gives the following totals:

	MSN			SSN	
Home	Institution	Total	Home	Institution	Total
771	252	1,023	715	389	1,104

Grand total 2,127

Table 3.8 compares the rate per 1,000 in each age group with the figures for Salford in 1961.[2]

In the case of the mildly subnormal the total figures for Salford and Sheffield are quite close. In both cases the figures were limited to those known to the Mental Health Service. The outstanding difference is in the fifteen to nineteen age group. The key factor here is probably the difference in date. The Salford figures are for 1961, the Sheffield ones for 1968. It has been seen already, in the section on the mildly subnormal at home, that since 1960 many fewer mildly subnormal children have been reported to the Mental Health

Service by the Education Department. This more selective policy has had a very marked effect on the numbers of mildly subnormal on the books of the Mental Health Service, and does much to account for the difference between Sheffield and Salford in the rates for this age group. This change in policy affected those aged twenty-three or less in 1968, and therefore it has affected the twenty to twenty-nine age group as well, though to a lesser extent.

Table 3.8   Prevalence rate of subnormality per 1,000 in each age group

	MSN Sheffield	Salford	SSN Sheffield	Salford
	1968	1961	1968	1961
0–4	0·00	0·15	0·34	0·89
5–9	0·06	0·36	3·70	1·62
10–14	0·46	0·29	3·66	2·55
15–19	0·78	8·63	2·55	3·62
20–29	2·83	4·16	3·98	3·44
30–39	5·00	1·83	3·32	3·77
40–49	3·43	2·56	2·23	2·47
50–59	2·70	1·04	1·58	1·70
60+	1·29	0·60	0·83	0·52
All age groups	2·12	2·06	2·29	2·24

In all the older age groups the Sheffield figures are higher than those for Salford. This is due to the inclusion in the Sheffield figures of those who have been discharged and are no longer active cases, and their exclusion from the Salford figures. It needs to be borne in mind that the numbers of mildly subnormal are subject to considerable variation, depending on definition and administrative practice, and any rates will reflect this as much as any theoretical absolute prevalence.

The rates for the severely subnormal are more even. In the main, the Sheffield figures show the same pattern as the Salford ones. The higher rates for Sheffield in the five to nine and ten to fourteen age groups could be related to administrative procedures and provision of facilities such as training centres. Provision of junior training centre places was increased considerably in Sheffield in 1963, when the Norfolk Park Junior Training Centre was opened, which provided a total of 140 places.

The Salford and Sheffield figures are quite close for all age groups from twenty to twenty-nine and upwards, but there is a puzzling dip in the Sheffield rates for the fifteen to nineteen age group for which there is no obvious explanation. It is accepted generally that the number of severely subnormal known in the fifteen to nineteen age group is very close to the actual number, as the vast majority will have been reported—only 4 per cent of the severely subnormal in Sheffield were reported after they were sixteen. Kushlick (1968, p. 372) found:

> that the prevalence rates of recognized severe subnormality in Salford remained constant from the age group fifteen to nineteen until the age of forty when it began to fall due to deaths among these subjects.

The difference between the Salford and the Sheffield rate for the fifteen to nineteen age group (Salford: 3·62; Sheffield: 2·55) is all the more puzzling because the Sheffield rates for two earlier age groups are 3·70 (ages five to nine) and 3·66 (ages ten to fourteen). In fact the Sheffield figures remain constant not from the fifteen to nineteen age group, as in Salford, but from the five to nine age group up to the age of forty, except for the fifteen to nineteen age group. Table 3·9 compares the Sheffield figures with those for Middlesex and Wessex. These figures are taken once again from Kushlick (1968).

Table 3.9   Comparison of prevalence rates of severe subnormality in younger age groups, where all subjects are likely to be known

	Middlesex (Goodman and Tizard, 1962) 1960	Salford (Kushlick, 1961) 1961	Wessex (Kushlick, 1964) 1964	1964	Sheffield 1968
			County boroughs	Counties	
10–14	3·61	2·55			3·65
15–19		3·62	3·54	3·84	2·55

The higher figures for the younger (ten to fourteen) age group, which are comparable with the Middlesex figures, suggest that the lower figures for the fifteen to nineteen age group, which contradict not only these but other studies, are a quirk which may be due to some now unknown administrative decision. There is no reason to think that severely subnormal children were less likely to have been born in Sheffield between 1949 and 1953.

Apart from this one age group the figures for Sheffield are comparable with those for Salford, and where there is a marked variation, a difference in administrative practice appears to provide the most likely explanation.

4 How the subnormal were reported

The mildly subnormal

The great majority of the mildly subnormal were reported to the Mental Health Service at about the age of sixteen, that is when they left ESN school. The section in the previous chapter on the mildly subnormal at home touched on the age at which they were reported, but this was omitted from the section on the mildly subnormal in hospital.

The pattern of the ages at which the two groups were reported is rather different and women tended to be reported later than men. About eighteen appears to be the critical age for distinguishing between the age at which the different groups were reported, as table 4.1 shows.

Table 4.1   Age at which mildly subnormal reported

Age reported	Home Male No.	%	Female No.	%	Institution Male No.	%	Female No.	%
Up to 18	365	93·4	283	80·2	43	69·4	31	54·4
Over 18	26	6·6	70	19·8	19	30·6	26	45·6
Total	391	100·0	353	100·0	62	100·0	57	100·0

χ^2 on whole table = 75·223   p = 0·001 χ^2 Home/Inst. = 46·579
p=0·001

The two most striking figures, and the most significant statistically, are the small proportion of males at home (7 per cent) and the large proportion of females in an institution (46 per cent) who were reported when they were over eighteen.

The noticeably higher age at which those now in an institution tended to be reported indicates that the two groups must differ in some respect, even if only in who reported them. It is unlikely that anyone over eighteen would be reported by the Education Department. The next step therefore is to see which agency or which people reported the mildly subnormal to the Mental Health Service. This is shown in table A1 (see appendix A). The two chief sources of referral were the Education Department and the Ministry of Social Security (or one of its predecessors: the National Assistance Board, the Public Assistance Committee or the Unemployed Assistance Board). The predominance of the Education Department is marked. Fewer females than males were reported by the Education Department and fewer of those in hospital than those at home. Conversely, more females than males were reported by the Ministry of Social Security and more of those in hospital than those at home.

In the population at large it is men rather than women who tend to get into trouble with the police, and this is true of the mildly subnormal. Those reported by the police or prison authorities were the second largest group among the males now in an institution (11 per cent). It can be seen that the women tend to be reported by the Ministry of Social Security, whereas the men tend to be reported by the police. The only other agency to report any number is some other service of the local authority. Included in this figure are those reported by a children's home through the Children's Department. Six of the seventeen males and four of the seventeen females at home and one of the four males in an institution were accounted for in this way.

We have seen already that the mildly subnormal in hospital tend to be reported later than those at home, and this is significant statistically. If we compare the agency which reported those notified up to the age of eighteen with the agency which reported those notified over the age of eighteen, we find, naturally enough, that the Education Department reported the overwhelming majority of those reported up to the age of eighteen (87 per cent of those at home and 85 per cent of those in hospital). But the main point of interest is those who were reported when they were over eighteen. They were reported by a wide variety of different people and agencies, of whom the Ministry of Social Security was the most important. The figures for those who were reported by the Ministry of Social Security (or rather the Public Assistance Committee) are given in table 4.2. This pattern makes one possibility seem very likely. Those who were under nineteen, and especially those under seventeen, when they were reported, were reported either as a matter of routine up to 1960 or after that as a precaution. Those who were reported after eighteen would be reported in most cases because some crisis had arisen.

They were found to be subnormal and so admission to a subnormality hospital appears to have been the way in which the crisis was resolved in quite a number of cases.

There remains the interesting question of why so many women were reported by the Ministry of Social Security or one of its predecessors. On the back of one of the old forms for admitting a mental defective person to an institution were the various circumstances which 'rendered a person being a defective liable to be dealt with under petition' (that is a petition to have them admitted to an institution). One of the circumstances was that 'she is in receipt of poor relief at the time of giving birth to an illegitimate child or when pregnant of such a child'. Clearly this would only affect the women, but unfortunately this neat way of explaining why there were more women in this group will not do, because this particular 'circumstance' went out even before the Poor Law was abolished, finally, in 1948, besides which only two of the eleven women who were reported by the Ministry of Social Security and were in an institution had had illegitimate children.

A more plausible explanation is that these were people who were affected by the Depression. This is given strong support when the year in which they were reported is considered. None of them was reported later than 1945. Three were reported between 1921 and 1928. Thirty-six were reported between 1931 and 1939 and seventeen were reported between 1940 and 1945. Nine were reported in 1931, the greatest number in any single year. The pattern in many cases was that the father would lose his job and apply for relief. When the relieving officer investigated he would discover that one member of the family over the age of sixteen was not earning. Some explanation had to be given for this[1] and if the person concerned 'appeared to be mentally defective', in all probability he would be ascertained as such and a satisfactory reason would have been provided as to why he was not earning.

But why more women than men? A local government official recalled that, between the wars, the workhouses were full of women, and thought that it was even more difficult for women than for men to get work in Sheffield during the Depression. This could account for it. It is impossible to check, as the relevant records were destroyed during the Second World War, and the figures that are available do not separate the sexes.

This suggests that those reported by the Ministry of Social Security, or rather the Public Assistance Committee, fall into a different category from the rest. Had social conditions been different and had there been no Depression, it is very likely that most of them would never have been reported. This may well be true even of most of those in an institution, because nine out of the thirteen were only admitted because of the death or illness of a parent. Under other circumstances they might well have gone into an old people's home, but only two of them did, and then only after the label of mental defective had been attached to them.

In view of the rather special position of those reported by the Public Assistance Committee there is a strong case for considering them separately. If they are deducted from those who were reported over the age of eighteen the difference is considerable. This is shown in table 4.2.

Table 4.2   Mildly subnormal reported over age of eighteen by Public Assistance Committee and other agencies

| | Home | | Institution | |
	Male	Female	Male	Female
Reported by PAC	8	35	2	11
Not reported by PAC	18	35	17	15
Total	26	70	19	26

The figures for those not reported by the Public Assistance Committee strengthen the contention that, in the case of the men, those reported after eighteen were reported because of some crisis, and so were much more likely to go into hospital than were those reported earlier. The number of men at home and in hospital was almost the same, but the eighteen men from the home group were only 4·5 per cent of the total, whereas the seventeen men from the institution group were 27 per cent of the total.

A much higher proportion of the women who had not been reported by the Public Assistance Committee were at home. Some clue as to why there should be a higher proportion of women than men at home can be gained by looking at the reasons which precipitated their admission to hospital. Eleven of the seventeen men were admitted because of some behaviour problem, but only five of the fifteen women were admitted for this reason. This does suggest that in many cases, with the men, it was a problem of behaviour which led to them being reported in the first place. The difference in the number of men and women reported by the police is one indication of this. Ten men, five at home and five of them in hospital, were reported by the police, but only one woman.

It is difficult to suggest any positive reasons why there should be more women than men at home in this group, apart from the assumption that the women were more likely to be useful in the home. It may be also that the women were more likely to be reported as a purely precautionary measure, because of the possibility of their being exploited, especially sexually. The greater number of women than men in the home group who were reported by their family may lend some support to this suggestion.

The severely subnormal

The severely subnormal were considerably younger than the mildly subnormal when they were reported, as they were reported to the Mental Health Service most frequently when they were excluded from the educational system. This has been mentioned in the previous chapter in the section on the severely subnormal at home.

There is no marked difference between the ages at which the sexes were reported. Females both at home and in an institution tended to be reported a little later than males, but this was not at all pronounced.

Table 4.3 compares the age at which those at home and those in hospital were reported.

Table 4.3   Age at which severely subnormal reported

	Home No.	%	Institution No.	%
0–3	27	4·0	29	13·0
4	84	12·5	18	8·1
5	123	18·2	31	13·9
6–10	194	28·8	85	38·1
11–15	155	23·0	24	10·8
16	72	10·7	19	8·5
More than 16	19	2·8	17	7·6
Total	674	100·0	223	100·0

χ^2 on whole table = 53·840   p = 0·001
χ^2 on more than 16 against the rest = 10·040   p = 0·01

It can be seen that those in hospital were reported rather earlier than those at home. This fits in with what might be expected. The more severely handicapped the child was, the more likely he was to be reported early, and also the more likely to need admission to hospital. This is particularly obvious in the case of those who were reported very early, before the age of four. By the age of ten, 64 per cent of those at home had been reported, but in the case of those in hospital the proportion is 73 per cent.

This tendency for the severely subnormal in hospital to be reported earlier than those at home is the reverse of what holds for the mildly subnormal. In their case those in hospital tended to be reported later. There is however a small group of the severely subnormal who follow the pattern of the mildly subnormal. There were seventeen men in hospital who were reported over the age of sixteen (8 per cent of the total in hospital). There were nineteen at home who were reported over the age of sixteen, and they are only 3 per cent of the total at home. This raises the same question as with the mildly subnormal—are they a distinct group? Can the agency that reported them tell us anything about them? Table 4.4 shows the agency which reported the severely subnormal at home and in hospital, and divides them by the age they were reported. There is no difference of any importance between the sexes.

Table 4.4 Agency reporting severely subnormal by age reported

	Under 17 Home	Institution	17+ Home	Institution
Education Department	610 (93·3%)	171 (83·4%)	2	1
Family	7	5	1	4
Other local authority service	13 (2%)	11 (5·4%)	0	0
Police or prison	1	1	0	1
Hospital or G.P.	16 (2·4%)	11 (5·4%)	0	4
MSS, etc.	4	3	13	3
Other	3	3	2	3
Sub-total	654	205	18	16
Not known	1	1	1	1
Total	655	206	19	17

The predominance of the Education Department as an agency among those who were reported before the age of sixteen is even more marked among the severely subnormal than among the mildly subnormal. The reason for this is that most of the severely subnormal were excluded from the educational system and when this happened they had to be reported to the Mental Health Service. This being so, it is necessary to explain why the figure is not 100 per cent. The explanation lies in the way the information was coded. The agency which first reported the subnormal to the Mental Health Service was the one which was entered. In most, if not all, cases of those reported up to sixteen years old the Education Department would have reported them as well. Thus, those reported by another local authority service, for instance a children's home or a health visitor, are likely to have been noticed before the child was of school age.

When we turn to those aged seventeen or more when they were reported, there is the same outstanding feature as was found with the mildly subnormal, namely, the high proportion reported by the Ministry of Social Security or, if the same is true of the severely subnormal as of the mildly subnormal, the Public Assistance Committee. The explanation is the same. The three in hospital were reported between 1934 and 1938, and those at home were reported between 1931 and 1945. All but three were reported in the 1930s. (The seven reported by the Public Assistance Committee before they were seventeen were also reported during the same period.) The distribution of the sexes among those reported by the Public Assistance Committee over the age of sixteen was more even than was the case with the mildly subnormal. Eight of the thirteen at home and two of the three in hospital were women. The ages at which they were reported range from twenty to thirty-eight. Even though these people were classed as imbeciles when they were reported, it is quite possible that they would never have come to the attention of the authorities but for their families having to apply for out-relief. Two of the three people in an institution only went in because of the death or illness of the person looking after them.

If this group of people, who were reported by the Public Assistance Committee and who seem to fall into a different category from the rest, is deducted from those persons reported over the age of sixteen, we are left with only six at home but fourteen in hospital. This suggests that the point made in respect of the mildly subnormal is even more relevant in the case of the severely subnormal. Those reported up to the age of sixteen will be reported as a matter of course. Those reported after sixteen will be reported because some crisis has arisen and in more cases than not it appears that the crisis was resolved by admission to an institution.

5 Factors which precipitated admission to hospital

Introduction

In the course of reading many of the files of those in hospital, it became clear that there was a key factor which had tipped the balance and led to admission. The most obvious was when the mother or the person in charge of the subnormal died or fell ill and the subnormal had to be admitted. This factor would not always have been self-evident from the other data, and so a specific entry was made for the factor which appeared to precipitate admission. It is only the *precipitating* factor, the one which actually led to the subnormal being admitted. It is not the only factor. For instance, if the subnormal was behaving very badly and started hitting his mother, this might be the precipitating factor. But the fact that the mother was getting old might be an important contributory one. It is only possible to show one precipitating factor.

The total number of different precipitating factors coded was twenty-seven, but they fall quite naturally into the five groups shown in table 5.1. Some of these categories have been grouped together in the detailed tables because in practice the distinction did not seem to be a real one.

Table 5.1   Precipitating factors in admission to hospital

Precipitating factor	MSN No.	%	SSN No.	%	Total No.	%
Behaviour or management	58	50·9	93	42·7	151	45·5
Death or illness of parent or parent figure	37	32·5	66	30·3	103	31·0
Social reasons	16	14·0	31	14·2	47	14·2
Nursing problem	1	0·9	19	8·7	20	6·0
Other	2	1·7	9	4·1	11	3·3
Sub-total	114	100·0	218	100·0	332	100·0
Not known	6		5		11	
Not known as % of total	5·0		2·2		3·2	
Total	120		223		343	

In the five sections which follow, each of these groups of pre-cipitating factors is considered in turn. The aim is to give some idea of the human realities behind these labels.

Behaviour or management

Table 5.1 shows how important a factor this is. It accounts for nearly half of all those who have gone into hospital. It was behaviour rather than management which was dominant. There were a few, thirteen in all, where the problem was one of management not associated with a serious behaviour disorder. The case notes record in one such case:

> The sister-in-law told the mental welfare officer that Andrew is getting on her nerves. When he is in the house he is very noisy, humming all the time and if he has to visit the bathroom at night he switches all the lights on and bangs the doors.

One older subnormal woman kept wandering away from home and getting lost. In addition to these thirteen, there were eight cases where the problem was one of management connected with epilepsy.

But such cases are a small minority in this group. Table 5.2 shows how the group is made up in detail.

Table 5.2   Details of 'Behaviour or management' factor

Category	MSN	SSN	Total
Problem of management not connected with serious behaviour disorder	6	7	13
Management associated with epilepsy	2	6	8
Aggressive behaviour	7	14	21
Aggressive and destructive behaviour	6	28	34
Behaviour and inadequate parental control	9	10	19
Behaviour and bad home conditions	5	3	8
Anti-social sexual behaviour	8	4	12
Crime or contact with police	6	3	9
Behaviour problem with younger sibs	0	6	6
General behaviour problem	9	12	21
Total	58	93	151

The two largest categories are 'Aggressive behaviour' and 'Aggressive and destructive behaviour'. These two categories accounted for fifty-five out of the 151 admitted as a result of some problem of behaviour or management.

This is hardly surprising. The mental welfare officer wrote of one visit to a severely subnormal man who was twenty-six at the time: 'John not too good this visit, he was very destructive and restless. His mother says when he is in this mood he tears things up and throws things of value on the fire.' Four months later he was admitted. In another case the Medical Officer of Health, writing to the Regional Hospital Board to try to obtain a hospital bed for a young man of sixteen, referred to a previous letter and continued:

> Since that date the mother, a widow, has reported that Philip has smashed the television set and attacked her on numerous occasions, causing actual bodily harm. He has now begun to struggle violently in the street when being taken to the bus for conveyance to the training centre and during these struggles he has kicked her very severely and has inflicted a deep cut on the face.

Another example is a strong tall man on the borderline between mild and severe subnormality who was intelligent enough to lead his parents, especially his mother, a fearful dance at home. He was twenty-seven years old when he was admitted. The mental welfare officer reported to the consultant psychiatrist:

> Edward has been throwing things at the electric light and breaking many other things in the house. He is shouting and waking the neighbour's baby up. He has ripped much of his clothing and his mother produced two vests and a jersey to prove this. He is taking his trousers and underpants off and refusing to put them on again. He wets himself from time to time. His mother has also caught him thumping the cat viciously.

Six months later the case notes relate:

> Today the G.P. reported the subnormal as being completely out of hand. He has been trying to harm himself by scratching at his neck and wrists and when the police had been called to a disturbance at the house the subnormal proceeded to half strangle the cat in their presence, grinning broadly all the time.

In another case a mildly subnormal man had lived with his parents quite peaceably for many years, then, when he was thirty, there was an incident of indecent behaviour. He was put on probation and returned home. It was seven years after this that the mental welfare officer wrote in the case notes:

> Brother and sister called at this office requesting urgent institutional care for subnormal. He has been in one of his tantrums since Sunday and his aged parents are afraid of him and unable to do anything with him. He has struck out at his father who is seventy-six years of age and suffers from a cardiac condition and is liable to collapse at any time; the mother is seventy years of age and registered as a blind person. Subnormal himself has had no food for two days and will not allow his parents to get any themselves. He has twice this week thrown all the food in the house on the fire. He is tearing his clothes to pieces and is generally destroying the home.

The worst cases tended to fall into the two categories of 'Aggressive behaviour' or 'Aggressive and destructive behaviour'.

Another category of some importance (nineteen cases) was 'Behaviour and inadequate parental control'. In these cases it was still the subnormal's behaviour which was the precipitating factor, but it appeared from the file that the parents' inability or reluctance to cope with the subnormal's behaviour was an important contributory factor. For instance, there was the boy whose school report said: 'At home he frequently tears the bed clothing. He is very destructive; will scratch the mortar out of the walls and often breaks the crockery.' The psychiatrist's report said of the mother: 'Her husband has left her. She lives with her aged parents. She is filthy, smells, drinks and is of poor moral standard. The mother is in my opinion of weak intelligence and character.'

Another case concerned a boy who was ten years old when he was admitted. The case notes indicated that it was a poor home and the father was illiterate. The Medical Officer of Health wrote: 'His conduct is not good. He throws stones, is difficult to manage and sometimes plays truant from the centre. These attacks nearly always follow a domestic crisis of which there are many.'

A further example serves to illustrate how difficult it is to distinguish inadequate parental control from the sheer difficulty of controlling the behaviour of some of the subnormals. In the face of the behaviour that some of them exhibited, very few parents would be 'adequate'. This severely subnormal boy was nine when he was admitted. The mother was illiterate. The mental welfare officer wrote in November: 'He is definitely beyond his mother's control.' In December he wrote:

> Visited following phone call from police, also fire brigade, stating that subnormal was on the rooftops again, this being about the fifth occasion during the past four or five weeks. The P.C. had been in the house for about four hours when I arrived. Subnormal was in a very dirty state and his clothes were all torn and his mother stated that she could not control him.

He used to get on to the roof in various ways. Sometimes he climbed out of the bedroom window; on another occasion he broke away from his mother when she was taking him out. His roof-climbing exploits were made more alarming by the fact that he was subject to major epileptic fits.

This category was often hard to distinguish from 'Behaviour and bad home conditions' (total of eight cases). One case where the house was described as 'very dirty and smelt very foul' was actually coded under 'Inadequate parental control', as the mother had been in prison several times for prostitution and other offences.

The precipitating factor in twelve cases was 'Anti-social sexual behaviour'. Ten of these were female and only two men. This ranged from completely promiscuous behaviour to 'The main problem is her constant lack of modesty which is upsetting people in the district.' While women accounted for most of those where the precipitating factor was 'Anti-social sexual behaviour', eight out of nine cases where the precipitating factor was 'Crime or contact with the police' were men. This is really self-explanatory. The record was the boy who was the subject of thirty-three police reports over a period of six months. In several instances the case was dropped by the police on the understanding that the subnormal would be sent to hospital; in others a court order was made directing that the subnormal should be admitted to hospital.

If the subnormal's behaviour was disturbed, the presence of other children was sometimes the critical factor. The medical report on a severely subnormal boy of eleven read: 'Very excitable—extreme temper: injures other children. Very troublesome in house as there are twins of four and a boy of six in danger.' In another case the mental welfare officer reported that the mother of a severely subnormal boy of eight was very distressed and 'she told me that Harry had hit his younger brother in the eye with a poker and that the child had had to be admitted to the Children's Hospital'. There were only six cases in this category, 'Behaviour problem with younger sibs', though the presence of younger children was certainly a factor in some other cases where the subnormal's behaviour was difficult.

The remaining category of 'General behaviour problem' was used where a more specific coding was difficult to make. There were twenty-one cases. Some of these cases come quite close to other categories, especially 'Aggressive behaviour' or 'Aggressive and destructive behaviour'.

There is much overlapping between the different categories and in view of this it is better to consider these cases under the general heading of 'Behaviour or management'. The sub-headings that have been described give some idea of the range of behaviour that this covers.

Death or illness of parent or parent figure

This was the second most common factor leading to admission to hospital, 31 per cent of the total being admitted because of this. Table 5.3 shows the detailed breakdown of this group.

Table 5.3　Details of 'Death or illness of parent or parent figure' factor

Category	MSN	SSN	Total
Death of mother or mother figure	18	30	48
Death of father or father figure	7	6	13
Parent or parent figure old, ill or infirm and cannot cope	12	30	42
Total	37	66	103

It was the death of the mother, or sometimes the mother figure (generally an aunt or sister of the subnormal), which accounted for nearly half of this group. The need for admission in these cases was so urgent that generally it happened extremely quickly. In a few cases the subnormal might stay a few days with a brother or sister or some other relative, but if that relative refused to be responsible for him, the authorities had no alternative but to admit the subnormal.

Thirteen subnormals were admitted following their father's death. In six cases the subnormal was living alone with his or her father, and the father's death made admission essential. In other cases the father's death deprived the mother of her husband's help, on which she depended, and so led to the subnormal's admission. This was so in the case of Geoffrey, a severely subnormal man who was twenty-nine years old when he was admitted. The mental welfare officer reported:

> Mrs C. is now very frightened of the subnormal and feels that she can no longer control him. His father was able to do so, but since his death that controlling influence has gone and the subnormal has become very difficult.

The distinction between the mother or the father dying and the subnormal having to be admitted to hospital, and the parents being ill and unable to look after him, was, in some cases, only a distinction of time. The case of Janet, a severely subnormal mongol aged thirty-five when she was admitted, illustrates this. An entry by the mental welfare officer in 1948 reads:

> Janet is in severe pain today (gallstones) and apparently has attacks about every six weeks which are increasing in severity. Mother is in poor general health and quite upset about Janet's condition.

A laconic entry next year says: 'Visited Janet by request—aged mother dying and no relative will accept responsibility for defective.'

The reluctance, refusal or unsuitability of relatives to care for the subnormal was a recurrent theme. The mother of one severely subnormal had 'a heart condition and disc trouble and was not considered by the doctor or the mental welfare officer to be capable of looking after her daughter though she was willing to do so'. She had one older sister, but 'the older sister has other responsibilities and is unwilling to take Mary on as well and lives too far away to take her to the Occupation Centre'. In another case the mother had entered hospital suffering from diabetes, hypertension, gangrene and had had one foot amputated. She was not expected to be discharged. There had been one helpful sister but she had died a short while previously and there was no one else willing or able to look after Joan.

In almost all these cases where admission to hospital was precipitated by the death or illness of the person looking after them, it was hard to see any alternative to permanent residential care. The age of which many of this group were admitted is striking, as will be seen in the sections on the factors precipitating admission and the age admitted later on in this chapter.

Social reasons

This factor came third in importance; 14 per cent of the total went into hospital for some reason included under this heading. It covers a wider range than the previous two general factors, as can be seen from table 5.4.

Table 5.4   Details of 'Social reasons' factor

Category	MSN	SSN	Total
Physical condition of subnormal and bad home conditions	2	2	4
Unsatisfactory home conditions	8	9	17
No home	4	8	12
Inadequate parental control or care	2	6	8
Parents' anxiety about other children	0	4	4
Family crisis unrelated to subnormal	0	2	2
Total	16	31	47

The first three categories all cover a rather similar state of affairs. The file said of one girl's mother:

> Mr A. has spent two short periods in prison on larceny charges recently. Mrs A. left with full family responsibilities has found it increasingly difficult to manage the children and affairs.
> She is not enjoying good mental health herself.

In another case the father asked if his seven-year-old boy could be placed in an institution, as he, his wife, the boy and their baby were all living in one room. Both of these cases were coded as 'unsatisfactory home conditions'.

The same coding was given in the case of a mildly subnormal boy of four about whom the Medical Officer of Health wrote to the Regional Hospital Board saying:

> When visiting yesterday the welfare officer was shown a small, dark and filthy room off a larger bedroom which is said to be the subnormal's mother's (she is subnormal herself). On that date she admitted to cohabiting with a coloured man but

denied promiscuous intercourse with others. This denial did
not convince the officer.

The category 'Inadequate parental control or care' was used
sparingly, because often the parents were contending with so
impossible a situation that such a judgment seemed unjust. However,
it appeared reasonable to use it when the psychiatrist's report said
of an eight-year-old boy, classified as an idiot:

> He stands no chance of mental development in this appalling
> house run by a mother who is herself obviously defective and a
> father who is unstable, a drinker and might well go insane
> in the near future.

The same could be said of the home background of a severely
subnormal epileptic boy who was ten years old when he was admitted.
The initial report on the home said:

> This is a very poor set up. Parents are mentally defective.
> Mother unable to manage house and family, mixed up with
> other men, clears off for days. Father in regular employment—
> drinks a lot.

Two years later the mental welfare officer wrote: 'Philip continues
to be a problem, his mother lets him run wild and has no idea of
controlling him, he is destructive and just about unmanageable.'
Two years after that there is a letter from the National Society for
the Prevention of Cruelty to Children, in which the Inspector
reported:

> 9.25 p.m. On visiting I found that the father was out at work.
> On investigation I discovered that the mother had left the home
> at about 7 p.m. and had locked the child in the bedroom; he
> had been seen leaning out of the bedroom window and crying
> for his mother by various people who had informed the police.
> I would like to point out at this stage that this kind of thing
> has happened before and on one occasion when the parents
> were missing, one child of the family fell out from the same
> window Philip was leaning out of and broke his leg.

Some of those who were admitted because they had 'no home'
were living in a children's home before they were admitted, but one
or two were older people whom circumstances had left stranded

and there was nowhere else for them to go. For instance, one woman was living-in as a domestic. The job finished and she was left without a home.

The final two categories concern the family in a slightly different way. The parents' anxiety about the other children differs from that shown by them under the category, 'Behaviour problem with younger sibs' (see p. 61), in that a behaviour problem was not to the fore and it was more a matter of the time that was taken caring for the subnormal, and the general effect on the other children. The mother of a mongol girl of twelve wrote to the Mental Health Service saying:

> We think that Michael (her younger brother) should now start to take his education seriously, but it is very difficult with Susan (the subnormal) at home, as she will just not allow him to concentrate. We know that she is considered 'high grade' but in spite of this she can be very difficult in the home at times.

The following year the school medical officer wrote to the Medical Officer of Health:

> Dr M. has sent a report about a boy Michael J. who has been reported by the teacher on account of deterioration in his school work and lack of concentration. His mother is very sensible and she attributes this to his sister who is a mongol and ineducable and persistently torments the boy so that he is becoming nervous and irritable. The parents are now anxious for Michael's sake for the girl to go into an institution permanently.

All four in this category were severely subnormal. The two cases of 'Family crisis unrelated to subnormal' were both marital crises, not totally unrelated to the subnormal but not strictly connected with him.

Nursing problem

This category applied almost entirely to the severely subnormal. There was only one mildly subnormal in this group. In nineteen cases the precipitating factor was a 'Nursing problem'. The twentieth case was a mongol who required a lot of attention and whose admission was precipitated by the birth of a mongol sister.

Other

This was a very mixed collection as might be expected. It is made up as shown in table 5.5.

Table 5.5   Details of 'Other' factors

Category	MSN	SSN	Total
Better care of subnormal	1	1	2
Request of parents	0	2	2
Other	1	6	7
Total	2	9	11

The mildly and severely subnormal compared

So far this chapter has been concerned to give substance to the groups of precipitating factors. Little mention has been made of the different problems for the mildly and severely subnormal. A brief consideration of table 5.1 shows that the proportions admitted because of the death or illness of a parent or parent figure and for social reasons are very similar. The main difference is the higher proportion of mildly subnormal where the precipitating factor was behaviour, and the correspondingly lower proportion of mildly subnormal admitted where the precipitating factor was a nursing problem. One might expect the severely subnormal to provide most of the nursing problems, and this was the case. The difference between the proportions admitted for reasons of behaviour is very nearly made up by the severely subnormal admitted because of a nursing problem. The proportion of mildly subnormal admitted for behaviour or a nursing problem is 52 per cent and the proportion of severely subnormal admitted for the same reasons is 51 per cent. Apart from the presence of those severely subnormal admitted because of nursing problems and a corresponding reduction in the number admitted because of behaviour problems, there is no striking difference between the factors precipitating the admission of the mildly and severely subnormal respectively.

The factors precipitating admission of the mildly subnormal and the age admitted

In chapter 3, the age at which patients were admitted to hospital was discussed at some length. The question arises of whether people who were admitted at a particular age tended to be admitted for a particular reason. The precipitating factor makes it possible to examine this. The pattern of age at admission of the mildly subnormal is very different from that of the severely subnormal, and so the mildly and severely subnormal are considered separately.

Figure 3 shows the age at which the mildly subnormal were admitted. On the basis of this diagram, those in hospital were put in four groupings of age on admission, nought to nineteen, twenty to thirty-four, thirty-five to forty-nine, and fifty plus. These groupings of age on admission to hospital have been used in figure 11.

The predominance of 'Behaviour or management' is most obvious, accounting for just over half the admissions. Table 5.1 shows the exact proportions. The numbers admitted for reasons of behaviour or management are consistent for the first three age groups, nineteen, eighteen and seventeen respectively. It is only in the small group of those admitted when they were aged over fifty that the number drops. There are only four, and two of these were problems of management without any serious behaviour problem.

The main difference between those admitted in the nought to nineteen bracket and those admitted between twenty and thirty-four is the smaller number in the older group admitted for social reasons, the balance being made up by those admitted because of the death or illness of their parents. It is this latter group which accounts for the big jump in those admitted between thirty-five and forty-nine. The admission of exactly half (twenty-two) was precipitated by the death or illness of a parent (or parent figure). It has been pointed out in chapter 3 that the second peak in the age structure of those in hospital, those aged between forty-five and fifty-four, was due to those admitted when they were aged between thirty-five and forty-nine (see figure 4). It can be seen from figure 11 that the increase is due in large part to the death or illness of the person looking after the subnormal. As might be expected, the majority of those admitted when they were aged fifty or over were admitted for this reason.

The factors precipitating admission of the severely subnormal and the age admitted

As in the previous section the groupings of age at which the severely subnormal were admitted to hospital are those discussed in chapter 3 (see pp. 44–5). Note that the age brackets are different from those used for the mildly subnormal, and the pattern is rather different. The diagram, figure 12, is slightly deceptive in that it makes it look as though the twenty to twenty-nine group go down and then the numbers admitted go up, but a glance at figure 8, which shows the age at which the severely subnormal were admitted, corrects this impression. The thirty plus group includes those admitted right up to the age of sixty-five or more.

There was only one mildly subnormal where the precipitating factor was a nursing problem, but among the severely subnormal this factor was more important. It occurred most often among those who were admitted before they were ten years old. There were ten cases in this group, but it was only in the group who were oldest on admission that no one was admitted for this reason. All those admitted as a result of a nursing problem were severely disabled. This is consistent with the tendency to earlier mortality of those admitted before they were ten, which can be seen in figure 9.

Social factors also figure largest in this youngest age group. In such cases the combination of a difficult home background and looking after a severely subnormal child appears to produce a crisis situation quite early. Eighteen out of the thirty-one where the precipitating factor was some social problem were admitted before they were ten years old. Considering the deprived background from which many of these people came, described in the section on 'Social reasons' earlier on in this chapter, this is understandable.

'Behaviour or management' was the precipitating factor in just under half the youngest group, but in the ten to nineteen bracket, it accounts for 62 per cent. The proportion admitted for reasons of behaviour remains high (exactly 50 per cent) in the twenty to twenty-nine age group, but drops to 14 per cent among those admitted when they were thirty years old or more. In this oldest group the vast majority were admitted because of the death or illness of a parent or parent figure. The numbers of those admitted for this reason increase strikingly from 2 per cent of the youngest group to 79 per cent of the oldest group.

It *might* be possible to provide some sort of treatment or help at home for those admitted for reasons of behaviour or management, or for social reasons, or even because of a nursing problem, but those admitted because of the death or illness of a parent figure must have some form of residential care provided.

The definition of 'children'

In the last two sections the relationship between the age and the reason for which patients were admitted to hospital has been examined. Whereas there is no one reason for admission which is limited to a single age group, the pattern does change as the age at which the patient was admitted increases. The age at which the patient was admitted is clearly of importance in several ways. This has been taken into account in the way in which 'children' have been defined.

It has been mentioned in chapter 1 that the information from the files about those in hospital was of their *home* circumstances at the time they were admitted to hospital. In the following chapters adults and children are considered separately where this is appropriate. The definition of a child *at home* is someone who was under the age of sixteen on 1 September 1968. But for those *in an institution* the definition is different. It is a person who was under sixteen *at the time he was admitted to hospital*.

This means that subnormals at home who were children in 1968 are compared with subnormals in hospital who were adults in 1968 but were children when they were admitted. The alternative would be to compare adults at home with adults in hospital, some of whom were children when they were admitted and for whom the details relate to the time when they were children. Naturally this has had the effect of increasing the number of 'children' in hospital. Table 5.6 compares the number of children first, as defined simply by their age at 1 September 1968 and second, as defined by their age on admission to hospital. Children at home are not affected by this.

Table 5.6　Children and adults—institution only

| | (Children = aged less than 16 on 1.9.68) | | (Children = aged less than 16 when admitted) | |
	MSN	SSN	MSN	SSN
Children	3	30	13	95
Adults	117	193	107	128
Total	120	223	120	223

Throughout the text, when children in an institution are referred to, it is always the second definition that applies, the age at which they were admitted, unless it is stated specifically that the chronological definition is being used.

6   Social class

Introduction

On the old forms they made no bones about it. The person filling in one of the early education forms had to decide whether the child's background was 'very superior, superior, average, inferior or very inferior'. In our more egalitarian day the issue of social class is not less important, only more confused. The consideration of social class has had to be based rather narrowly on the father's socio-economic group. There are, of course, many other indications of social class, such as type of housing, style of life, education of children, social expectations and so on but, apart from the first, none of these data was readily available from the files. Consequently, this chapter is, of necessity, limited to the clues to the social background of the families given by the father's socio-economic group and, to a lesser extent, the families' housing.

Some difficulties considered

The socio-economic group of the family was decided by what job the father did. Even if the father was dead, the job he used to do was still taken as the most accurate indicator available of the socio-economic group in which the family should be placed. The only exception to this was when the subnormal was living permanently with another relative and the socio-economic group of the man of the house was known. In this case his job determined the socio-economic group in which the family was placed.[1]

Unfortunately there was a lot of cases where there was no record of what the father's job was. This may be explained in part by the number of cases reported during the Depression, when, time and time again, under the heading 'Father's Occupation' were written the letters 'O.O.W.', that is, 'Out of Work'. There were other cases where it was simply lack of information. These pose a difficult problem in an important table. Table 6.1 excludes the unknowns but shows what percentage they are of the total.

Table 6.1 Socio-economic group of father or father figure

	MSN Home No.	%	MSN Institution No.	%	MSN Total No.	%	SSN Home No.	%	SSN Institution No.	%	SSN Total No.	%
Professional	4	0·7	1	1·3	5	0·8	27	4·8	10	5·6	37	5·0
Intermediate	22	4·0	5	6·7	27	4·4	71	12·6	20	11·3	91	12·3
Skilled	161	29·5	19	25·7	180	29·1	193	34·2	69	39·0	262	35·4
Semi-skilled	113	20·7	12	16·2	125	20·2	100	17·7	25	14·1	125	16·9
Unskilled	241	44·2	34	45·9	275	44·4	170	30·1	53	29·9	223	30·1
H.M. Forces	4	0·7	3	4·0	7	1·1	3	0·5	0	0	3	0·4
Sub-total	545	99·8	74	99·8	619	100·0	564	99·9	177	99·9	741	100·1
Not known	201		46		247		110		46		156	
Not known as % of total	26·9		38·0		28·5		16·6		21·0		17·4	
Total	746		120		866		674		223		897	

The high proportion where the socio-economic group was not known is striking. It seems likely that those cases where the socio-economic group was not known would tend to come from the lower end of the social scale, as the skilled, semi-skilled and unskilled were more likely to be described as out of work. Also, it seems more likely that the father's job would be known if he was in the professional or intermediate categories. In order to see if the cases where the socio-economic group was not known have distorted the picture seriously, a cross-tabulation was done with type of housing.

The method adopted was to use a simple manual/non-manual division. The professional and intermediate groups were classed as non-manual and the rest as manual. A table was drawn up showing the numbers of manual and non-manual people in each type of housing—council, urban or suburban. The table also shows the number of cases in each type of housing where the socio-economic group was not known. The cases were redistributed between the manual and non-manual groupings according to the proportion of manual and non-manual in each type of housing in each standard group. Table A2 in appendix A shows how this was worked out. The result of this redistribution is shown in table A3.

It is now possible to get a better idea of the distortion that the unknowns have produced. Table 6.2 shows the difference in the proportions of non-manual fathers, with the top line showing the unadjusted figures and the bottom line the adjusted figures which take account of the unknown cases classified by type of housing.

Table 6.2 Percentage of non-manual fathers according to adjusted and unadjusted figures

% of non-manual fathers	MSN			SSN		
	Home	Institution	Total	Home	Institution	Total
Not adjusted	4·8	8·4	5·2	17·5	16·9	17·3
Adjusted	4·7	7·7	5·1	16·6	16·3	16·5

The percentages for the figures that have not been adjusted have been re-calculated to treat the ten cases in H.M. Forces as not known. This is how they were treated in the adjusted figures.

As had been anticipated, the adjusted figures reduce the proportion in the non-manual category. However, the reduction is slight and it seems reasonable to treat the figures in table 6.1 as worthy of discussion.

There is one other possible bias in the population in the survey. The higher socio-economic group moves from one area to another more frequently than those groups further down the social scale. It could be that there was a disproportionate number of people from the professional and intermediate groups among those who moved into Sheffield from another local authority area. These people have not been included in the standard groups. This was explained in chapter 2. However, when these ninety-four cases are included, the difference they make is very small. The biggest difference they make to any group is 1 per cent. It seems fair to assume that the absence of this group has caused no serious bias.

A consideration of the class distribution of the subnormal

Table 6.1 made the difference between the mildly and severely subnormal quite clear. Only 5 per cent of the mildly subnormal were in the professional and intermediate groups compared to 17 per cent of the severely subnormal. If the dividing line is put between the skilled and semi-skilled groups, only 34 per cent of the fathers of the mildly subnormal were skilled or above, but the proportion among the severely subnormal was 53 per cent. Dr Kushlick has been quoted already in chapter 2 as saying (1966, p. 75):

> It has long been known that in industrial societies, parents of severely subnormal children are evenly distributed among all the social strata in the society, while those of the mildly subnormal subjects come predominantly from the lower social classes.

In table 6.3, the percentages for the mildly and severely subnormal are compared with the percentage of economically active males in Sheffield. These figures confirm the generally accepted view expressed by Dr Kushlick that the mildly subnormal 'come predominantly from the lower social classes'. This is especially marked in the unskilled group, where the proportion for Sheffield as a whole is 10 per cent; but for the mildly subnormal it is 44 per cent.

It is the severely subnormal who pose the problem. They are not evenly distributed among all social strata. They are underrepresented heavily in the professional group, quite heavily in the intermediate, and noticeably in the skilled. They are overrepresented heavily in the unskilled group. It is not easy to decide why this should be the case. In order to examine this, the distribution of the father's socio-economic group in various groups in the population surveyed was studied. Table 6.4 presents the evidence in simplified form. The first row gives the group concerned and the second row the number in that group excluding cases where the father's socio-economic group was not known. The third row shows the percentage of that group that had fathers in non-manual jobs. The fourth row will be explained later.

Table 6.3   Comparison of socio-economic groupings for Sheffield C.B. with mildly subnormal and severely subnormal population

	MSN %	SSN %	Sheffield C.B.* %
Professional	0·8	5·0	12·9
Intermediate	4·4	12·3	18·4
Skilled	29·1	35·4	42·0
Semi-skilled	20·2	16·9	16·0
Unskilled	44·4	30·1	10·1
H.M. Forces	1·1	0·4	0·1
Other	—	—	0·5
Total	100·0	100·1	100·0

* Extracted from Sample Census (1966). County Table for Yorkshire, West Riding. Table 4, 'Economically active males by area and socio-economic group'.

The key figure in table 6.4 is the proportion of non-manual workers in Sheffield. This was 31 per cent. The proportion of non-manual fathers in the groups shown in the top row is compared with this percentage. The bottom row indicates whether the difference between the percentage of non-manual workers in that group and the percentage for Sheffield is statistically significant or whether it could have happened by chance. So in column 2 all the severely subnormal are taken together. The number, which excludes cases where the socio-economic group of the father was not known, is 741; of these 17 per cent fell into the non-manual category, and this percentage is significantly lower than the percentage for Sheffield. One would not expect a difference of this size to occur by chance. It is significantly different from the percentage for Sheffield and so 'Yes' appears in the fourth row.

The same is true when the severely subnormal are divided into adults and children (columns 3 and 4). There is a lower proportion of non-manual fathers than was expected. The proportion of non-manual fathers among the children is, however, considerably higher than among the adults. This difference is important and will be referred to later.

The next four columns (5, 6, 7 and 8) divide the adults and children into those in hospital and those in an institution. In the case of both groups of adults (columns 5 and 6) and the children in an institution (column 8) the difference is greater than can be explained by chance but the proportion of children at home (column 7) with non-manual fathers comes just within the limits of what might be expected by chance.

The next column (column 9) takes the figures for mongols to see whether this more specific group can provide clearer evidence. They too fall within the range of what might be expected by chance, and this figure includes adults as well as children. If one takes mongol children only, the proportion with non-manual fathers rises to 28 per cent.

The final two columns (10 and 11) take those whose IQ was less than 40. The figures are rather low because the IQ was not known in a considerable number of cases. There will, of course, be a number of mongols in this group. The reason for taking only those with a lower IQ was to exclude those on the borderline between mild and severe subnormality. We have seen already that the mildly subnormal are weighted heavily towards the lower end of the social scale. It might be expected that these borderline cases would be weighted in the same way, though to a lesser extent. Column 10 gives the figures for both adults and children, and the proportion of non-manual fathers is considerably lower than can be explained by chance. However, when the children are taken by themselves, the proportion of non-manual fathers is not significantly different from the proportion for Sheffield.

Can these figures explain the lower proportion of non-manual fathers among the severely subnormal in Sheffield or must the even class distribution of the severely subnormal be queried?

It appears from these figures that mongols may well be evenly distributed among all classes, but the fact that they are a distinct group makes it difficult to argue from them to the whole population of subnormals.

One finding is quite consistent and that is the greater proportion of non-manual fathers among the children of every group. (The only

Table 6.4 Percentage of non-manual fathers among various groups of severely subnormal compared with percentage for Sheffield

Col. no.	1	2	3	4	5	6	7	8	9	10	11
Group	Sheffield	Total SSN	Total adults	Total children	Adults at home	Adults in institution	Children at home	Children in institution	Total mongols	Total IQ less than 40	Total children IQ less than 40
Total numbers in group ignoring unknowns	153,190	741	525	213	376	149	185	28	166	191	73
% of non-manual fathers	31·3	17·3	15·0	23·0	13·9	18·1	24·9	10·7	25·3	18·8	24·7
Difference significant at 5% level to % for Sheffield		Yes	Yes	Yes	Yes	Yes	No	Yes	No	Yes	No

Note: Children in institutions are defined chronologically in this table because in this instance it is the actual age which is important, not the age on admission to hospital. This distinction is explained on page 70.

exception to this is among the small number of children in an institution.) Why should this be? The only hypothesis which appears to be reasonable is that this is a reflection of the increasing size of the middle class. The socio-economic group of many of the fathers dates from between the wars or even earlier. At this time the middle class was considerably smaller than it is now. For instance, in 1931 23 per cent of occupied males in Great Britain were in non-manual jobs, but by 1966 the proportion had risen to 34 per cent.[2] The consistency of the difference between adults and children makes it seem very likely that this explains at least part of the discrepancy between the proportion of people in the non-manual class in Sheffield and among the severely subnormal.

This still leaves a discrepancy. The proportion of all children with non-manual fathers is just outside the limits which could be expected by chance at the 5 per cent level. It is true that when the children are divided between those at home and those in an institution, those at home fall just within the limits of what can be accepted as due to chance, but it is not obvious what justification there is for making this division.

The reason for considering only those with an IQ below 40 has been explained already. In this group the proportion of children with non-manual fathers falls quite easily within the 5 per cent confidence limits, whereas this is not true of severely subnormal children as a whole. This does suggest that the general statement about the even class distribution of the severely subnormal should be modified to say that this is only partly true of cases on the borderline between mild and severe subnormality who will tend to have a higher proportion in the manual classes, though a smaller proportion than those who are clearly mildly subnormal.

Another explanation for the discrepancy is that it may be due to mobility. The argument would go like this: the higher social classes are the most mobile, therefore more of them with their severely subnormal children are likely to have left Sheffield and therefore to have been excluded. They will have been replaced by other parents with severely subnormal children, mostly from the higher social classes moving into Sheffield, but some of these parents may have placed their severely subnormal children in hospital before they moved to Sheffield. This means that these severely subnormal people were not admitted to hospital from Sheffield and therefore were not included in the figures. But there is a clear answer to this argument. Where a severely subnormal person was admitted to hospital while he was living in Sheffield and his parents moved subsequently, he was still included in the survey, so these two factors should cancel one another out.

It is true that the figures in table 6.4 do not include the ninety-four cases which moved into Sheffield from another local authority area, but if they are included they increase the proportion of non-manual fathers for all the severely subnormal by only 0·2 per cent from 17·3 per cent to 17·5 per cent. The percentage for children at home is increased by the same amount from 24·9 per cent to 25·1 per cent. In no case does this come anywhere near tipping the balance between the proportion being significantly different or not. Furthermore, a total of fifty-three severely subnormal people moved into Sheffield from another local authority area, but a total of only fifty-two both mildly and severely subnormal were excluded because they had left Sheffield. Any bias this gives should increase the proportion of non-manual fathers.

Another possibility is to look for an administrative answer. A new and much improved junior training centre was opened in 1963 which provided far better facilities for the education and training of severely subnormal children than was available anywhere else in Sheffield. This may have provided the incentive for parents and doctors to report severely subnormal children to the Mental Health Service who were not reported before, and may have added a few cases from non-manual families to the severely subnormal children.

Two factors have been suggested which can go some way to explaining the much lower proportion of non-manual fathers among the severely subnormal than there are in Sheffield. The phenomenon of the increasing proportion of the population in the middle class does something to reconcile the actual figures. The difference when those with an IQ in the 40s are excluded suggests a modification to the statement about the even class distribution of the severely subnormal.

The quotation from an article by Kushlick (see pp. 31, 74), which appeared in 1966, about the even class distribution of the severely subnormal, reflects a widely held opinion, and one followed by Pauline Morris in 1969. However, in a later article Kushlick (1968, p. 389) suggests, though his position is not altogether clear, that this may be subject to qualifications and that severe subnormality 'is more prevalent among the lower social classes'. One example of the complex of medical and social factors which may contribute to this is low birth weight, as is indicated in a further extract (ibid.):

> Low birth weight may cause severe subnormality although it is
> possible that the factor causing the low birth weight also causes
> the severe subnormality. . . . Because low birth weight is more
> common among lower social class births [Baird, 1962] this is
> one possible cause of the excess of severely subnormal subjects
> among children from low social class families.

But it is unlikely to be very important numerically.

The findings of this study support the view that the severely
subnormal are not distributed evenly. It must be admitted that these
Sheffield figures need to be treated with some reserve. First of all
the evidence is second hand. It was collected by a variety of people
for a different purpose and there is some doubt about its accuracy,
though generally the description of the father's job was quite precise.
Second, and more serious, is the very large number of unknowns. It is
true that it was possible to check on this to some extent by the cross-
tabulation with housing, but this involved making assumptions
about the distribution in different types of housing of cases where the
socio-economic group was not known.

In view of these limitations, it is probably best to consider these
Sheffield figures as a useful indicator rather than firm fact. As such
they put a serious question mark against the assumption that the
severely subnormal are distributed evenly among all social classes.
This is all the more interesting as a study in Aberdeen (Birch *et al.*,
1970) found that the severely subnormal *were* distributed evenly.
The definite concentration of the severely subnormal at the lower
end of the social scale in the Sheffield figures must at least make
it open to question whether this is true generally.

Is social class related to admission to hospital?

We have seen that there is a clear distinction between the mildly and
severely subnormal in terms of socio-economic group. There was no
such clear-cut distinction between those at home and those in
hospital. Table 6.5 shows the proportion of each socio-economic
category at home. All those whose socio-economic status was not
known and the few in H.M. Forces have been disregarded in this
table.

In the total column the gradual increase in the proportion at home
from the professional category, with the lowest percentage, to the
semi-skilled, with the highest percentage, and a slight dip down to

the unskilled, looks interesting. However, it does not approach significance. If the professional category, the one with the lowest proportion at home, is taken against all the rest, the same is true, and if the semi-skilled category, the one with the highest proportion at home, is taken against the rest, the same is still true.

Table 6.5   Percentage of each socio-economic grouping at home

	MSN	SSN	Total
	%	%	%
Professional	80	73	74
Intermediate	81	78	79
Skilled	89	74	80
Semi-skilled	90	80	85
Unskilled	88	76	83
Overall	88	76	82

Note: There were only four in the professional grouping among the mildly subnormal at home, and one in hospital.

Table 6.4 showed a marked difference between the proportions of the severely subnormal from non-manual families at home and in an institution, when they were divided between adults and children. However, children were defined in table 6.4 as being less than sixteen years old on 1 September 1968, because in the earlier discussion it was the chronological factor which was important. Now that it is the relationship between class and admission to hospital that is being considered, it is the age at which people were admitted which is important. When adults and children in an institution are redefined by age admitted, the proportion of non-manual adults in an institution drops from 18 per cent under the chronological definition to 13 per cent under the age admitted definition. This is very close to the figure for those at home, which is 14 per cent. In the case of children, the proportion in the non-manual category goes up from 11 per cent under the chronological definition to 21 per cent under the age admitted definition. This is quite close to the figure for children at home, which is 25 per cent. The difference is not at all significant.

The data can show no significant relationship between socio-economic grouping and admission to hospital. The most that can be said is that a few more persons in the semi-skilled category do seem to remain at home, but even this does not approach significance.

7   Housing and money

Type of housing

The categories of housing which were used were very broad ones—council housing, working-class urban housing and suburban housing. These three categories were divided into houses, flats, or rooms, but the numbers in flats or rooms were so small that these sub-divisions have been ignored.

It was hoped that these results might throw some light on such questions as whether an old industrial working-class area like Attercliffe had a higher proportion of subnormals at home: and if this was the case, whether the indication might be that these areas have preserved the extended family and network of friends who support the subnormal and his family and so increase the chances of his staying at home.

The number of unknowns is high. The files were often vague, or completely blank, about the type of housing. If the information was not available in the file, the matter was not pursued because of the time factor. There is no reason to think that the unknowns come from any particular group. The results are shown in table 7.1.

Table 7.1 Type of housing

	MSN Home No.	%	Institution No.	%	SSN Home No.	%	Institution No.	%
Council	278	49·4	29	30·2	281	50·4	60	31·6
Working-class urban	253	44·9	51	53·1	177	31·7	93	48·9
Suburban	32	5·7	16	16·7	100	17·9	37	19·5
Sub-total	563	100·0	96	100·0	558	100·0	190	100·0
Not known	183		24		116		33	
Not known as % of total	24·5		20·0		17·2		14·8	
Total	746		120		674		223	

χ^2 (MSN) = 21·243   p = 0·001 χ^2 (SSN) = 22·804   p = 0·001
Note: The unknowns for the MSN at home include two coded as 'no fixed abode'.

Table 7.1 shows how the four standard groups were distributed among the three types of housing. Table 7.2 shows the percentage of mildly and severely subnormal from each type of housing who were at home.

The differences in table 7.2 as a whole are significant for both the mildly and severely subnormal. Among the mildly subnormal, the proportion of those living in council housing who were at home is strikingly high, and the proportion in suburban housing is strikingly low. These two groups are the most significant statistically. The proportion in the working-class housing is very close to the overall proportion. The small group of mildly subnormal in suburban housing is slightly out of place by the mere fact of being mildly subnormal and living in suburban housing. Too much importance should not be attached to the high proportion in hospital, because eight out of the sixteen were admitted owing to the death or illness of a parent.

Table 7.2   Mildly subnormal and severely subnormal at home in different categories of housing

	MSN %	SSN %
Council	90·5	82·4
Working-class urban	83·2	65·5
Suburban	66·7	72·0
Overall	85·4	74·6

The pattern for the severely subnormal is different. Many more of them lived in suburban housing, and the percentage of these who were at home was very close to the overall percentage. The contrast comes between those in council houses and those in working-class urban areas. The original coding did not distinguish between pre- and post-war council housing, which is regrettable. Recent council building in Sheffield has a style and distinctiveness about it which makes it very different from the rather dreary council estates built between the wars. However, almost all the council houses have better amenities than almost all the old nineteenth-century working-class housing, much of which is due for demolition. There is a marked difference between the proportions at home from these two types of housing. The old working-class housing has the lowest proportion of severely subnormal at home (65 per cent) and the council housing has the highest proportion at home (82 per cent). These figures have to be modified to a certain extent when the cases where the subnormal was admitted to hospital because of the death or illness of a parent are considered. Such cases were more likely to come from the old working-class housing but the proportion at home from council housing remains significantly higher even when account is taken of this.

This reverses the suggestion about working-class housing made at the beginning of this section. In its place it might be suggested that the policy of slum clearance and redevelopment has undermined the former cohesion of the old urban areas. In contrast, the council estates are now well established and families have begun to have kin living near at hand. (The Dagenham study showed the extent to which this has taken place (Willmott, 1963).) It could be that this affects not only the pre-war estates but also the newer post-war ones. In the case of the latter it would seem that the larger stock of council housing and the policy of the housing committee has enabled members of the wider family to live fairly close to one another when they want to. In two of the families which were visited the Housing Department had made it possible for a daughter to live near her mother.

Neither the data from the files nor those from the visits are adequate to test this theory, though they do lend some support to it. Whatever theories may be put forward to explain it, it is certainly true that among council tenants a significantly higher proportion of families with a subnormal member managed to keep him at home than did families in the old working-class housing.

Standard of housing

A three-point classification was used: 'good', 'adequate' or 'bad'. The standard was not very demanding. A house described as 'fairly clean and reasonably well furnished' or 'reasonably clean and tidy' was coded as 'good'. A house described as 'poorly furnished and untidy' was coded 'adequate', as was another where the case notes said: 'the house was scruffy but they appeared happy together'. A house described as 'bad' had to be very bad. For instance, an NSPCC inspector described one such house in the following terms: 'The living conditions are foul in the extreme, the solitary bed used by parents and children defies words. Perhaps "foul urine soaked mass" would be a fair description.' Later, the medical officer visited and reported: 'I visited with Miss D. and found the house indescribably foul and stinking.'

In every case the standard refers not to the structural state of the house but to the way in which the family looked after it. Table 7.3 gives the figures for the mildly subnormal and table 7.4 the proportion of each category at home, so, for instance, 88·2 per cent of those whose housing came into the category 'good' were living at home.

Table 7.3   Standard of housing of mildly subnormal

	Home No.	%	Institution No.	%
Good	412	68·8	55	56·7
Adequate	149	24·9	25	25·8
Bad	38	6·3	17	17·5
Sub-total	599	100·0	97	100·0
Not known	147		23	
Not known as % of total	19·7		19·2	
Total	746		120	

$\chi^2 = 15\cdot050$ p = 0·001
χ^2 on Good and Adequate against Bad = 14·342   p = 0·001

Table 7.4   Standard of housing of mildly subnormal. Percentages of each category at home

	%
Good	88·2
Adequate	85·6
Bad	69·1
Overall	86·1

Table 7.4 shows quite clearly that the important distinction is between the houses where the standard was described as bad and the rest. This bears out an impression received during the reading of the files. It appeared that some of the social workers visiting the families did not take account of the 'grind' of looking after the subnormal and also that they imported middle-class standards into their accounts of the tidiness and general appearance of the home. It was this impression which led to the middle category being called 'adequate'. The results seem to justify this description, as it is only in the 'bad' category that there is a significant difference between the

home and the institution groups. Even in this category it needs to be remembered that thirty-eight out of the fifty-five were at home. The following case is one where a severely subnormal man in his fifties was living with his father and aunt, both of whom could be described as slow-witted. There had been a series of crises and a public health inspector had described the house as one of the worst he had seen for some time. It seems from the file that the public health authorities fumigated the house and gave the family some help in cleaning it up. After this the mental welfare officer wrote:

> Washing is constantly about the house and cooking seems to take place in steps as a continuous process, meals being prepared serially as it were, with potatoes cooked at one stage and meat at another, all being finally assembled round about evening. The patient himself is always dressed in the same way. He wears a balaclava helmet, blue suit, a woollen pullover and heavy duty workman's boots, and does not seem to make any concessions to temperature, being clad in the same way on warm and cold days. It is evident that the patient's father has made such efforts as he can to clean up the home. Colour washing has been carried out in a haphazard way in most of the rooms. It is difficult to imagine that any form of improvement is possible. The subnormal's aunt told me plaintively that I visited much too frequently and that if I would leave her for a couple of months she would be able to 'get down to it'.

The last entry in the file was about fifteen months later and read: 'House in deplorable state, but they appear quite happy.'

Such a case helps to make the point that even very low standards in the home do not by any means lead to a subnormal being admitted to an institution. The figures show simply that in cases where a social worker considered the standards of cleanliness, etc. in the home were unusually low, there is a definite though not very strong association with admission to hospital.

The pattern with the severely subnormal is much the same as with the mildly subnormal. The main difference is the smaller proportion where the standard of housing was described as bad. The figures are given in tables 7.5 and 7.6.

The dividing line is once again between the adequate and the bad categories. This difference is clearly apparent in the table showing the percentage of each category at home, and is significant. As in the case of the mildly subnormal, there is a discernible, though not a strong, association between low standards of cleanliness within the home and admission to hospital.

The effect of dividing those cases in an institution who were admitted because of the death or illness of a parent from the rest is interesting. Hardly any of those admitted because of the death or illness of a parent came from a household where the standard was bad. There were only two mildly subnormal cases and one severely subnormal case of this. All the other cases came from those who had been admitted for some other reason. The association with admission is not strong, but it helps to fill in the picture and shows a very marked difference between those admitted because of a parent's death or illness and the rest.

Table 7.5   Standard of housing of severely subnormal

	Home No.	%	Institution No.	%
Good	474	80·6	139	69·8
Adequate	93	15·8	41	20·6
Bad	21	3·6	19	9·5
Sub-total	588	100·0	199	99·9
Not known	86		24	
Not known as % of total	12·8		10·8	
Total	674		223	

$\chi^2 = 14·659$ p $= 0·001$
$\chi^2 =$ Bad standard against the rest $= 11·007$ p$=0·01$

Table 7.6   Standard of housing of severely subnormal. Percentages of each category at home

	%
Good	77·3
Adequate	69·4
Bad	52·5
Overall	74·7

Money

The distinction which has been drawn here is of necessity a crude one. The financial circumstances of a family were coded as 'about MSS level' if they appeared from the evidence in the file to rely entirely or almost entirely on Ministry of Social Security benefit. In most cases this was quite easy to decide. In many of the families who came into this category the father was retired or the mother was a widow. In other cases the father might be chronically ill and the family relying on sick pay. A family did not have to be drawing benefit to be put in this category. The definition was 'about MSS level', so if the father was doing a low paid manual job and the family was hard up, it too would fall into this category. If, on the other hand, the father was in regular employment and there was no evidence of any hardship, then the family was coded 'above MSS level'. Table 7.7 gives the results.

Table 7.7   Financial circumstances

	MSN Home No.	%	Institution No.	%	SSN Home No.	%	Institution No.	%
Above MSS level	447	69·6	43	40·2	456	72·8	113	57·1
About MSS level	195	30·4	64	59·8	170	27·2	85	42·9
Sub-total	642	100·0	107	100·0	626	100·0	198	100·0
Not known	104		13		48		25	
Not known as % of total	13·9		10·8		7·1		11·2	
Total	746		120		674		223	

χ^2 (MSN) $= 35\cdot136$ p $= 0\cdot001$
χ^2 (SSN) $= 17\cdot511$ p $= 0\cdot001$

Roughly a third of the mildly subnormal at home had incomes about MSS level, but in the case of those in hospital the proportion goes up to nearly 60 per cent. The percentages in table 7.8 underline this point. Of those above MSS level, 91 per cent were at home, but for those about MSS level the proportion drops to 75 per cent.

The pattern is the same with the severely subnormal. The overall proportion about MSS level is lower but this is a reflection of the higher proportion of the severely subnormal in the higher socio-economic groups. The proportion of families about MSS level at home is very similar to the proportion Tizard and Grad found among their home sample. The figure for Sheffield is 27 per cent: Tizard and Grad (1961, p. 59) found 25 per cent whose income level was 'poor', which was defined as less than 10 per cent above the National Assistance Board level.

Table 7.8 Financial circumstances. Percentages of each category at home

	MSN %	SSN %
Above MSS level	91·2	80·1
About MSS level	75·3	66·7
Overall	87·5	76·0

The proportion of severely subnormal living about the level of MSS benefit is much higher among those now in hospital. Exactly one-third of the severely subnormal whose family's income was about MSS level were in hospital, compared with one-fifth of those whose income was above this level.

In this case it is particularly important to take account of those who were admitted to hospital because of the death or illness of a parent. Table 7.9 gives the figures.

Table 7.9 Financial circumstances of those in institution divided by precipitating factor (P.F.)

	MSN		SSN	
	Above MSS level	About MSS level	Above MSS level	About MSS level
P.F. Not death or illness of a parent	35	39	94	44
P.F. Death or illness of a parent	8	25	19	41
Total	43	64	113	85

Among the mildly subnormal there was a significantly greater proportion of those about MSS level in hospital from both those admitted because of the death or illness of a parent and those admitted for some other reason. This is not so in the case of the severely subnormal. Among those admitted for some other reason there was no significant difference between the financial circumstances of those at home and those in hospital. There was, however, a very decisive difference between the home group and those admitted because of the death or illness of a parent, of whom over two-thirds were living at MSS level. But the critical factor here was not money but the age of the parents. The parents of this group were older and more likely to be on pension, and so in turn more likely to die or be ill and unable to look after their subnormal. The high proportion of those living at MSS level is simply a reflection of this. Shortage of money may not have helped but it was not the decisive factor.

In the case of the mildly subnormal there is an association between poor financial circumstances and admission to hospital which is independent of the age of the parents.

Conclusions

In this chapter the type of housing, the standard of housing and the families' financial circumstances have been considered, but one of the most important points to emerge has been the age of the parents. It was only where the parents tended to be younger, those where the subnormal was not admitted because of the death or illness of a parent, that there was any association between a low standard of cleanliness in the household and admission to hospital.

In contrast to this, the association between admission to hospital and poor financial circumstances occurs in the case of the severely subnormal only among those admitted on the death or illness of a parent. This can be seen to be a reflection of the age of the parents. This was not the case among the mildly subnormal, where there was a discernible association between lack of money and admission to hospital even though it was not a very strong one.

The age of the parents modified but did not alter the finding that those in council housing were more likely to stay at home than those in the old urban housing. This was especially marked in the case of the severely subnormal. Among those in suburban housing, there was, overall, no clear difference either way.

8   The family background

Arnold was the second child of a family of seven. He was excluded from special school and ascertained as an imbecile. His father, who was a labourer, died when Arnold was about twenty-five. The mother then went out to work as a cleaner to provide an income for the family, while one of her daughters stayed at home to look after Arnold and to keep house. He could be left alone for short periods and would go out for walks alone but had to be assisted with dressing, shaving, etc. After the eventual marriage of all his siblings he was left living with his mother, who still worked but arranged for him to be looked after during the day by one of his sisters. After the breakdown of her marriage, one of his sisters returned to live at home, which made things easier to organize. Arnold's mother died when he was about fifty years old and the tenancy of their corporation house was granted to his sister, on the understanding that she would look after Arnold. This sister works part-time and Arnold makes frequent visits to other members of the family living near by.

It was the cohesion and support of his family which made all the difference to Arnold. In this chapter the subnormal's family and the individual members of it are considered, in order to try to see which aspects of the family's life were critical to whether he was admitted to an institution or not.

Whom the subnormal was living with

This was seen to be a critical question, and so a very detailed list of fifty-four categories was used. When it came to analysing the material, it was obvious that this was much more detailed than was necessary, and the categories have been grouped.

Naturally many more children were living with their parents than were adults. Table 8.1 gives the figures for the children. The figures for the mildly subnormal are too small for any conclusions to be drawn but the pattern seems similar to that of the severely subnormal. The vast majority of the severely subnormal, both those at home and those now in hospital, were living with their parents, but the proportion at home who were living with their parents was significantly higher. Among those in hospital a correspondingly higher proportion (20 per cent) come into the 'other' category. Of these nineteen, four were living with their mother and stepfather, two with their mother and grandparents, seven were in a children's home and the remainder were with some other relative. It is hardly surprising that there were more in an institution in this group.

Table 8.1   Whom the subnormal was living with—children

	MSN Home No.	Institution No.	SSN Home No.	%	Institution No.	%
Parents	11	7	195	87·1	67	70·5
Mother	1	1	16	7·1	9	9·5
Other	4	5	13	5·8	19	20·0
Total	16	13	224	100·0	95	100·0

χ^2 on whole table (SSN) = 16·185   p = 0·001
χ^2 on Other against the rest (SSN) = 14·896   p = 0·001

The picture is very different in the case of the mildly subnormal adults. The figures are shown in table 8.2. The categories have been put in three groups. The groups are homogeneous in that there is no significant difference at the 5 per cent level between the proportions at home and in hospital within the group. In group A a higher proportion than expected was at home: in group B there was no statistically significant difference either way: in group C there was a higher proportion than expected in hospital.

The presence of those who were living with their husband or wife in group A is no surprise. Those subnormals who get married will tend to be the most able and will often be on the borderline of 'normality'. It is surprising, though, to find those who were living with their mother and 'other than the subnormal's father' in this group. These thirty-three are made up as follows:

Mother and stepfather	25
Mother and maternal grandparent	1
Mother and married sib	7

That none of this group should be in hospital is really very striking. This is the exact opposite of what one might expect, especially when one considers that twenty-five of the thirty-three were living with their mother and stepfather.

When we look at group B there is another surprise. Those who were living with their parents fall into this neutral group. A higher percentage of those who were living with their parents was at home, but the difference is not significant. In this same neutral group as the parents were those who were living with the mother (where there was at least one other person living in the same household in addition to the subnormal and his mother), and cases where the subnormal was living by himself or was in sole charge of the household.

Table 8.2   Whom the subnormal was living with—mildly subnormal adults

	Home No.	%	Institution No.	%
(A) Spouse	166 ⎤	22·8	4 ⎤	3·8
Mother and other than subnormal's father	33 ⎦ 199	4·6	0 ⎦ 4	—
(B) Parents	208 ⎤	28·6	21 ⎤	19·8
Mother-household of more than two	58 ⎬ 324	8·0	10 ⎬ 40	9·4
Self	58 ⎦	8·0	9 ⎦	8·5
(C) Mother and subnormal only	43 ⎤	5·9	16 ⎤	15·1
Father or father and other than the subnormal's mother	36 ⎬ 204	5·0	10 ⎬ 62	9·4
Sib and no parent	76	10·4	19	17·9
Other relative	28	3·8	11	10·4
Other	21 ⎦	2·9	6 ⎦	5·7
Sub-total	727	100·0	106	100·0
Not known	3	1	1	
Total	730		107	

χ^2 on whole table = 49·303   p = 0·001
χ^2 on A v. B v. C = 48·955   p = 0·001

Cases where the subnormal was coded as living with his mother have been split according to whether the household consisted of just the subnormal and his mother or whether there were other people in the household as well. It can be seen from the table that cases where there were other people in the household fall into the neutral group B but those cases where the household consisted of just the subnormal and his mother fall into group C, where there were more than expected in hospital. The size of the household was the crucial factor in these cases. We shall see in the next section on the size of the household that households of only two were especially vulnerable. The other categories making up group C do not present any surprises.

The pattern is different in the case of the severely subnormal. Table 8.3 divides the figures into the same three groups as the mildly subnormal: group A, where there was a higher proportion than expected at home; group B, where there was no significant difference either way; and group C, where there was a higher proportion than expected in hospital.

Very few of the severely subnormal were married but all twenty-seven that were married were at home. Unlike the mildly subnormal adults, the severely subnormal adults were more likely to be at home if they were living with their parents. Nearly half of the severely subnormal adults at home were living with their parents. The difference between the proportion of mildly and severely subnormal who were living with their parents may be due to nothing more complex than that more of the mildly subnormal were married. If the proportion of those married and the proportion of those living with their parents are added together, we can see that 51 per cent of the mildly subnormal adults at home and 55 per cent of the severely subnormal adults at home were either living with their parents or with their spouse.

The number in the neutral group B is much smaller than with the mildly subnormal because those living with parents have moved up into group A.

The interesting feature in group C is that both categories living with their mother were in this group, where more than expected were in hospital. Where the household was more than two, the proportion in hospital was less than where the household consisted of only the subnormal and his mother, but they both fall into this last category. In this case it is not possible to argue, as was argued in the case of the mildly subnormal, that this is due to the size of the household. The difference between the smaller and larger household suggests that this was a factor but it cannot be the only one. The difference between the two is not significant but the tables for both the mildly and the severely subnormal (tables 8.2 and 8.3) do suggest that once the subnormal's mother loses the support of her husband, whether the husband is the father of the subnormal or not, she finds it more difficult to cope. It is fair to presume that the severely subnormal as a whole are more of a burden than the mildly subnormal, and it is worth noticing that, in the case of the severely subnormal, the category of mother and other than the subnormal's father (generally stepfather) has moved down from group A to group B, and the category of mother in a household of more than two has moved down from group B to group C. On the other hand, those living with their parents have moved up from the neutral group B, where they were with the mildly subnormal, to group A in the case of the severely subnormal. This suggests that the presence of both parents is a positive factor in the severely subnormal remaining at home, an assertion which cannot be made for the mildly subnormal adults.

Table 8.3 Whom the subnormal was living with—severely subnormal adults

	Home No.		%	Institution No.		%
(A) Spouse	27	245	6·0	0	41	0
Parents	218		48·6	41		32·3
(B) Sib and no parent	48		10·7	15		11·8
Mother and other than subnormal's father	16	69	3·6	3	19	2·4
Self	5		1·1	1		0·8
(C) Mother-household more than 2	35		7·8	14		11·0
Mother and subnormal only	55	135	12·2	30	67	23·6
Father or father and other than subnormal's mother	27		6·0	12		9·4
Other relative	18		4·0	11		8·7
Sub-total	449		100·0	127		100·0
Not known	1			1		
Total	450			128		

χ^2 on whole table $= 25 \cdot 755$ p $= 0 \cdot 001$ χ^2 on A v. B v. C $= 24 \cdot 441$ p $= 0 \cdot 001$

None of the few severely subnormal who were married and only four of the mildly subnormal who were married was in hospital, but this is a clear case where the relationship between being married and staying at home is one of association rather than cause. Those who are married will be the more able and therefore less likely to go into hospital anyhow.

Those living with their father or their father and someone other than the subnormal's mother (most of them were living with their father), those living with some other relative and those who fall into the 'other' category all come into group C, with a higher proportion than anticipated in hospital. This applies to the mildly and severely subnormal. This is much as might have been expected. Less expected, however, is the transition of those living with a sib and no parent from the hospital-biased group C in the case of the mildly subnormal to the neutral group B in the case of the severely subnormal. It is not possible to say why this is the case but this category is one of some importance in spite of the comparatively small numbers in it. The crucial factor in whether the subnormal will have to go into hospital eventually will in many cases depend on whether his brothers or sisters are prepared to have him. We have seen already in chapter 5 that the major precipitating factor among those who were admitted to hospital when they were older was the death or illness of their parents. In some cases there was no relative to care for them, in others the relatives were not prepared to care for them. The subnormal's sibs are especially important because they will probably be nearer his age, and in consequence are more likely to be able to care for the subnormal until the end of his life than is a relative who is a generation older.

Therefore it is of interest to see how many subnormals who could be living with a sib were in fact doing so. In order to find this out all subnormals whose parents were dead were taken and then those who had no sibs and also those who were married were excluded. This left 235 cases. The detailed table (table A4) will be found in appendix A.

The mildly subnormal at home were divided evenly between those living with a sib and those not doing so. It is interesting to notice that roughly twice as many women as men were living either with a sib or with some other relative or friend. Among those in hospital out of a total of thirty-nine, roughly one went straight into hospital on his parent's death for every two that were living with some other relative when they were admitted and every three that were living with a sib when they were admitted.

Among the severely subnormal there is a much more definite pattern. Over 85 per cent of those at home who could be living with a sib were doing so. Especially striking is the fact that there was only one woman out of the twenty-three who could be living with a sib who was not doing so. Of those in hospital just over half (seventeen) went straight in following the death of a parent, no sib being able or willing to take them on. Of the remainder, two-thirds were living with a sib and one-third with some other relative when they were admitted. It is significant that once again only one of the nine women who could have been living with a sib was not doing so at the time she was admitted.

Just over half of all the severely subnormal who could be living with a sib were living at home with either a brother or sister. This means that probably well over half of those who could be expected to look after their subnormal sib were doing so. There was often no indication in the file as to whether the brothers and sisters who had been mentioned earlier in the records were still alive. In those cases where the subnormal was not living with one of his sibs there may well have been a totally convincing reason why he or she could not look after him; the sib might have died or emigrated or been in poor health himself.

Those who were not living with a sib have been described as 'living with another relative or friend'. Many were living with an aunt or uncle or stepfather or stepmother, and three of the mildly subnormal women at home were living with their own child or children, but the largest single category is those who were living by themselves. In the home group this accounted for six of the mildly subnormal men, twenty-four of the mildly subnormal women and three of the severely subnormal men.

The evidence suggests that a high proportion of the brothers and sisters of subnormals whose parents had died and who were in a position to care for their subnormal sib were doing so.

Size of the household

The importance of the number of people living in the household has been mentioned already. The number recorded is the number of people living in the household on 1 September 1968 or on the latest date recorded in the file before that; it is not the size of the family. The number includes the subnormal, and so a household of one means the subnormal was living by himself. Table 8.4 gives the figures for the children, both mildly and severely subnormal.

Among the severely subnormal there is no significant difference in the size of household between those at home and those in hospital.

There were very few mildly subnormal children but over half of those in hospital came from households of seven or more. The difference between these large households and the rest is significant. It seems very likely that these were cases where the mother simply could not cope. In three out of the seven cases the factor which precipitated admission to hospital included bad home conditions or inadequate parental control. It was unusual for the mildly subnormal to be reported before the age of sixteen. The large average size of the families with a mildly subnormal child in hospital does suggest that they were an unusual group, and some of them would probably fall into that ill-defined but real group of 'problem families'.

Table 8.4   Size of the household—children

	MSN Home No.	Institution No.	SSN Home No.	%	Institution No.	%
1, 2 or 3	1	2	32	14·8	14	16·3
4, 5 or 6	12	3	152	70·4	56	65·1
7+	2	7	32	14·8	16	18·6
Sub-total	15	12	216	100·0	86	100·0
Not known	1	1	8		9	
Total	16	13	224		95	

χ^2 on 7+ against less than 7 (MSN) = 6·075   p = 0·02
χ^2 on whole table (SSN) = 3·502 NS

In the case of the adults it can be seen that these larger households were not associated with hospital admission; it was the small households that were most vulnerable. Table 8.5 gives the figures for both mildly and severely subnormal adults.

The same point emerges from the figures for both the mildly and the severely subnormal—the vulnerability of households of two. This means a household consisting of just the subnormal and the person in charge of him. Among the severely subnormal the high proportion in hospital was very pronounced. There is no significant difference between the proportion at home and the proportion in hospital in households of any other size. The only significant difference is in households of two. Why should this be? The first question to ask is why those in hospital who had been living in households of two were admitted.

Among the mildly subnormal twenty-one out of the twenty-eight admitted from a household of two were admitted because of the death or illness of a parent or parent figure, and among the severely subnormal forty out of the forty-eight were admitted for this reason.

Table 8.5   Size of the household—adults

	MSN Home No.	%	Institution No.	%	SSN Home No.	%	Institution No.	%
1	38	5·9	8	8·1	4	0·9	1	0·8
2	113	17·7	28	28·3	79	18·2	48	39·3
3 +	488	76·4	63	63·6	350	80·8	73	59·8
Sub-total	639	100·0	99	100·0	433	99·9	122	99·9
Not known	91		8		17		6	
Total	730		107		450		128	

χ^2 on full table (MSN) = 15·706   p = 0·001
χ^2 on Row 2 against Rows 1 and 3 (MSN) = 6·230   p = 0·02
χ^2 on full table (SSN) = 25·906   p = 0·01
χ^2 on Row 2 against Row 3 (SSN) = 24·826   p = 0·001

It is clear that a large proportion were admitted from these small households simply because of the death or illness of the only person looking after them. Among households of any other size the proportion who were admitted because of the death or illness of a parent was much lower. These small households are the result of brothers and sisters getting married and moving away, the subnormal's father dying and a mother who is probably getting old finally being unable to care for her subnormal child any longer, whether because of death or illness. Where the precipitating factor was the death or illness of a parent the majority of the cases were living in households of two— twenty-one out of thirty-seven mildly subnormal and forty out of sixty-two severely subnormal.

The greater likelihood of admission from small households tallies with the findings of the PEP study (Moncrieff, 1966). It would be interesting to know the reason why those from small households were admitted. The only clue that is given is that one-sixth of the admissions were accounted for by the death of a parent.[1]

Size of the subnormal's family

This section is concerned not with the size of the household in which the subnormal was living but with how many brothers and sisters he had. It was quite impossible in the case of most adults to check whether the brothers and sisters were still alive, and so these figures represent the size of the family in which the subnormal was brought up in his early years. They also give as accurate an indication as it is possible to obtain from the files of the number of sibs the subnormal has at present and the help that may be available from that quarter.

The figures for the mildly subnormal adults show very little difference between those at home and those in hospital, and no difference that approaches significance. The most striking feature of the families of the mildly subnormal is the number of large families. Nearly one-fifth of all the mildly subnormal had at least four brothers or sisters, whereas the equivalent figure for the severely subnormal is less than one-tenth; just over 60 per cent of the mildly subnormal had at least three brothers or sisters, but only 45 per cent of the severely subnormal. However, the size of the families of the mildly subnormal adults is *not* associated in any way with admission to hospital. The size of the families of the mildly subnormal children *is* associated with admission to hospital. In this case most of the siblings will have been at home and the seven large families are, with one exception, the same as the seven large households discussed at the beginning of the previous section.

The figures for the severely subnormal are slightly more revealing. The only significant difference between those at home and those in hospital was among those who had three or more older sibs, for whom the figures appear below. The percentages are of the total number in that column (i.e. 11·5 per cent of the children at home had three or more older sibs).

	Children		Adults	
	Home	Institution	Home	Institution
Having 3 + older sibs	25 (11·5%)	1 (1·1%)	57 (12·8%)	26 (21·0%)

The difference is significant in both cases. Why is it that among the children with three or more older sibs there should be more at home than expected, and the exact reverse be the case among the adults? Among the adults almost one-third of the total number with three or more older sibs are in hospital. The following explanation appears reasonable. While the subnormal is still a child the chances are that at least some of his older sibs will be at home and able to help look after him. Once he is an adult the chances are that most if not all of his sibs will be living elsewhere. In addition, the fact that the subnormal is the youngest of a fairly large family means the mother will be quite old. It could be that in the case of the adults the high proportion in hospital is primarily a reflection of the age of the mother, who may by now have died, or is ill and so unable to look after the subnormal. The fact that eighteen out of the twenty-six adults in hospital were admitted because of the death or illness of a parent indicates that this was the case.

A look at the members of the subnormal's family

We have looked at whom the subnormal was living with, how many brothers and sisters he had and how big the household was. It is now time to consider the people who made up those households, especially the parents or the people looking after the subnormal.

The main burden of looking after the subnormal falls on the parents, and one would imagine that if the parents were not fit in any way, this would increase the chances of the subnormal having to go into an institution. It was therefore important to find out about the physical health of the parents or relatives looking after the subnormal. Discovering information from the files about the parents' health was not always easy. In many cases it was a matter of searching for clues. The category of 'nothing adverse known' means that evidence in the file indicated that there was nothing seriously wrong with the parent's health. But the mother's health was coded 'fair' when a case note said: 'the subnormal's mother is booked to enter hospital for a gynaecological operation. She has been waiting since June and her medical condition is deteriorating.' So frequent references that the mother or father 'has not been well' or 'who is in poor health' meant that their physical health would also be coded as 'fair'. The same applied to such remarks in the case notes as 'the father has been ill for some time' and 'mother up and about though suffering from angina'. In all cases such references would have to be quite recent before health was coded as 'fair'. The same difficulty did not apply where the parent's health was obviously bad, such as the case where the subnormal's mother was suffering from disseminated sclerosis or where the case notes said: 'father is suffering from a severe cardiac condition'.

Tables 8.6 and 8.7 give the figures for the physical health of the mother or the mother figure. The mother figure is used to describe any woman other than the mother who was in charge of the sub-normal. In the discussion rather than write 'mother or mother figure' on every occasion 'mother' will generally be used to cover both. A large number of cases appears in the 'not applicable' row. For those at home this is owing to where there was no mother figure, for instance where the subnormal was living alone or with an unmarried brother. Where the subnormal was married the mother figure or father figure was the spouse. In the case of a married subnormal woman her husband was treated as the father figure and the entries for the mother figure were coded 'not applicable'. In the case of a married subnormal man the same principle operated. This accounts for a considerable number of cases of those at home where there was no mother figure, especially among the mildly subnormal.

The reason for the rather large number of cases where there was no mother figure is rather different in the institution groups. In some instances it was because, as in the home group, there was no mother figure, and the subnormal was living, for example, with his father. However, in many cases the reason was that the mother had just died and naturally her physical health was coded as 'not applicable'.

Table 8.6   Physical health of mother or mother figure—children

	MSN Home No.	Inst. No.	SSN Home No.	%	Institution No.	%
Nothing adverse known	14	10	207	95·0	68	80·0
Fair	1	1	11	5·0	15	17·6
Bad or in hospital	0	0	0	0	2	2·4
Sub-total	15	11	218	100·0	85	100·0
Not known	1	1	2		1	
Not applicable	0	1	4		9	
Total	16	13	224		95	

χ^2 on row 1 against rows 2 and 3 (SSN) = 16·306   p = 0·001

Table 8.6 gives the figures for the physical health of the mothers of the children. It can be seen that among the severely subnormal, when the mother's health was only fair, there was an association with admission to hospital.

When we turn to the adults the position is more complex. If a straightforward table was drawn up, it would show that where the mother's health was bad there was a clear association with admission to hospital in the case of both the mildly and the severely subnormal adults. But such a table would give only half the picture. The distinction has been made already, for instance in relation to the size of the household, between those who were admitted because of the death or illness of a parent and those who were admitted for some other reason. This is a distinction of some importance and is critical in this instance.

Table 8.7   Physical health of mother or mother figure—adults

	MSN Home No.	%	YIG No.	%	OIG No.	SSN Home No.	%	YIG No.	%	OIG No.
Nothing adverse known	436	87·7	45	84·9	7	343	85·8	50	83·3	5
Fair	53	10·7	8	15·1	3	53	13·2	9	15·0	6
Bad or in hospital	8	1·6	0	0	7	4	1·0	1	1·7	18
Sub-total	497	100·0	53	100·0	17	400	100·0	60	100·0	29
Not known	37		4		1	8		3		1
Not applicable	196		13		19	42		4		31
Total	730		70		37	450		67		61

These two groups differ in many ways, as will be seen in the next chapters. The mean age on admission of those who were admitted because of the death or illness of a parent was higher (MSN = 44·1 years old, SSN = 38·7 years old) than of those who were admitted for some other reason (MSN = 32·4 years old, SSN = 23·5 years old). It is their age and their parents' age which is the critical factor.

In view of this they will be referred to as 'the younger institution group' and 'the older institution group'. In the tables they will be referred to by their initials (YIG and OIG). In some tables it makes no difference if those in an institution are divided in this way, and so they have been left undivided.

In table 8.7 it is easy to see why these two groups have to be divided. There is little difference between those at home and the younger institution group among both the mildly and severely subnormal. The difference is concentrated almost entirely in the older institution group. They account for almost every case where the mother's health was bad and the majority of the cases where the mother's health was coded 'not applicable' (generally because she had just died). This distinction is what one would expect from the very definition of the older hospital group. The point still remains that where the health of the mother or the woman looking after the subnormal was bad, very few families were able to keep a severely subnormal adult at home. Among the mildly subnormal there were more cases at home where the mother's health was bad (eight) than there were where she was in hospital (seven). It could well be that in some of these cases the subnormal was looking after her mother.

There is one interesting difference between the adults and children. There was very little difference among the adults between the proportions at home and the proportions in hospital where the mother's health was fair. But among the severely subnormal children there were fifteen in this category in hospital and only eleven at home. One explanation might be that severely subnormal children are more difficult to look after, and therefore a lower threshold in terms of the mother's physical health operates. Those who were admitted while children did tend to be more severely handicapped than those who were admitted when they were older. From this it might be possible to argue that those who were admitted while they were children demanded a higher degree of fitness from their mothers. However, fifty-three mothers in only fair health were still looking after a severely subnormal adult at home. This does suggest that once a severely subnormal person has reached adulthood he may in the majority of cases make fewer physical demands on his mother, though there were a few cases where the exact opposite was true. Finally, among the older institution group, it was the failing health of the mother, rather than the specific demands of the subnormal, which was the key factor in admission.

The physical health of the father or father figure was much less important. In a third of all the cases there was no father figure. Among the mildly subnormal there was hardly any difference between the health of the fathers of those at home and those in hospital. Among the severely subnormal there were eight fathers with bad health whose subnormal was in hospital, but only three where the subnormal was at home. In six out of the eight hospital cases the subnormal fell into the older institution group. Except in a small minority of cases it does not seem that the physical health of the father was anything like as decisive a factor as that of the mother.

The information that was gathered about the mental health (this referred to mental illness only) of the mother or mother figure and the father or father figure proved to be unusable. The difficulties of devising sufficiently stringent criteria with which to classify the information from the files were too great. Even if this had been possible there remained the larger question of the reliability of such assessments of mental health based on the opinions of a large number of people whose competence to make such assessments varied considerably. In only one case, the adult severely subnormal, did the results show a significantly higher proportion in an institution, and it is clear that the physical health of the parents was a factor of greater importance.

Information was also gathered about whether the subnormal's mother was herself subnormal. An additional category was introduced between 'nothing adverse known' and 'known to be subnormal'. This is the rather vague category of 'dim'. The only justification for this loosely defined category is that it seemed appropriate in many cases. The following are some examples of cases where the mother was considered 'dim': 'The old mother is a simple and incompetent woman who cannot cope with her feeble-minded daughter's difficult ways.' 'There is of course, the fact that the mother herself is not very intelligent.' 'The mother is, in my [the regional psychiatrist's] opinion, of weak intelligence and character.' No claim can be made of any great precision for this category but the claim is made that the results do give an indication of the number of mothers who were not very bright. Those whose mothers were 'dim' were no more likely to be in hospital than those whose mothers were not, indeed, overall, a higher proportion with 'dim' mothers was at home. What is striking is the considerable number of mildly subnormal whose mothers were described as 'dim' or who were known to be subnormal. It amounted to nearly a fifth (19 per cent) of all the mothers of the mildly subnormal where it was possible to make a coding. The proportion in the case of the severely subnormal was considerably lower (12 per cent).

It is the severely subnormal children who provide the one significant difference between the home and the institution groups. It has been seen that where the mother was considered to be 'dim', there was no difference at all between the two groups, but where the mother was known to be subnormal, there were nine severely subnormal children in an institution and none at home. The precipitating factor in the case of seven of these was a social one, for instance unsatisfactory home conditions or inadequate parental care, and in the remaining two it was behaviour. It does not require much imagination to see why admission to hospital was needed in these cases.

The figures for the adults (table A5 in appendix A) show how, among those in hospital, all the mothers who were known to be subnormal and very nearly all the mothers described as 'dim' were in the younger institution group. It would seem that the less able mothers were not competent to look after their subnormal for as long as most of the mothers of the older institution group had done. In fact the older institution group not only had proportionally fewer 'dim' mothers than the younger institution group but also fewer than the home group. It was old age, not incompetence, which had defeated the mothers of the older institution group.

We have just seen what a high proportion of the mothers of the subnormal, in particular the mildly subnormal, could be called 'dim'. The number of subnormals with subnormal sibs was even larger. No distinction was made between whether the sibs were educationally, mildly or severely subnormal. Many of these will never have been classified as subnormal, especially those who left school after 1960. There is no significant difference at all between those at home and those in an institution. The interest lies in the figures themselves. There were quite a number of families where there were more than two subnormals (8 per cent of the mildly subnormal adults and 5 per cent of the severely subnormal adults). The family where there were seven subnormals was exceptional. Only five of them were actually on the books of the Mental Health Service. If, however, we simply take the percentages of all those with one or more subnormal sibs, there were very nearly a quarter of the mildly subnormal adults (23·5 per cent) with at least one subnormal sib. In view of what is known about the often deprived background of many of the mildly subnormal, this proportion is not altogether surprising. What is rather surprising is the proportion of the severely subnormal with one or more subnormal sibs (19 per cent). This is most likely a reflection of the tendency, which was noticed in the chapter on social class (chapter 6), for the severely subnormal to be over represented in the lower socio-economic groups. Also in that chapter a greater proportion of fathers with non-manual jobs was found among the severely subnormal children than among the adults, so also here a smaller proportion of the severely subnormal children had subnormal sibs (9 per cent) than had the adults (19 per cent). This may be due in part to the fact that some of their sibs were subnormal but had not yet come to official notice, or that some of their sibs as yet unborn would be subnormal. Whatever reasons may be advanced to explain it, it is striking that nearly one mildly subnormal adult in four and one severely subnormal adult in five had a brother or sister who was subnormal to some extent.

So far this section has considered various individual members of the family. In addition an attempt was made to evaluate the relationships within the family, as revealed by the file. This was subject to the same sort of difficulties that have been mentioned already with regard to the subnormality of the mother. In many cases there was nothing said one way or the other in the file, and these cases were coded 'not known', which appears in the table as 'inadequate information'. This category can be considered as virtually the same as 'average'. Any other coding, whether 'good', 'fair', 'bad' or 'very bad', was only given when there was positive evidence to merit such a coding. In the table 'bad' and 'very bad' have been amalgamated. This was easier to decide than the gradings of mental illness or subnormality of the parents because the whole tenor of some files made it quite clear whether the family was a happy one or not.

The two examples from the files which follow were both coded as 'good' family relationships.

John has a good positive relationship with his mother. She is an alert and cheerful ex-nurse. She has good insight into John's condition and understands and has made provision for his future problems.

This is an untidy but happy home, although Mrs R. appears to be exasperated with the care of a large family of boys, she can pull herself out of it and has a very good attitude to Arthur.

The description of relationships as 'fair' indicates a rather unhappy state of affairs. For example, the husband of one subnormal woman was described as 'rather a bully' and he was also 'on bad terms' with his mother-in-law. In another case the case notes recorded: 'Apparently the father is bitterly disappointed over the boy and resents his presence in the house.' Later in the same file it was stated: 'Domestic situation still very strained'. A third case of an imbecile mongol girl also illustrates family relationships which can only be described as 'fair'.

Mr B. does not show any interest in Mary and from what I have gathered does not show much interest in his wife. Each weekend he goes out and Mrs B. is left to cope with Mary and her aged father of 91.

The following cases are examples of 'bad' family relationships.

Mrs D. blamed her husband for much of Peter's troublesome behaviour. She alleged that he hits and kicks Peter. She also said her husband recently struck her across the face for shaking one of the younger children.

There were frequent references in Mark's file to a greater or lesser extent of marital disharmony and friction. For instance, the mental welfare officer reported on one occasion:

> Mark's mother again resurrected the details of her husband's extra-marital activities. I feel she has a certain pleasure in talking about these things and takes every opportunity to do so.

David, the subnormal, was married and the mental welfare officer reported:

> There is constant friction in the home, mainly between husband and wife. Mrs A. has left her husband on several occasions and appears to be frightened of him.

The figures are given in tables 8.8 and 8.9. There was a significantly greater proportion of subnormals in hospital from families with relationships that were fair or bad in every group except one (not taking into account the few mildly subnormal children). The pattern was very similar for the severely subnormal children in hospital and both the mildly and the severely subnormal younger institution groups. It was the mildly subnormal younger institution group that had the highest proportion with poor family relationships, just over a third. The proportion of the mildly subnormal older institution group with poor family relationships was considerably lower, but there was still a significantly higher proportion in hospital. However, among the severely subnormal older institution group, the proportion in hospital was hardly different from that of those living at home, with whom they had more in common than the younger institution group. The families of over half of both these groups had good family relationships.

Table 8.8   Family relationships—children

	MSN Home No.	Inst. No.	SSN Home No.	%	Institution No.	%
Good	10	2	106	47·3	24	25·3
Inadequate information or average	4	5	96	42·9	44	46·3
Fair	2	2	16	7·1	17	17·9
Bad	0	4	6	2·7	10	10·5
Total	16	13	224	100·0	95	100·0

χ^2 (SSN) = 23·791   p = 0·001

Table 8.9 Family relationships—adults

	MSN Home No.	%	YIG No.	%	OIG No.	%	SSN Home No.	%	YIG No.	%	OIG No.	%
Good	258	35·3	12	17·1	9	24·3	264	58·7	18	26·9	33	54·1
Inadequate information or average	388	53·2	34	48·6	19	51·4	157	34·9	32	47·8	23	37·7
Fair	57	7·8	19	27·1	6	16·2	23	5·1	9	13·4	4	6·6
Bad	27	3·7	5	7·1	3	8·1	6	1·3	8	11·9	1	1·6
Total	730	100·0	70	99·9	37	100·0	450	100·0	67	100·0	61	100·0

χ^2 on Home against YIG (MSN) = 33·084 (rows 3 and 4 amalgamated) p = 0·001
χ^2 on Home against OIG (MSN) = 6·016 (rows 3 and 4 amalgamated) p = 0·05
χ^2 on Home against YIG (SSN) = 36·719 (rows 3 and 4 amalgamated) p = 0·001
χ^2 on Home against OIG (SSN) = 0·559 (rows 3 and 4 amalgamated) NS

Family relationships are something that it is impossible to measure accurately, but even these rough approximations from the files have made it clear that they are important. This measure of the quality of family relationships appeared to be generally consistent with the factors which precipitated admission to hospital. This suggests that the results given are a finding of substance despite the difficulties of precise definition.

Some further details about the subnormal's family

Legitimacy   The number of the subnormal who were illegitimate was not high. Five per cent of all the mildly subnormal were illegitimate and 4·9 per cent of the severely subnormal. This is comparable with the rate in the general population. But illegitimate children were more likely to go into hospital. The difference between the proportions at home and the proportions in hospital was definitely significant among the mildly subnormal adults (ten out of forty-one were in hospital) and the severely subnormal children. Exactly half of the twenty illegitimate severely subnormal children were in hospital.

Age of mother when the subnormal was born   It is well known that older mothers have a much higher risk of bearing a subnormal child than have younger mothers. This is especially true of mongols. This can be seen in tables A6 and A7 in appendix A. Thirty-three per cent of the mothers of the severely subnormal were over thirty-four years old when their subnormal child was born. Even among the mildly subnormal, 24 per cent of the mothers were over thirty-four years old when their subnormal child was born. There were three mothers over fifty at the time of their child's birth. In one case it was the mother's twentieth child. In both cases there was a far higher proportion in the oldest age group than among the general population, where only 11 per cent of mothers were over thirty-four when their child was born (see table A8).

However, the main interest of these figures from the point of view of this study is how the age of the mother at the birth of her subnormal child was related to admission to hospital. In the case of the mildly subnormal adults the differences between the proportion in the different age groups at home and in the two institution groups are not significant. Among the severely subnormal there is an interesting contrast between the children and the older institution group. The difference between the home group and the institution group is significant in both cases but in opposite directions: of the severely subnormal children whose mothers were *under* thirty when they were born, more than expected were in hospital; but of the severely subnormal adults from the older institution group whose mothers were *over* thirty-four at the time of the subnormal's birth, more than expected were in hospital. Those aged between thirty and thirty-four when their children were born mark the watershed where the proportions at home and the proportions in hospital are fairly even. There is no significant difference between the proportions in the different age groups between the adults at home and the younger institution group.

It is easy to explain why many of the adult severely subnormal in the older institution group whose mothers were older when they were born were in hospital. Their mothers were older and therefore more likely to have died or be ill and unable to look after them. This led to their admission and presence in this group. This is one more obvious reflection of the critical importance of the age of the mother.

It is less obvious why more severely subnormal children whose mothers were younger when they were born should have gone into hospital. One clue is that many of the subnormals born to older mothers will be mongols. Kushlick has made an interesting suggestion about the social consequences of the association between increasing maternal age and the incidence of mongolism. He writes (1968, p. 390):[2]

> First, half of all cases of mongolism are born to mothers aged over thirty-six, an age by which most families will be completed and this is likely to mean that the most difficult stage of child rearing, the early years, will continue well into the parent's middle age. On the other hand, it means that mongol children will be more likely than other severely subnormal children to be born to experienced mothers who have raised other normal children. This may be a possible explanation for the suggestion that most mongol children have an easy and happy disposition.

This can provide a reasonable explanation for half of the problem, that is why more severely subnormal children born to older mothers were at home and more severely subnormal adults born to older mothers were in hospital, but it does not explain why more children born to younger mothers should have been admitted to hospital. This finding is made more significant by the fact that the PEP study found just the same (Moncrieff, 1966, p. 22). Although the children were not considered separately, half of those persons in hospital were aged under sixteen when they were admitted and a further quarter were aged between sixteen and twenty years.

Part of the answer may be the reverse of Kushlick's argument, that is that these mothers were younger and inexperienced and so were less likely to be able to cope with the problems of care and management that arose. There is another factor which fits in with this. In the section 'Size of the subnormal's family' we saw that there was a similar pattern if the severely subnormal person had three or more older sibs. More were at home as far as the children were concerned; more were in hospital as far as the adults were concerned (see p. 100). The younger mothers would tend not to have older children who could help. On the contrary, any other children, whether they were older or younger than the subnormal, would probably be young and need a fair amount of looking after themselves. The probability of this is shown by the fact that no other combination of older and younger brothers and sisters was associated with the subnormal staying at home. The only combination associated with the child staying at home was if he had at least three older siblings.

The differences between the various groups in the proportions at home and the proportions in hospital, according to the mother's age when the subnormal was born, provide circumstantial evidence of the importance of the mother's age and health, her experience and the help that older brothers and sisters give.

Employment of the parents   The employment of the subnormal's father or father figure contains no surprises. The only point of interest is that out of the nine mildly subnormal children in hospital who did have a father figure, five of the fathers were unemployed.

The figures for the employment of the subnormal's mother or mother figure are more interesting. Among the severely subnormal children, very few of the mothers of those in hospital went out to work at all (9 per cent) and only one did so full-time. A higher proportion of the mothers of those at home did go out to work (23 per cent), mainly part-time, and the difference is definitely significant. The higher proportion of those in hospital whose mothers were unable to go to work is related to a considerable extent to their child's disability. The precipitating factor in the admission of fifty-eight out of the seventy-eight whose mothers were unable to go out to work was either the subnormal's behaviour or a nursing problem. It is not difficult to understand why their mothers were unable to go out to work. In some cases the decisive factor is likely to have been whether the child went to a training centre or not.

With the adults the pattern is rather different for the mildly and the severely subnormal. Among the mildly subnormal, a smaller proportion of the mothers of the older institution group (only three) were going out to work (13 per cent) than the home group (20 per cent). This was due very largely to the age of the mothers, many of whom were pensioners. But an even lower proportion of the mothers of the younger institution group were going out to work (12 per cent) and this cannot be explained by their age. It may be that the care of their subnormal prevented them from doing so. The figures are too small to draw any firm conclusions.

Among the severely subnormal older institution group, it is clear that the small proportion of mothers going out to work (5 per cent) was due very largely to the age of the mothers, but the younger institution group (19 per cent working at least part-time) did not differ significantly from the home group (23 per cent working at least part-time). Although these figures reveal no significant difference, the mother going out to work was an important issue in some of the visits, and will be discussed later.

Conclusions

The recurring theme throughout this chapter has been the vital importance of the age and physical health of the mother. It has been seen that it is this which underlies other differences between the home and the hospital groups which appeared to be significant. It was shown that this was the critical factor underlying households which consisted of just the subnormal and one other person, generally his mother.

When the physical health of the mother was discussed, it became clear that those adults who were admitted to an institution because of the death or illness of a parent had to be considered separately from those admitted for other reasons. When this was done, it was seen that this older institution group accounted for most of the people in hospital where the mother's health was bad.

This important distinction showed how very few of the mothers of the older institution group were mentally 'dim' compared with the younger group, and how many more of the younger institution group had poor family relationships. There was hardly any difference at all between the family relationships of the older severely subnormal institution group and the home group.

The physical health of the father or father figure was not important but the section on whom the subnormal was living with did indicate that, at least in the case of the severely subnormal, the presence of the husband of the woman who was looking after the subnormal appeared to make it more likely for the subnormal to remain at home. Another important issue considered was the high proportion of subnormals whose parents were dead who were living with their sibs.

The critical importance of the age of the parents, especially the mother, affected almost every subject touched on in this chapter. Its importance is underlined still further in the next chapter.

The subnormals themselves

This chapter describing the subnormals themselves has been delayed until now deliberately to make the point that they do not exist in isolation. On the contrary, the extent of their handicap can only be understood fully when it is put into its social setting. Nevertheless, what the subnormals can or cannot do and the way they behave is of critical importance, and is the subject of this chapter.

IQ and mongolism

Much has been said about the reliability or otherwise of the IQ test, but it is at least a yardstick, and so a note was made of the IQ given in the files. The IQ which was taken was that nearest to the date of ascertainment. Such a second-hand IQ is clearly of only limited value, especially when it covers such a wide period of time. A few of the tests will have been carried out during the First World War. They do, however, give a rough idea of the distribution of intelligence within the different groups. The number of unknowns is very high, so the figures can only be treated as a guide. Among the adults, both mildly and severely subnormal, they show a tendency for those at home to be well represented at the top of the range. Those in hospital are more evenly distributed, but among the severely subnormal, especially the children, there is some concentration at the bottom end of the scale.

The figures are more reliable when it comes to the number of mongols. There were only two unknowns in the whole population surveyed. Table 9.1 gives the number of mongols in each group and what percentage they formed of each group. Thus, for instance, there were seventy-four severely subnormal mongol children living at home, and they were 33 per cent of all severely subnormal children at home.

This gives a rate per 1,000 in the five to fifteen age group of 1·17/1,000, which is very close to Goodman and Tizard's rate for Middlesex in 1960 in the age group seven to fourteen of 1·14/1,000 and Kushlick's rate for Wessex in 1964 in the age group fifteen to nineteen of 1·18/1,000 in the counties and 1·15/1,000 in the county boroughs (Kushlick, 1968, p. 391). The very much lower rate for the adults, only 0·30/1,000, reflects the much earlier mortality of mongols only a decade or two ago.

Table 9.1   Mongols

| | Children | | | | Adults | | | |
| | MSN | | SSN | | MSN | | SSN | |
	Home	Institution	Home	Institution	Home	Institution	Home	Institution
No. of mongols	3	0	74	6*	5	0	83	26*
No. as % of total	18·8	–	33·2	–	0·7	–	18·6	–

* See note 1

In order to calculate these rates the chronological figures have been used.[1] Of more direct relevance to the present study is the significantly greater proportion of mongol children at home than in hospital. The most likely explanation of this is the suggestion that mongols tend to be quite docile and well-behaved. This suggestion does receive a good deal of support from this study. This is discussed in chapter 8 on page 111 f. and in note 2 on page 389 f. The reason that there is not a similar difference among the adults is probably due to their mothers tending to be older when they were born and so dying or becoming infirm and unable to continue looking after the subnormal.

The subnormals' physical abilities and disabilities

Walking   This was thought to be important, especially among the severely subnormal adults, where it was felt that problems of lifting might well loom large. The results are given in tables 9.2 and 9.3. The numbers of the mildly subnormal whose walking was defective were insignificant. In the case of the severely subnormal the results were the reverse of what had been anticipated. The difference between the adult home group and hospital groups does not reach the level of significance in either case, but among the children the difference is clearly significant where the child was severely handicapped or totally unable to walk. How is this to be explained? Two complementary reasons appear likely. First, some of those who were admitted while they were children will have been multiply handicapped, and their handicap in walking was one aspect of this. Thirteen out of the twenty-two in hospital who were unable to walk were admitted because of a nursing problem. All those admitted for this reason were very severely handicapped. Second, if the subnormal was unable to walk or his walking was very shaky but he had reached adulthood and was still at home, the chances are that he and his family had come to terms with his disability and were able to cope with it.

Table 9.2   Walking – children

	MSN Home No.	Inst. No.	SSN Home No.	%	Institution No.	%
No defect or slight defect	14	13	183	82·4	62	66·7
Severe	2	0	10	4·5	9	9·7
Total disability	0	0	29	13·1	22	23·6
Sub-total	16	13	222	100·0	93	100·0
Not known	0	0	2		2	
Total	16	13	224		95	

χ^2 on whole table (SSN) = 9·544   p = 0·01
χ^2 on row 1 against rows 2 and 3 (SSN) = 9·426   p = 0·01

Talking   The number of mildly subnormal who were handicapped in talking was insignificant. The chief interest lies in the severely subnormal where the situation is different for the children and both the younger and older institution groups.

Among the children there was a significantly greater proportion in hospital only when they were unable to speak at all. Nearly a quarter of those at home could not talk, but for those in hospital the proportion was nearly a half. There is not much difference between the actual figures: there were exactly 100 severely subnormal children who could not talk at all. Fifty-five of them were at home and forty-five in hospital.

There was no significant difference between the adult home group and the younger institution group, but there was when the adults at home were compared with the older institution group. There was a significantly greater proportion in hospital where the subnormal had any speech defect at all. This may seem surprising until it is remembered that the position of the older institution group was fundamentally different from the others. The question was not whether the mother would let her subnormal child go into hospital or not but whether a relative would take him into her household and look after

Table 9.3 Walking – adults

	MSN Home No.	%	YIG No.	%	OIG No.	%	SSN Home No.	%	YIG No.	%	OIG No.	%
No defect or slight defect	719	98·5	69	98·6	34	91·9	421	93·6	61	91·0	53	86·9
Severe	9	1·2	1	1·4	3	8·1	15	3·3	4	6·0	5	8·2
Total disability	2	0·3	0	0	0	0	14	3·1	2	3·0	3	4·9
Sub-total	730	100·0	70	100·0	37	100·0	450	100·0	67	100·0	61	100·0
Not known	0		0		0		0		0		0	
Total	730		70		37		450		67		61	

χ^2 on Home against OIG (SSN) = 3·559 NS

him. It appears that any speech defect in the subnormal reduced the chances of a relative taking on the subnormal.

Deafness and blindness Only a tiny proportion was deaf, just over 2 per cent, and there was no significant relationship with admission to hospital, except for the severely subnormal children. Ten of them were deaf, five were at home and five in hospital. It was the same with blindness. It was only among the severely subnormal children that a significant number were blind. There were twelve severely subnormal blind children at home (eight of them also had little or no speech) and thirteen in hospital (ten of them also had little or no speech). The difference is significant but in many cases the blindness was part of a multiple handicap.

Continence Continence was naturally important, but in this case, unlike that of walking, the difference between the severely subnormal children and adults followed a more obvious pattern.

The number of mildly subnormal who were incontinent at all was small. The proportion in hospital was much higher than the proportion at home, and most of these were in the younger institution group of whom 19 per cent were incontinent to some extent. The number of severely subnormal who were incontinent was considerably greater. In the case of severely subnormal children a much higher proportion of those at home were fully continent (53 per cent) than of those in hospital (20 per cent). Where the child was partially incontinent there was no difference between those at home and those in hospital, but there was a marked difference if the child was totally incontinent. Over half of those in hospital were totally incontinent (51 per cent), but only 16 per cent of those at home. In fact the majority of those who were totally incontinent were in hospital. There were thirty-five at home and forty-seven in hospital.

There was very little difference between the severely subnormal younger and older institution groups. Of the severely subnormal adults at home, 88 per cent were fully continent, but only 63 per cent of the adults in an institution. The distinction between those at home and those in hospital came where there was any incontinence at all. The actual numbers were fifty-three at home against a total of forty-six in hospital.

The difference between the children and adults is very understandable. Incontinence in children is more acceptable than it is in adults. Many of the children who were partly incontinent would be learning and becoming better controlled. In the adults any incontinence probably meant incontinence for good, which is a daunting, expensive and exhausting prospect for the parents or the person looking after the subnormal. It is easy to appreciate why a relative would be reluctant to take on a subnormal if he was incontinent.

Epilepsy   Epilepsy affected the mildly subnormal, to some extent, as well as the severely subnormal. It affected children's admission to hospital at a less severe level than it affected some of the adults. Among the severely subnormal children, and it appears true of the mildly subnormal as well, there was a significantly higher proportion in hospital if they had fits at not less than monthly intervals. Of the children at home, 9 per cent had fits at least monthly, compared with 29 per cent of those in hospital. Among the severely subnormal adults in hospital almost all the cases of severe epilepsy were in the younger institution group, and it was only when the fits occurred weekly or more often that they were associated with admission to hospital. Twelve of the younger institution group (18 per cent) had fits with this frequency. The severely subnormal older institution group differs very little from the home group. The mildly subnormal adults follow the same pattern, though it is not as marked and the numbers are small.

The number with frequent fits is small when one gets to the adults, and the fact that only one of the severely subnormal older institution group and only sixteen (4 per cent) of the adults at home had fits frequently makes it seem that where a subnormal had epileptic fits at least weekly he was likely to be admitted before he had reached middle age.

General physical condition and mental illness   Information was coded about the subnormals' general health, but apart from indicating that about 15 per cent of all groups had only 'fair' health, the results did not reveal much or produce any significant difference between the home and the hospital groups. The sort of condition that was described as 'fair' health was persistent bronchitis or a minor heart complaint.

But with mental illness, the association with admission to hospital is unmistakable. The numbers are small but, overall, there were more who were mentally ill in hospital than there were at home. Table 9.4 gives the figures. The subnormal was only coded as mentally ill if the evidence of his illness was very clear indeed. The most common evidence accepted for this was if the subnormal had been admitted to hospital specifically because of mental illness. In other cases the coding was based on evidence from the file. The following examples give an idea of the sort of evidence that was taken to justify this coding of 'clear evidence of mental illness'.

Table 9.4   Mental illness

| | Children | | | | Adults | | | | | |
| | MSN | | SSN | | MSN | | | SSN | | |
	Home	Institution	Home	Institution	Home	YIG	OIG	Home	YIG	OIG
Mentally ill	1	0	3	4	20	17	5	8	11	3
Mentally ill as % of total in that group	6·2	–	1·3	4·2	2·7	24·3	13·5	1·8	16·4	4·9

X^2 on Home against YIG (MSN) $= 67·884$ p $= 0·001$
X^2 on Home against YIG (SSN)$= 37·345$ p $= 0·001$

A mildly subnormal man who was also epileptic was described as 'aggressive and violent at times'. The Medical Officer of Health wrote about him:

He is very confused and has delusional ideas which might at any time cause him to make trouble for himself and others. He has also deteriorated very markedly in health and it would appear that some action to keep him under hospital supervision is necessary.

The man was still at home in September 1968.

The file on a mildly subnormal woman of nineteen was more specific. The Medical Officer of Health wrote to the Superintendent at Middlewood (Mental) Hospital: 'my opinion is that this girl is in a state of toxic confusion with schizoid excitement superimposed on subnormality.' The discharge report three years later diagnosed 'schizophrenia in a mental defective'. Unfortunately her subsequent behaviour at home continued to be very disturbed.

The mental welfare officer recorded in the case notes of a severely subnormal girl of fifteen:

Father went to the office with a letter from his G.P. to Dr Esher requesting him to see the child and suggest treatment. He says she is deteriorating, banging her head, and is now troubled by voices which bother her.

Later that year the mental welfare officer wrote: 'It is obvious to me that Phyllis is extremely hallucinated. All the time I was there she was continually laughing, looking around and muttering to herself.' Shortly after this she began to have out-patient psychiatric treatment.

The concentration of cases in the younger institution group among both the mildly and severely subnormal indicates that mental illness affected the young adults primarily. Broadly speaking the distinction between the mentally ill who stayed at home and those who had to go into hospital was simply that among those in hospital their illness was connected with a behaviour problem and among those at home it was not.

Dressing and feeding

These two basic skills were chosen to indicate how much the subnormal was able to look after himself. An additional reason for choosing them was that it was generally possible to find the necessary information in the file. The two categories at each end of the scale 'feeding or dressing by self' and 'not at all' are self explanatory. 'Can with help' meant in the case of feeding that the subnormal could at least eat with a spoon unaided. If he needed his meat cutting up he was still coded as 'can with help' because he was not able to feed entirely by himself. The same principle was applied to dressing. If the subnormal was able to put most of his clothes on but needed help with some clothes and buttons he would be coded 'can with help'. This same coding was given even if all the help that was needed was tying bows, because this indicated that he was not able to dress completely by himself.

The number of mildly subnormal unable to dress or feed themselves completely independently is very small so we will concentrate entirely on the severely subnormal. There is a significant difference between those at home and those in hospital in all three groups of the severely subnormal, but the association with admission is at two different levels. It was only complete inability to dress which was associated with admission for the children (60 per cent of those in hospital but only 33 per cent of those at home could not dress themselves) and the younger institution group (17 per cent could not dress themselves at all compared with 5 per cent of the adult home group). However, for the older institution group there was a definite association with admission, even if the subnormal only needed some help with dressing. Only 18½ per cent of the severely subnormal adults at home needed help with dressing, but among the older institution group the proportion rose to 42 per cent. This appears to be another instance where the criteria a relative may apply before taking on a subnormal whose mother had died have had their effect, and some of the more able subnormal were admitted in this older institution group as a result.

The pattern is slightly different with feeding. The number of mildly subnormal affected is again minute. Among the severely subnormal children it was once again only complete inability which was associated with admission to hospital (49 per cent of those in hospital compared with $17\frac{1}{2}$ per cent of those at home) but in the case of both the younger as well as the older institution group there was a clear association with admission to hospital, even if the subnormal only needed help with feeding. This applied to 26 per cent of the younger and 28 per cent of the older institution group, compared with 9 per cent of the adults at home. Inability to feed oneself indicates a lower level of ability than inability to dress oneself. Most children start feeding themselves before they start dressing themselves. Also, it is more acceptable to have to feed a child than it is to have to feed an adult. Both these points may explain why the level at which feeding and dressing were associated with admission to hospital differed for the younger institution group.

It can be seen that many of the severely subnormal, especially the children, lacked these basic social skills, and that this lack was associated strongly with admission to hospital. This was especially noticeable where the subnormal was unable to feed himself.

Behaviour

The behaviour of the subnormal was considered in three different areas; at home, at training centre or at work, and in the locality. By far the most important of these was behaviour at home. Behaviour was the most important single factor leading to admission to hospital, dwarfing all others. Its importance stands out unambiguously in tables 9·5 and 9·6. Common sense might suggest that this would be the case. The actual figures confirm it decisively. In every group there were well over twice as many with a serious behaviour problem who were in hospital as there were at home. The original coding was a fourfold one. The problem was coded 'none', 'slight', 'moderate' or 'severe'. The distinction between 'none' and 'slight' was not clear, nor was that between 'moderate' and 'severe', but the distinction between 'slight' and 'moderate' was much more clear cut, and it was this level that distinguished between the home and hospital groups. The following examples of the different categories cover behaviour both inside and outside the home.

Slight behaviour problem   A severely subnormal woman living at home with her mother had an IQ of 48. The mental welfare officer reported: 'Jean is getting more difficult to handle and although Mrs Wilde says she is quite good at Pitsmoor [senior training centre], when she is at home she is very restless and dashing about the house all night.'

A note on Joan, a severely subnormal woman, said: 'Very aggressive at times towards relatives, locks doors, will not let people into the house: resents interference in the house. But the general position is that she is not much trouble.'

A note made at the time of coding the file mentioned below gives an idea of the boundary between a 'slight' and 'moderate' problem. 'Christopher was generally very little trouble in his very good home but when his father died he seems to have tried to become "boss" and on several occasions threatened and actually struck his mother. As she was extremely ill with a heart complaint, he was soon admitted to hospital.' (This was coded as 'slight behaviour problem', though a coding of 'moderate' was considered as, in themselves, the attacks were quite serious.)

Moderate behaviour problem   Martin, a severely subnormal boy living in a poor home, was the oldest of seven children. He was nine at the time of this report:

> Two neighbours came into the office today to make complaints about Mrs D. They stated that Martin is continually hitting and throwing stones at two little girls aged about six years old. Often neighbours are troubled in the same way, but Mrs D. makes no attempt to stop him. Martin is a nuisance generally and drivers of cars who know him will not bring them into the street because he lets the air out of the tyres and throws stones through the glass. These two people are afraid that he will do some harm to their children as he has been known to kill at least three cats.

Diana, a mildly subnormal woman of twenty-five, was also mentally ill. She was the oldest of three children. In 1967 the mental welfare officer recorded what her mother had told him:

Diana was discharged last Saturday and has been unmanageable since. Put her fist through the window Saturday evening – cut wrist. Exposing herself and takes off underclothes. Wandering around at night . . . at the moment Diana is locked in the house, as mother cannot restrain her, and is trying to break down the door.

In another case the notes record a complaint from a neighbour that 'Philip has again called at their home, wanting to fight.' The complaints had been made regularly over the previous twelve months.

Another man shouted out and exposed himself sexually on many occasions but there was no record in the file of any assault. His behaviour was therefore coded as a 'moderate' problem. If there had been any sort of actual interference it would have been coded as a 'severe' problem.

Severe behaviour problem   Ethel was a mildly subnormal woman in her early forties, living with her brother, sister-in-law and their two small children. The mental welfare officer reported in 1957:

Ethel has been a source of constant trouble at home getting drunk and having to be fetched out of public houses. At such times she has become very violent. Attacked her mother during her last illness. She is dirty in her habits and would defecate in the living room in front of the children, refusing to use the W.C. She ill-uses the children [both under five], sexually as well, and is violent at times.

Shortly after this, she was admitted to hospital.

The difficulty of deciding between the coding of a 'moderate' and a 'severe' problem has been mentioned already. The case above was coded a 'severe' behaviour problem in the locality and a 'moderate' behaviour problem at home, and illustrates why the two categories were eventually put together.

The file on a severely subnormal boy of seven who lived alone with his mother said of him: 'Kicks and strikes those about him, throws knives and tries to strangle his mother. Set house on fire on two occasions. Very destructive.'

In the case of a severely subnormal woman of thirty-six, the mental welfare officer reported: 'When we arrived at the house she was at the window bellowing like a bull, and her father was trying to comfort her.'

The following quotation is taken from a letter which was written in the early 1950s. It was written by the Deputy Medical Officer of Health to the Board of Control. It is reproduced to give some idea of the appalling situations that some parents have to endure. Unfortunately it is not the only example of such a state of affairs.

I have to draw your attention to the extremely urgent need for institutional treatment of this mentally defective child, a boy of eight years, who has been ascertained as an imbecile [epileptic]. I visited his home and saw the defective together with his mother and father. The child is very well developed physically, but suffers from a spastic hemiplegia (he was a rhesus baby), although this does not impede his activity materially. He was stark naked and apparently this is his normal condition as he removes his clothes as soon as they are put on him. He had one epileptic seizure while I was present. During the time I was in the house he micturated into a cup he took from the china cupboard and threw the contents round the room. He also took a saucer from the cupboard, filled it with water from the tap, and poured the contents over the kitchen table. Apart from these acts, he divided his time between masturbating and screaming. He is completely beyond control and his parents are absolutely at the end of their tether. I am quite satisfied that unless he can be taken into institutional care very quickly a tragedy will occur in this household, either the father will murder the boy, or the mother will commit suicide. (The mother's arms are scarred and bruised from wrist to shoulder, where the boy has pinched and bitten her.) The house is a three roomed back-to-back type, as clean as it can be under the circumstances, but pools of urine have dripped through the bedroom floor and stained the ceiling of the living room.

The figures for behaviour at home are given in tables 9.5 and 9.6. Some examples have been given to show what is meant by the different categories of behaviour problem. The two speak for themselves. Among the children and younger institution groups, both mildly and severely subnormal, the proportion with 'moderate' or 'severe' behaviour in hospital is vastly greater than for those at home. Only a few with behaviour problems were still at home. It is understandable that it is behaviour at home which was critical. There was no escape for the family from this.

The overwhelming proportion of those in hospital with 'severe' behaviour problems among the children and younger institution groups makes the few with serious behaviour problems in both the older institution groups all the more striking. The reason is easy enough to see. Those with serious behaviour problems did not generally stay at home for long. If they presented a serious behaviour problem they were admitted while they were comparatively young. There is a limit to the time a family can stand the strain imposed on them by such behaviour.

Table 9.5   Behaviour problems at home – children

	MSN Home No.	Institution No.	SSN Home No.	%	Institution No.	%
None or slight	14	4	191	92·7	40	44·9
Moderate or severe	1	7	15	7·3	49	55·1
Sub-total	15	11	206	100·0	89	100·0
Not known	1	2	18		6	
Not known as % of total				8·0		6·3
Total	16	13	224		95	

$\chi^2 = $ (MSN) 9·669   p $= 0·01$
$\chi^2 = $ (SSN) 83·499   p $= 0·001$

Behaviour problems in the locality and to some extent at training centre or at work were also quite important. There was only one adult in either of the older institution groups who presented a serious behaviour problem. The presence of a behaviour problem in the locality was the more important factor, more important than even behaviour at home in the case of the small group of mildly subnormal children in hospital. Eight of these thirteen presented a 'moderate' or 'severe' behaviour problem in the locality. This may account for how they came to the attention of the authorities before the age of sixteen. Sixteen is the age at which most mildly subnormal were first reported to the Mental Health Service. In the other groups, except for the mildly subnormal adults at home, the numbers with 'serious' behaviour problems in the locality were lower than the number with similar problems at home, but there was still a majority in hospital. Seventeen of the mildly subnormal younger

Table 9.6 Behaviour problems at home – adults

	MSN Home No.	%	YIG No.	%	OIG No.	%	SSN Home No.	%	YIG No.	%	OIG No.	%
None or slight	671	98·0	26	44·8	32	88·9	431	96·9	26	41·9	56	93·3
Moderate or severe	14	2·0	32	55·2	4	11·1	14	3·1	36	58·1	4	6·7
Sub-total	685	100·0	58	100·0	36	100·0	445	100·0	62	100·0	60	100·0
Not known	45		12		1		5		5		1	
Not known as a % of total	6·2		17·1		2·7		1·1		7·5		1·6	
Total	730		70		37		450		67		61	

χ^2 on Home against YIG (MSN) = 259·881 p = 0·001
χ^2 on Home against YIG (SSN) = 184·633 p = 0·001

institution group presented a serious behaviour problem, compared with eighteen of the mildly subnormal adults at home, but at the other end of the scale, among the severely subnormal children, there were only three at home to twenty-five in hospital.

The numbers who presented a serious behaviour problem at training centre or at work were smaller again. The number of cases to whom this did not apply was high, because many did not go out either to work or to a training centre. The difference between the home and hospital groups was only significant among the severely subnormal children.

One boy underlined the importance of distinguishing between behaviour at home and behaviour at the training centre. Leslie appeared to be quite a serious behaviour problem in and around his home but not at Norfolk Park Training Centre. This bad behaviour seemed to be a product of his unsatisfactory home environment. The NSPCC reported one August: 'During the past holiday period Leslie has been allowed to run wild; his behaviour has deteriorated, the police have been called to the home many times with complaints of excessive use of foul language by the boy, severe aggression to children and animals and causing no end of trouble to the neighbourhood in general.' But in November of the same year a psychiatrist reported on him: 'the boy is a well developed lad who is well controlled at the Centre – his attitude is quite normal for a subnormal lad. He likes affection but is not demanding – is interested in what is available here within the limits of his intelligence (IQ 50–60) and away from the unbalanced background of his home life, he could be a quite well trained and well-behaved subnormal adult who might well earn his living.'

Slightly more men than women manifested serious behaviour problems, but there were only two categories where the difference was marked. There were more males with 'severe' behaviour problems among the severely subnormal in hospital. In the case of the children, sixteen boys but only five girls presented a 'severe' problem: the equivalent figures for the adults were eleven men compared with four women. There were also eleven boys at home with 'moderate' behaviour problems, but only three girls. The same pattern of slightly more males than females presenting serious behaviour problems was also true of behaviour outside the home.

It is probably true that once a family was confronted with a subnormal member whose behaviour made life extremely difficult, the mental welfare officer did not minimize the problems in his attempts to get a hospital bed for the subnormal. Such beds were scarce and only went to the most urgent cases. This may have had the effect of exaggerating the difficulties, but the difficulties were real enough none the less, and it remains true that the presence of serious behaviour problems was the most important single factor associated with admission to hospital.

Contact with the law

This is connected closely with the previous section on behaviour. The table has been given the title of 'criminal record' but in many cases this meant no more than some contact with the police. In general, more mildly than severely subnormal had come up against the police, and more of those in hospital than those at home.

Only a tiny proportion of the severely subnormal children at home, two out of 224, had any 'criminal record', but slightly more of those in hospital, nine out of ninety-five. The mildly subnormal children in an institution make the connection between behaviour and 'criminal record' very clear. Eight out of the thirteen mildly subnormal children in hospital had presented a serious behaviour problem in the locality. Five of these same eight also got themselves into trouble with the police.

The figures for the adults show how important it is to distinguish the older and younger institution groups. Both the mildly and the severely subnormal older institution groups have a lower proportion with any 'criminal record' (MSN 16 per cent, SSN 8 per cent) than not only the younger institution groups (MSN 49 per cent, SSN 35 per cent) but also their respective home groups (MSN 27 per cent, SSN 12 per cent). A significantly higher proportion of both the younger institution groups had a 'criminal record', but from table A9, in appendix A, it can be seen that the less serious categories account for the majority of the cases, especially among the severely subnormal. The mildly subnormal adults who were dealt with more severely are worth attention. Nineteen of those who had been sent to hospital on a court order were living at home in 1968 and two of these had been in one of the high security special hospitals (Rampton or Moss Side). Only five were still in hospital.

It is misleading in many cases to think of the subnormal having committed a crime, though he had in some cases. This is apparent when the type of 'offence' is considered. There is an overall pattern which is similar for all four groups – roughly 35 per cent trivial matters or petty stealing, 35 per cent some sexual 'offence', 6 per cent threatening behaviour and 12 per cent running away from home. The main departures from this pattern were the higher proportion of mildly subnormal at home, nearly half, whose only 'offence' was trivial, and the higher proportion of mildly subnormal in hospital who had committed some sexual 'offence'. This applies to the severely subnormal at home as well, and a larger proportion of the severely subnormal in hospital had run away. These deviations from the general pattern, though interesting, are not significant except for the last.

The word 'offence' has been used in inverted commas. The reason for this is especially clear if the sexual 'offence' of 'sexually assaulted' is considered. This refers to the person who was assaulted not the person who did the assaulting. Seventeen out of the total of eighteen in this category were, naturally enough, women. The reason these cases have been shown is that the assault brought them into contact with the police and in time past it led on a number of occasions to the woman being admitted to an institution. In one case a woman of twenty-eight, described as low-grade feeble-minded, was living with her sister and brother-in-law. She was assaulted sexually by her brother-in-law and *she* was sent into an institution. She was admitted in 1947 and she was still in an institution in 1968.

The same is true of 'running away'. This is hardly a crime, but it did bring the subnormal into contact with the police and it is interesting that nine of the twenty-nine severely subnormal adults in hospital who had committed some offence had run away from home. It was very likely just one aspect of unruly behaviour in and around the home.

The difficulties of using the word offence in the case of subnormals are underlined when one or two instances are considered in a little more detail. A mildly subnormal man was accused of acting in an indecent way. The mental welfare officer wrote:

> It has been reported that when the subnormal was at the cinema he acted in an indecent way with the woman next to him. He was charged and appeared in court and was remanded in custody pending an examination by the prison doctor. I can hardly believe that the subnormal was guilty of this. During the time he has been under supervision he has behaved very well and his parents say he is very truthful.

Ill-founded or not, this was coded as 'exhibitionism', which also covered sexual exposure and minor sexual interference. The difficulty in this case was made worse by the fact that the man had a severe speech defect.

The same sort of problem can be seen in the case of Harry, a mildly subnormal man of twenty, who was charged with indecent assault of a girl of seven. According to his mother this 'indecent assault' seemed to amount to 'he is accosting young girls in the street and tickling their legs'. In this case Harry's 'offence' was coded 'sexual assault'. It points to a difficulty which many subnormals face, though it does not apply directly in this case. Behaviour which, in the case of ordinary young men, might be looked on as simply 'being fresh with the girls' in the subnormal's case may be blown up into 'sexual assault'.

The fourth category of sexual offence was 'prostitution'. This covers prostitution itself but far more common was promiscuous sexual behaviour. This doctor's report was one of the comparatively few cases where money came into it.

> This simple minded girl is becoming a severe problem at home. She will stay in bed all day rather than go to work, wets her bed, won't change into night clothes and generally defies the authority of her people. She will have sexual relations with anyone who will take her and always earns enough money for her wants by these means.

When considering the 'criminal' record of the subnormal, it needs to be remembered that they form a very small proportion of the whole. Adults involved in any sort of sexual 'offence' were less than 1 per cent of the total. Of the total of twenty-one whose 'crime' was described as 'threatening behaviour', only one went so far as actually to commit a violent crime. All the other 'crimes' involved running away or some trivial offence.

This section is really a commentary on the previous section on behaviour and in so far as the subnormal's 'crime' is related to admission to hospital, this is covered effectively under the all-important heading of the subnormal's behaviour.

Supervision needed

Many of the consequences of what has been discussed so far in this chapter are epitomized in the single factor – how much supervision does the mother or the person in charge of the subnormal have to exercise? This is one important measure of the impact the care of the subnormal had on his household and in particular on his mother.

The coding was not easy to decide. The question was rarely answered directly by the file and it had to be deduced from the clues that were available. The category of 'can be left all day' did not really apply to the children. This coding was given when it was apparent that the subnormal was left all day or, more commonly, when it appeared from the file that there was no feature of his temperament or behaviour which made this impossible. This quotation from the file of a mildly subnormal man of forty-six is an example of the sort of evidence that would be used to support such a coding. 'He is a big hefty man and still seems rather dull mentally and just answers yes or no. He is quite satisfied to sit at home by the fire for most of the day and has few or no interests at home.' A further quotation, this time from the file of a mongol woman of twenty-six, is another of the snippets of evidence that were taken to suggest that 'can be left all day' was the most suitable coding: 'The subnormal was in bed when I called this morning—her mother had gone shopping.'

The next category was 'can be left for an hour or so'. If the mother was able to leave the subnormal for long enough to go for a reasonable shopping expedition, though not able to leave him over a meal time, this was the coding given. Frequently the evidence was more oblique than this, and if the file suggested that while the subnormal needed a fair amount of care and attention yet at the same time was generally stable and well behaved, 'can be left for an hour or so' was considered the appropriate coding. The following quotation is one example of this. 'He is dull mentally and childish for his years (nineteen). Well behaved and easily controlled and amused but he needs care and supervision.' This note from the file of a severely subnormal woman who was also epileptic is typical of the rather elusive evidence from which the coding had to be made in some cases: 'Fanatically jealous, especially of children visiting the home. Has a mania for housework, never rests. Moody, but quiet and well behaved when alone with her aunt.'

In practice 'can be left for an hour or so' was often used as a definition when the category 'can be left all day' and that of 'can be left for a few minutes' were both inappropriate. This latter category meant that the mother was very tied, as is suggested by the notes on a severely subnormal boy of seventeen: 'He is an excitable epileptic and should not be left alone for long periods.' Sometimes there would be a fairly specific indication that the subnormal could not be left for long, as in the quotation above. More often what the file had to say about the subnormal's temperament and behaviour was the main evidence, for instance: 'Very difficult to manage at times, sullen and moody.' Another example shows how the balance of evidence led to this coding. The boy was severely subnormal from a very poor home: 'He is most disobedient and violent in the home. Is destructive and makes his mother's life a misery.' The mental welfare officer wrote a little later: 'He is now seven years of age. He is a small, robust, aggressive subnormal who is relatively well controlled at the training centre.'

This last example comes very close to the last category of 'constant supervision'. While behaviour often figures large in the subnormal needing constant supervision, sheer physical incapacity can make the same demand. The mental welfare officer reported of one twenty-one-year-old severely subnormal girl: 'according to the mother she is unruly, disobedient, aggressive and destructive. She kicks and bites and tears her clothes, will not wash herself, refuses to go to bed before 2 a.m. etc.' Another case of a mildly subnormal boy is quite specific: 'He responds very well but needs constant supervision and training.'

The other main group that needed constant supervision was the very severely handicapped, for instance the child of three of whom it was written: 'She is doubly incontinent, blind, spastic . . . and quite unable to do anything for herself.'

Having defined what is meant by the various categories, it is now possible to consider the figures themselves. Table 9.7 sets out the

Table 9.7   Supervision needed—children

	MSN Home No.	Institution No.	SSN Home No.	%	Institution No.	%
Left all day	2	1	1	0·5	0	0
Left one hour	5	2	34	15·2	2	2·2
Left few minutes	8	3	117	52·5	16	17·2
Constant super-vision	1	6	71	31·8	75	80·6
Sub-total	16	12	223	100·0	93	100·0
Not known	0	1	1		2	
Total	16	13	224		95	

χ^2 on rows 1, 2 and 3 against row 4 (SSN) = 62·897   p = 0·001

figures for the children. The dividing line between the home group and the hospital group comes between those who can be left for a few minutes and those who need constant supervision. This is true of both the mildly and the severely subnormal, but as there are so few mildly subnormal, the discussion will concentrate on the severely subnormal. The difference is clearly significant. More who needed constant supervision were in hospital than were at home: seventy-one at home and seventy-five in hospital. The proportion of severely subnormal children in hospital needing constant supervision was very high, just over four-fifths. This indicates the way the amount of supervision the subnormal needs draws together the consequences of all the other aspects of the subnormal's capacities and temperament.

The position is more complex when the adults are considered. The figures can be seen in table 9.8. The adults needed two additional categories—those who were either partly or wholly responsible for the household. Very nearly a quarter of the mildly subnormal at home were completely responsible for the household, the vast majority being those who were married or were living by themselves. A further eighth were partly responsible for the household, and would be those living with various relatives and taking a real part in the running of the household. This might mean that they were living with their father, as nineteen of them were, or that they took some of the responsibility for the household off the shoulders of a married sister, for instance. Naturally there were very few cases, only eight, where people in either of these categories were in an institution, but 270 of the mildly subnormal at home, that is over one-third, were at least partly in charge of the household. Most of the remainder of the mildly subnormal at home, slightly over half, could be left all day. Much of what has been written has had to concentrate on the subnormals' disabilities rather than their abilities, and so it is worth drawing attention to the fact that no less than 665 out of the 723 mildly subnormal at home for whom there was information on this question could be left all day. This is 92 per cent. Furthermore, a quarter of the total were completely in charge of the household. The difference between both the mildly subnormal hospital groups and those at home comes where the subnormal could only be left for an hour or so. However, more of the younger institution group needed quite close supervision. Nineteen could only be left for a few minutes or needed constant supervision. Fifteen of these were admitted as a result of a behaviour problem. None of the older institution group

Table 9.8 Supervision needed—adults

	MSN Home No.	%	YIG No.	%	OIG No.	%	SSN Home No.	%	YIG No.	%	OIG No.	%
Completely responsible	178	24·6	1	1·5	0	0	23	5·1	0	0	0	0
Partly responsible	92	12·7	4	6·0	3	8·1	16	3·6	0	0	11	18·0
Left all day	395	54·6	19	28·4	15	40·5	179	39·9	7	10·8	28	45·9
Left one hour	48	6·6	24	35·8	12	32·4	150	33·5	14	21·5	28	45·9
Left few minutes	8	1·1	15	22·4	7	18·9	55	12·3	25	38·5	20	32·8
Constant supervision	2	0·3	4	6·0	0	0	25	5·6	19	29·2	2	3·3
Sub-total	723	99·9	67	100·1	37	99·9	448	100·0	65	100·0	61	100·0
Not known	7		3		0		2		2		0	
Total	730		70		37		450		67		61	

χ^2 on Home against OIG on rows 1, 2 and 3 against rows 4, 5 and 6 (MSN) = 72·578   p = 0·001
χ^2 on Home against YIG on rows 1, 2 and 3 against rows 4, 5 and 6 (MSN) = 173·423   p = 0·001
χ^2 on Home against OIG on rows 1, 2 and 3 against rows 4, 5 and 6 (SSN) = 20·350   p = 0·001
χ^2 on Home against YIG on rows 1, 2, 3 and 4 against rows 5 and 6 (SSN) = 76·915   p = 0·001

needed constant supervision and a smaller proportion than that of the younger institution group could only be left for a few minutes.

The same pattern can be seen more clearly among the severely subnormal adults. Nearly half of those at home could be left all day and a few were even in charge of the household. This was a far higher proportion than that of either of the institution groups. But the level at which there was a greater proportion in hospital was not the same in both the institution groups. Among the younger institution group the proportion in hospital was not greater until the subnormal could only be left for a few minutes. Among the older institution group even if the subnormal could be left for an hour or so there was still a decisively greater proportion in hospital than at home.

This is not the complete picture. The proportion of the older institution group who needed constant supervision was, not significantly but very interestingly, lower than the proportion at home. This points to two complementary developments. First, severely subnormal children who need constant supervision tend to go to hospital; young, severely subnormal adults who can only be left for a few minutes tend to go to hospital; older adults who can only be left for an hour or so tend to have to go into hospital when their parents die, as relatives tend not to take them on. This produces the complementary effect that by the time severely subnormal adults reach middle age, very few who need constant supervision are at home and the numbers at home who can only be left for a few minutes have been reduced considerably. The severely subnormal show clearly the pattern which was there, but not so obvious, in the case of the mildly subnormal.

The amount of supervision that the subnormal needed is the best indication available of the extent to which the person in charge of him was tied. It is worth noting that among the mildly subnormal younger institution group there was a greater proportion in hospital when the subnormal could be left for an hour or so, but for the severely subnormal younger institution group it was not until the subnormal could only be left for a few minutes that the proportion was greater. This may be because it is more tolerable to accept severe restriction on one's freedom of action for someone who is obviously retarded than for someone whose handicap is less obvious.

The reason why there is an identical distinction between the severely subnormal younger and older institution groups need not be so speculative. The extent to which a relative will be prepared to accept restriction on her freedom of action is bound, on the whole, to be less than that which the subnormal's mother would accept. This is shown very clearly in the difference between the two adult severely subnormal institution groups.

The amount of supervision that the subnormal needed is not an independent variable. It depends on many aspects of the subnormal's condition and behaviour. It is a useful measure of the impact the subnormal's presence had on his household and the pressure to which the mother was subject. The finding that the greater the impact on the household and the heavier the pressure on the mother, the more likely the subnormal was to be in hospital is hardly astonishing. One of the most revealing aspects of the figures is the different points at which the various groups were affected. The large number of mildly subnormal who were in charge of their household is a useful reminder of the abilities of many subnormals; the number of subnormals who needed a great deal of supervision and yet were still at home is a useful reminder of the abilities of many parents.

The relative importance of the different factors

This chapter has considered the subnormals' physical abilities or disabilities, two basic social skills (dressing and feeding), their behaviour and the amount of supervision they needed. Very little attempt has been made so far to assess the relative importance of the various factors. The only criterion that has been used is whether the difference between the home and the hospital groups is statistically significant in respect of each factor. An attempt must be made to establish which factors are the most important.

This has been done by using either the phi test or the coefficient of contingency. This measure appears under 'Relative strength of association with admission' in table 9.9, which deals with the mildly subnormal, and table A10, which deals with the severely subnormal and can be found in appendix A. The measure comes between 0 and 1. A rating of 0·0000 would mean that there was no association at all with admission to hospital and the closer the rating gets to 1·0000 the stronger the association with admission to hospital. The technical aspects of the construction of this scale are discussed in appendix C. It is the placing of the various factors relative to one another which is of prime importance. The numbers given are the numbers at home and in hospital with that characteristic. For example, in table 9.9(a) there are fourteen with a moderate or severe behaviour problem at home and thirty-two in hospital in the younger institution group. Both the younger and the older institution groups are compared with the same one 'Home' group, which can be seen if the figures for 'Supervision needed' are compared. The same is true for table 9.9(b).

Table 9.9 *Relative strength of association with admission to hospital of physical characteristics and behaviour: mildly subnormal adults*

(a) *Younger institution group*

Strength of association with admission	Factor	Level at which associated with admission	Number	
			Home	Institution
0·5915	Behaviour at home	Moderate or severe problem	14	32
0·4685	Supervision needed	An hour or so, a few minutes or constant supervision	58	43
0·3496	Behaviour in locality	Moderate or severe problem	18	17
0·2924	Subnormal mentally ill	Clear evidence	20	17
Total in group			730	70

(b) *Older institution group*

Strength of association with admission	Factor	Level at which associated with admission	Number	
			Home	Institution
0·3090	Supervision needed	An hour or so, few minutes or constant supervision	58	19
Total in group			730	37

Table 9.9 shows the factors in order of importance for the mildly subnormal. Only those factors which were definitely significant statistically have been included. It can be seen that there is a very marked difference between the younger and the older institution groups. The younger institution group is dominated completely by behaviour. 'Supervision needed' and 'subnormal mentally ill' owe

their position on the list very largely to their association with behaviour. It was the behaviour of the younger hospital group which was all important.

By comparison there was only one factor definitely associated with the admission to hospital of the older institution group, the numbers in which were small: this was the amount of supervision they needed, and it was the only factor of any real importance.

Here is further evidence that these two groups are different and the only factor of substance affecting the admission of persons of the older hospital group was the death or illness of a parent. The amount of supervision they needed indicates the importance of this factor in whether a relative would take them on after their mother's death or not.

Among the few mildly subnormal children it was again behaviour which was the factor most strongly associated with admission. In their case, behaviour in the locality was more strongly associated with admission than was behaviour at home.

The pattern for the severely subnormal is more complex. It is set out in table A10. The table is divided into three parts. The left-hand section deals with severely subnormal children, the central section with the younger institution group (i.e. excluding those in an institution who were admitted because of the death or illness of a parent) and the right-hand section with the older institution group. The measure of the strength of association with admission is the same that was applied to the mildly subnormal.

Among the children and in the younger institution group, behaviour was clearly the most important factor, but the patterns within the different groups, especially the older institution group, are different in important ways.

The children had a greater number of physical disabilities which were associated with admission, and right down to the seventh factor, epilepsy, there was a greater number of cases with that characteristic in hospital than there was at home. There were two physical disabilities which were statistically significant among the children but not among the adults—that of defective walking and that of blindness. There is also the distinction, noted in the course of the chapter, that in the case of incontinence and feeding and dressing disabilities, a greater proportion of the children was in hospital only when the disability was total, but among the adults the difference was generally significant when the disability was only partial. However, with epilepsy the reverse was true. One could summarize the list of factors affecting the children by saying that, while behaviour was the most important factor, physical disabilities appeared to be more important than was the case with either of the adult groups. The severely subnormal children who were admitted to hospital form a clearly definable group, most of which had severe handicaps. Only nine out of ninety-five had none of the handicaps at the level shown in table A10. Those children who were not severely disabled physically almost invariably presented problems of behaviour.

The children at home were much less disabled. Just over two-fifths of them (ninety-eight out of 224) had none of the handicaps at the level shown in table A10, and also more of the children at home had only one disability (forty-four = 20 per cent) compared with the children in hospital (five = 5 per cent). The main difference is that those at home had far fewer behaviour problems.

Although many of the severely disabled children were in hospital, it is striking how many very seriously disabled children were still at home. If one excludes all cases where there was a behaviour problem, there were:

Two children in hospital with eight disabilities, and one at home.
Two children in hospital with seven disabilities, and five at home.
Six children in hospital with six disabilities, and fifteen at home.
Eight children in hospital with five disabilities, and eight at home.

The importance of the difference between the younger and the older institution groups has been referred to throughout this chapter. The difference between these two groups is made obvious in this table. Four of the five most important factors for the younger institution group—behaviour at home, behaviour in the locality, the subnormal being mentally ill, and epilepsy—have all disappeared from the older institution group's list. On these factors there was no significant difference between the home group and the older institution group. The second most important factor for the younger institution group, the amount of supervision the subnormal needed, is the second least important for the older institution group. Furthermore, even those factors in the older group that were associated with admission to hospital were not very strongly associated. There was a majority at home in every instance. The younger adults in hospital had many more behaviour problems and were more disabled generally than was the older institution group. Only fifteen out of the sixty-seven (22 per cent) in the younger institution group, but twenty-three of the sixty-one (30 per cent) in the older institution group, had none of the disabilities shown for either of the adult groups in table A10.

Naturally the adults at home were far less seriously disabled on the whole. Over two-thirds of them (68 per cent) had none of the disabilities listed for adults in table A10, and a further thirty-seven had only a minor disability, such as needing some help with dressing, a lesser degree of incontinence or needing some supervision.

Table A10 shows quite a firm pattern for admission, which fits in with figure 12 (see p. 367). This diagram showed how the precipitating factors were related to age on admission to hospital. Sheer physical disability was most marked among the children. The precipitating factor in many of the cases of severe physical handicap will have been a nursing problem. Quite soon, probably about the age of seven, behaviour takes over as the main reason for admission and remains the dominant one up to the age of about thirty, as can be seen in the younger institution group. A connected but separable group are those in adverse social circumstances of some sort. Where such circumstances lead to admission, they do so quite early on. Most of those who remain at home until they are thirty will only be admitted because of the death or illness of the person looking after them. Those persons in this group, who are admitted to hospital when they are older, tend to have the sort of disabilities which make them either too much of a burden for their aged parents, or too much for their relatives to take on. It makes good sense that the three factors which show up as being the most important in this older institution group are all to do with basic unavoidable functions—continence, feeding and dressing—and it is understandable that relatives should be unwilling to take on an adult of perhaps forty who needs substantial help of this nature. It is worth noticing that where there were adults with multiple disabilities at home, it was these three plus needing supervision which combined most frequently. Such people are clearly likely to need residential care when their parents die or become too old or ill to look after them.

Each of the sections in table A10 shows which factors were important for people once they had reached that age group. This means that while serious difficulty in walking was not associated with admission among the adults, nevertheless all those adults who were seriously handicapped in walking had remained at home during their childhood, during which period the disability was associated with hospital admission. This applies to all those physical disabilities which were strongly associated with admission among the children. All those families whose adult subnormal had any of these disabilities and was still at home had coped with him at home during the period when these disabilities increased the chances of his having to go into hospital. The three sections of the table indicate which factors are important at different stages of the subnormal's life. At the same time any factor which was important for a younger group has a certain relevance for those in the older group or groups.

These findings are broadly consistent with what was discovered in the PEP follow-up study (Moncrieff, 1966, pp. 18–20). Thirty-seven out of the original 150 severely subnormal people at home visited by Dr Grad had been admitted to hospital by the time of the follow-up study about eight years later. When the home circumstances recorded by Dr Grad of those still at home were compared with those who had been admitted to hospital, it was found that bad health in the subnormal, severe incontinence, limited locomotion in movement, no speech, and temper tantrums were associated with admission. These thirty-seven are best compared with the children and younger institution group. The disagreement about the importance of the subnormal's health may be due to the inaccuracy of the files. All the other factors were associated with admission in the case of the children, and incontinence and behaviour were associated with the admission of those in the younger institution group.

The disabilities used as a basis for deciding whom to visit

The details recorded about the subnormal's disabilities and behaviour appeared to be one of the most reliable pieces of information in the file. It is certainly true that the number of cases where there was no information about these aspects was generally low, much lower than in many of the other questions. It was this, plus the very clear association with admission to hospital of many of the factors that have been discussed in this chapter, which led to the decision to use these factors as the basis for deciding whom to visit. It was decided for a variety of reasons, which are discussed later on, to limit the visits to severely subnormal adults and to visit all those who had two or more disabilities. For this purpose the definition of these disabilities was slightly more rigorous than the level shown in table A10 —only complete inability to dress or feed was taken, and only semi-

or total incontinence. The only exception to the rule of visiting those with two or more disabilities was that those who needed constant supervision, but for whom none of the other disabilities was recorded, were also selected.

It was felt that the combination of comparative reliability of data, comparatively strong association with admission to hospital and undeniable relevance to the care of the subnormal made these factors the best ones to take. There were two other possibilities. These were family relationships and help from family or friends, but they were rejected on the grounds of being less reliable and having too high a proportion of unknowns. In two or three cases these criteria were misleading but, taken as a whole, they appear to have been sound and to have produced a list of families whom it was valuable to visit.

10 The help and services the subnormals and their families received

Howard was born a few years after the First World War. He was a mongol. He was excluded from school at the age of seven. In 1932 his parents refused the offer of a place in the Royal Albert Institution at Lancaster. At that time, in Sheffield, admission to some such institution was the only way that mentally defective children, who had been excluded from school, could receive any systematic training. In 1933 Howard's father wrote to the Mental Deficiency Committee:

> Howard is our only child and has, as you are well aware, a good home and we do not want to part with him, yet it seems that unless we let him go altogether there is no chance of him being taught anything which, to say the least, is very unfair and hard. If he could go, shall we say, to Sharrow Lane [centre for the physically handicapped] we would take and fetch him.

The first local authority occupation centre in Sheffield was opened in 1938. This was too late for Howard. He was admitted to hospital in 1939, and in 1968 he was still there. His mother died about the beginning of the war. The last entry in the file reads:

> Grandmother now aged eighty-three states that she has not seen her son (Howard's father) for years. He remarried. Neither she nor the aunts ever visit the patient. They have not time and the grandmother is crippled with rheumatism. The maternal relatives used to visit but it now appears that there is no-one to take any interest whatever in the patient.

What difference attendance at a training centre would have made to Howard is impossible to say, but there can be no doubt about the difference that attendance made to the mother of Frances. She wrote the following letter to Dr Holt, who carried out a survey of subnormal children in Sheffield (see p. 387):

> Dear Doctor,
>   I was so pleased to hear from you. It is nice to think someone is interested in our problems but since I saw you I am

quite a new woman: in fact my problems are now shared by half for Frances goes to Craddock Road Day Nursery from 9.30 to 3.30 five days a week. I can now almost live a normal life for I can do a normal hour's shopping, and for a year I have been working at my old trade. Lucky for me I learned a trade. The younger generation won't learn one, so my employer welcomes me to do any hours I want. Am I happy to be working with young people again! It does help my morale. Not only that but we have more money. Remember I told you my husband gave up all his pleasures so we could buy an old car to take Frances out; well now this very week we have a capital of £100 towards a better one next year, life has seemed worth living this last year. It is almost too good to be true. My health seems better too, to get that break I have never had for eight years. Oh, about John doctor, I wonder if you know where I can get in touch with some home outside Sheffield where the hospital send backward children for two weeks during the summer so my husband and I can spend a holiday with John alone because I know he often feels neglected and it would be heaven for him to get all the attention.

The two cases are not strictly comparable because Howard needed an ordinary training centre, whereas Frances attended a day nursery that was the forerunner of the special care unit for very severely disabled children. The letter from Frances's mother raises many important points. She shows clearly the difference that attendance at a training centre or special care unit can make to the life of the family. This chapter considers the education or training that the subnormals did or did not receive, what they did after school leaving age, and some of the other help and assistance they received.

Education

On 1 April 1971 responsibility for the education of severely subnormal children passed from the Department of Health and Social Security and the local health authority, to the Department of Education and Science and the local education authority. This meant that parents would no longer receive a letter telling them that their child was ineducable. However, in the period covered by the survey, severely subnormal children were generally excluded from the education system. Table 10.1 shows where the children received their 'education'. The special care unit for very severely disabled children was not opened until 1963. Before that, many of the severely handicapped children attended a nursery run by the local health authority. Frances, who was mentioned in the introductory section, was one who did so. Some continued to attend it after the special care unit was opened. Those who are down as 'excluded from an ordinary or ESN school' were excluded from school but never admitted to a training centre. If a child was excluded from a school and then was admitted to a junior training centre, he has been shown as being educated at a junior training centre.

Table 10.1   *Education—children*

	MSN Home No.	Institution No.	SSN Home No.	%	Institution No.	%
None	0	2	39	17·4	47	49·5
Junior training centre	13	2	149	66·5	23	24·2
Special care unit or nursery	1	0	30	13·4	18	18·9
Ordinary school or ESN school	1	3	3	1·3	1	1·0
Excluded from ordinary or ESN school	1	6	2	0·9	5	5·3
Other	0	0	1	0·4	1	1·0
Total	16	13	224	99·9	95	99·9

The most striking feature of table 10.1 is that virtually half of the children in hospital received no education, but less than one-fifth of those at home were not receiving any education on 1 September 1968.[1] In fact the contrast is even greater, because many of the thirty-nine at home who were not receiving any education were admitted to the new junior training centre which opened in February 1969. In September 1968, eighteen of the thirty-nine were on the waiting list for a junior training centre place and nine for a place in the special care unit.

There are three reasons which account for the large proportion of those in hospital who received no education. The first is the year in which they were admitted to hospital. It was pointed out at the end of chapter 5 that children in hospital were defined by being under the age of sixteen *at the time they were admitted*. This means that the ninety-five severely subnormal children in hospital were admitted any time between 5 July 1948 and 1 September 1968. Because of this, the proportion who received no education reflects in part the inadequate provision of the past.

The second reason is that a considerable number of the children in hospital were too severely handicapped to attend a junior training centre and places for them before the special care unit was opened were very limited indeed. There was still a shortage of places even after the unit was opened.

The third reason is that thirteen of the forty-seven who received no education were admitted before they were five, and so they never had the chance to receive any education before they were admitted to hospital.

The education of the mildly subnormal adults presents a very different pattern from that of the severely subnormal. The figures can be seen in table 10.2. Over three-quarters of those at home had attended either an ordinary school or an ESN school. The proportion was only slightly lower for those in hospital, and then mostly in the older institution group. The only other numbers of any size were those who were excluded from school. In order to get into this category at all, the child had to attend school for at least six months. If he did not do so, he would be coded as having received no education. If he did attend for at least six months but was excluded from school before he had completed his education and was not found a place in a junior training centre, he was shown as 'excluded from school'. The large numbers of mildly and severely subnormal adults in this category (21 per cent of all the adults) shows how grossly inadequate provision was in the past.

These two categories account for the vast majority of the mildly subnormal. There was no difference of any importance between the home and two institution groups, but it is worth noting that five out of the thirty-seven in the older institution group received no education.

There was a much greater variation in the type (or lack of) education that the severely subnormal received. There was also a clear difference between those at home and the older institution group, but not much difference between the home group and the younger institution group. The big difference was the much higher proportion of the older institution group who received no education. This does raise the question of whether those mothers who were determined to

Table 10.2 Education—adults

	MSN Home No.	%	YIG No.	%	OIG No.	%	SSN Home No.	%	YIG No.	%	OIG No.	%
None	12	1·7	1	1·6	5	14·3	91	20·5	19	28·8	26	45·6
Junior training centre	18	2·6	1	1·6	0	0	93	20·9	10	15·2	5	8·8
Special care unit or nursery	0	0	0	0	0	0	8	1·8	2	3·0	1	1·7
Ordinary school or ESN school	533	75·8	47	73·4	22	62·9	103	23·2	14	21·2	13	22·8
Excluded from ordinary or ESN schools	117	16·6	11	17·2	6	17·1	135	30·4	16	24·2	9	15·8
Other or home teacher or SN institution	23	3·3	4	6·2	2	5·7	14	3·2	5	7·6	3	5·3
Sub-total	703	100·0	64	100·0	35	100·0	444	100·0	66	100·0	57	100·0
Not known	27		6		2		6		1		4	
Total	730		70		37		450		67		61	

go on looking after their subnormal until they were physically unable to do so also tended to be the sort of mothers who would not let go of their children at all, even to attend a training centre. A much simpler explanation is that this reflects the poor provision of training centre places in the past. Very few of the older institution group attended a junior training centre. The number of those who were excluded from an ordinary school or ESN school was also smaller.

It is interesting that between a quarter and a fifth of all groups managed to stay the course at an ESN school. Ten of them (seven at home, three in hospital) even managed to remain at an ordinary school. In addition there is a rather puzzling finding that a considerably higher proportion of those who were excluded from school were at home. In view of the similar proportions of those at home and those in hospital who attended an ordinary or ESN school, this is difficult to explain.

The big difference between those at home and those in hospital is the higher proportion of the older institution group who received no education. This can be explained most plausibly by the inadequate provision of the past. It may be this that explains the larger proportion of those at home who were excluded from school. They would have been able enough to go to a junior centre, but there was not one when they needed it. The distortion produced by this inadequate provision is such that it would be hazardous to deduce anything further from these figures.

The careers of the mildly subnormal after school leaving age

The transition from school to work is not an easy one for many children. For the subnormal it is much more difficult. Tables 10.3(a) and 10.3(b) show how, by what education they received, the mildly subnormal were employed.[1] The total figures for their 'present' employment can be seen in the extreme right-hand column. The percentages show the proportions in each type of employment according to the education they received. The difference between the younger and older institution groups was not marked and so the figures for those in hospital have not been divided.

Very nearly two-thirds of the mildly subnormal adults at home were either in open employment or were housewives. Most of these had been to either an ordinary or an ESN school but some had been excluded from school after attending for a while. Those who attended an ESN school or ordinary school (eighty-one managed at an ordinary school) and then went into a job will have had only a fleeting contact with the Mental Health Service in many cases. Many of them would not be reported under the more selective policy of reporting which has been operating since 1960. Most of this group will be indistinguishable from the general population and be leading perfectly normal lives. The same is true of most of those who were excluded from school.

Out of the total of 471 who were either in open employment or were housewives, 101 were housewives. If the numbers of women who were either housewives or in open employment are added together, they amount to 56 per cent of all the mildly subnormal women at home. This is considerably lower than the proportion of men in open employment (74 per cent). One reason for this difference will be the amount of help the women gave at home. This is discussed a little further on.

A very much smaller proportion of those at home were in sheltered employment or at training centre. Forty-eight were attending a training centre and twenty-nine were in sheltered employment. It was very clear from both the files and the visits what a help the training centres were. Visits to the centres confirmed this impression. The people attending the centres appeared happy and contented and their attendance gave the life of their families a normality and stability which many of them would never have had without such help. The mildly subnormal attending training centre tend to be those on the borderline with severe subnormality.

Table 10.3(a) Present occupation by education: mildly subnormal adults at home

Present occupation	Ordinary school or ESN school		Excluded from ordinary school or ESN school		Education Junior training centre	Nothing	Other and not known	Total present occupation	
	No.	%	No.	%	No.	No.	No.	No.	%
Open employment or housewife	380	73·1	62	53·0	5	3	21	471	65·8
Sheltered employment or senior training centre	39	7·5	16	13·7	11	1	10	77	10·7
Nothing	101	19·4	39	33·3	2	8	18	168	23·5
Sub-total	520	100·0	117	100·0	18	12	49	716	100·0
Not known	13		0		0	0	1	14	
Total education	533		117		18	12	50	730	

Table 10.3(b)   Present occupation by education: mildly subnormal adults in hospital

Present occupation	Ordinary school or ESN school		Excluded from ordinary school or ESN school	Junior training centre	Nothing	Other and and not known	Total occupation	
	No.	%	No.	No.	No.	No.	No.	%
Open employment or housewife	10	14·5	2	0	0	1	13	12·3
Sheltered employment or senior training centre	12	17·4	1	1	0	2	16	15·1
Nothing	47	68·1	13	0	6	11	77	72·6
Sub-total	69	100·0	16	1	6	14	106	100·0
Not known	0		1	0	0	0	1	
Total education	69		17	1	6	14	107	

There were over twice as many mildly subnormal living at home and not going out to any employment as there were attending a training centre or sheltered employment. They make up nearly a quarter of those at home, but among the hospital group they are nearly three-quarters of the total. The numbers of those in hospital who were either in open employment or housewives, or attending a training centre or going to sheltered employment, were small. The figures for those in hospital are dominated by those who were not employed outside the home at all.

Tables 10.3(a) and 10.3(b) show that many of those not employed outside the home had attended either an ESN or ordinary school or been excluded from them. This suggests that many of them were functioning at a fairly efficient level. Why, then, were so many of them staying at home? Table 10.4 shows the extent to which those who were doing nothing outside the home helped in it. The table is divided by sex. It is both natural and obvious that the women were much more help than the men. This does something to explain why more women than men were not employed outside the home. The vast majority of the women at home were helping quite considerably. Rather fewer of the women in hospital were as helpful at home but over half of them were at least 'some help'.

The following examples show how the categories were defined. A statement in the file like 'I gather Jessie helps a good deal domestically' was coded 'some help', but 'Mary helps her mother a lot in the house and can do practically any domestic work' was coded 'considerable help'. Some of the men were also quite handy about the house. One lad who attended a senior training centre 'does quite a lot of chores when at home, washes up, cleans utensils, makes beds and is able to use the hoover around the house'. At the other end of the scale, 'she can only do odd jobs under strict supervision' was coded 'little help'.

Table 10.4   Helpfulness at home of mildly subnormal, by sex, not employed outside the home

| | Home | | Institution | |
	Male	Female	Male	Female
Some or considerable help	27	80	10	23
Slight or no help	10	5	13	13
Not known	28	18	11	7
Total	65	103	34	43

This does a good deal to account for the surprisingly large number whose education suggests a reasonable level of intelligence who were not employed outside the home. This is more relevant for the women than for the men, and is more marked among the women at home than among the women in hospital.

On the face of it, it appears a matter for concern that so many subnormals should have been sitting at home ever since they left school. This must be modified to some extent by the fact that many of them, especially the women, were a considerable help at home. Nevertheless, doubts remain about whether in many cases this was really in the subnormal's best interests. In a few cases they were treated as cheap labour. On a more positive note, the way in which some subnormals blossomed when they started attending a training centre makes it seem very likely that a good many of those staying at home would benefit considerably from attending a centre or possibly going out to work.

There is a clear association between admission to hospital and the subnormal not attending anything outside the home. What this association means is hard to say, but, even when account has been taken of the amount that many subnormals help in the home, it appears that having no employment outside the home does have some bearing on admission to hospital. No less than thirty out of the thirty-seven in the older institution group, who were admitted on the death or illness of a parent, were not employed outside their home. In the younger institution group the proportion was slightly lower, forty-seven out of seventy.

The careers of the severely subnormal after school leaving age

The use of the word 'career' may have seemed slightly inappropriate when applied to the mildly subnormal: it is in many ways even more inappropriate when applied to the severely subnormal. It is used deliberately, for why should the subnormal not have the aim and purpose in life which is indicated by the word career? One person in table 10.5 did manage a career which deserves the name. This was Arthur, who was mentioned in the Introduction. He retired after fifty years' service in a steel works.

Tables 10.5(a) and 10.5(b) follow the same pattern as the tables for the mildly subnormal.[1] The totals for the subnormals' present occupation are given in the extreme right-hand column. Those in hospital have not been divided into the younger and older groups, as the proportions in each category were very similar.

The number who were either in open employment or were housewives was naturally much lower than among the mildly subnormal but, nevertheless, one-fifth of those at home came into this category. Thirteen women were housewives and another twenty-three women were doing an ordinary job. In all, 16 per cent of the women at home were either housewives or in open employment. The proportion of men in open employment was rather greater (24 per cent). As in the case of the mildly subnormal, the same factor was operative here; the women tended to be more useful in the home. Most of the men were in labouring jobs and most of the women in a cleaning job or a repetitive manual job, such as buffing cutlery. Predictably enough, most of those in this category came from the top end of the educational scale. Only four of those in an institution had been in open employment.

The senior training centres catered for more of the severely subnormal than of the mildly subnormal. The difference that attendance at a training centre makes to the subnormals and their families has been mentioned in the last section. The activities of the training centres extend beyond working hours, including visits to swimming baths in the evenings, hiking and fishing trips at the weekends and holiday camps in the summer. Both in the files and during the visits

Table 10.5(a) Present occupation by education: severely subnormal adults at home

Present occupation	Ordinary school or ESN school		Excluded from ordinary school or ESN school		Junior training centre		Special care unit or nursery	Nothing		Other or not known	Total attends now	
	No.	%	No.	%	No.	%	No.	No.	%	No.	No.	%
Open employment or housewife	47*	46·1	34	25·8	7	7·6	0	1	1·1	1	90	20·3
Sheltered employment or senior training centre	18	17·6	33	25·0	68	73·9	2	14	15·4	6	141	31·8
Nothing	37	36·3	65	49·2	17	18·5	6	76	83·5	12	213	48·0
Sub-total	102	100·0	132	100·0	92	100·0	8	91	100·0	19	444	100·1
Not known	2		3		1		0	0		0	6	
Not known as a % of total		1·9		2·2								1·3
Total	104		135		93		8	91		19	450	

* Including one retired from steady open employment

Table 10.5(b) Present occupation by education: severely subnormal adults in hospital

Present occupation	Ordinary school or ESN school	Excluded from ordinary school or ESN school	Junior training centre	Education Special care unit or nursery	Nothing		Other or not known	Total attends now	
	No.	No.	No.	No.	No.	%	No.	No.	%
Open employment or housewife	2	2	0	0	0	0·0	0	4	3·2
Sheltered employment or senior training centre	5	3	12	1	4	9·1	5	30	24·0
Nothing	20	19	3	1	40	90·9	8	91	72·8
Sub-total	27	24	15	2	44	100·0	13	125	100·0
Not known	0	1	0	1*	0		1	3	
Not known as a % of total									2·3
Total education	27	25	15	3	44		14	128	

* Admitted to hospital from special care unit when aged sixteen

there were references to the unpopularity of the holidays when the subnormals were not able to go to the training centre. A slightly larger proportion of those at home attended training centre but the difference was not very great.

A hundred and forty-one of those at home were either in sheltered employment or attended a training centre. In only ten out of the 141 cases were the subnormals in sheltered employment. In all the other cases they were attending a training centre. It can be seen that most of those at the senior training centre had graduated from the junior training centre. This is where most of them stay. A very few go on to open employment. There were just four men who had gone to a junior training centre, then to the senior training centre and finally into open employment. The other three in open employment who had attended a junior training centre appear to have gone straight into a job.

The startling figures are those where the subnormal was attending nothing outside the home. This accounted for nearly half those at home and nearly three-quarters of those in hospital. It can be seen from tables 10.5(a) and 10.5(b) that a fair proportion of these people had spent at least some time at an ordinary school or ESN school, but almost as many received no education at all.

The number of those who had received at least some education is reflected in the number of people not employed outside the home who were a considerable help in it. The figures are given in table 10.6. Examples to illustrate the different categories have been given in the previous section.

Table 10.6 Helpfulness at home of severely subnormal not employed outside the home

| | Home | | Institution | |
	Male	Female	Male	Female
Some and considerable	27	72	12	16
Slight or no help	27	47	26	24
Not known	30	10	9	4
Total	84	129	47	44

There were considerably more women among those at home, and they tended quite naturally to be much more useful in the home than did the men. This is reflected in the lower number of women than men who were in open employment. Thirty-five of the women at home were a 'considerable' help. It is possible that some of these could have managed an ordinary job. It is interesting that there was no such predominance of women in the hospital group, and the women were not much more helpful than the men. Fifty of those in hospital were neither employed outside the home nor much help in it. The same was true of seventy-four of those at home. It is these rather large numbers of people who appear to be sitting at home doing very little that pose the biggest question. The two outstanding figures in table 10.5 which epitomize this question are those who were not employed at all outside the home and who also had received no education.

There were seventy-six at home in this position. If their past employment is considered we find that:

1 had previously been in open employment
2 had previously been in sporadic open employment
5 had previously attended a senior training centre
10 had previously attended a senior training centre sporadically
58 had previously done nothing.

There were forty in hospital who had been in this position before they were admitted:

2 had previously attended a senior training centre sporadically
38 had previously done nothing.

This means that there were fifty-eight people at home and thirty-eight in hospital who had received no education and were not employed outside the home and never had been. Out of the fifty-eight at home who had done nothing outside the home in the past, only fifteen gave any appreciable help, and thirty-six were little or no help. It is unlikely that the seven cases the extent of whose help was not known helped very much. Out of the thirty-eight in hospital who were in the same position when they were admitted, only eight gave much help and twenty-six were little or no help. In four cases the amount they helped was not known.

These subnormals who received so little help with their education, training and occupation are not the only ones that deserve examination. For instance, six out of the eight who had been either to a nursery or the special care unit when they were children were also sitting at home doing nothing. However, the group that has been discussed does act as a focus for the fact of the non-career of many of the severely subnormal.

It is not as if these families were without problems. Out of the thirty-six at home who were not employed outside the home and never had been in the past, who had received no education and were little or no help in the home, only eleven had none of the major disabilities discussed in the last chapter and fourteen were multiply handicapped with at least two of these disabilities. In the case of the twenty-six in hospital who were in a similar position, only three had none of the major disabilities and nineteen had at least two.

This curious situation, where severely handicapped people were among those who had received least help, underlines a serious gap in the present provision. The very seriously disabled children were catered for by the special care unit, but once they were sixteen they had to leave and there was no provision for these seriously handicapped adults apart from a hospital bed. The only exceptions to this were a few cases where arrangements were made for day care in hospital one or two days a week. Fortunately, the Sheffield Development Project should make good this serious gap in provision in the foreseeable future. This project is discussed in the final chapter.

The extent to which the severely subnormal did or did not attend a training centre depended on his disabilities, provision of training centre places in the past, how much he, or, more likely, she, was able to help in the home, and how much that help was needed. While in one case a reasonably high level of competence might enable a subnormal to attend a training centre, the different home circumstances of a person of similar abilities might mean that she helped at home instead.

The effect of this is that while there is a definite association between lack of employment outside the home and admission to hospital (and that association is equally strong for both the younger and older institution groups), it is not one of the most important factors. However, provision for adults does remain seriously inadequate, though the Sheffield Development Project does plan substantial improvements. In all fairness, it should be pointed out that the figures for the adults reflect the inadequate provision of the past. The number of severely subnormal children who receive no education is now very small indeed. But the figures for the adults do underline the importance of having a place available at the right time, because once a severely subnormal adult has become set in his ways, the offer of a place at a training centre later on is sometimes too late.

Short-term care

Short-term care is an arrangement whereby the subnormal goes into a hospital or hostel for any period between a week and a month while his parents either go on holiday or have a spell at home by themselves. Many parents find this break of immense value. Not all short-term care was successful, but, in general, it was, and there was mention on several occasions of subnormals looking forward to their 'holiday', by which they meant their period of short-term care. A mental welfare officer recorded that one mother, a widow, said of short-term care that: 'she was only really able to cope for the rest of the year by this very necessary break which she looked forward to annually'.

Short-term care for children who were not very severely handicapped was given most often in a special unit attached to a junior training centre. It had eight beds but at holiday times more were fitted in. For adults, a very few were admitted to the new local authority hostel, but for most of them it had to be a subnormality hospital. There was always considerable pressure on beds for short-term care during holiday periods and the mental welfare service were not always able to arrange a bed when the parents wanted it. Occasionally they were unable to arrange a bed at all. Generally this would be where the parents were only able to accept a limited range of dates or gave short notice.

The figures for short-term care need to be treated with some reserve. It is not certain that every time the subnormal went into short-term care the fact was entered in the file. Those in hospital received more short-term care than did those at home. As those in hospital were more disabled, their parents needed relief more urgently. The proportion that had received short-term care reflects how disabled the different groups were. Virtually half the severely subnormal children in hospital, 31 per cent of the severely subnormal adults in hospital, but only 17 per cent of the mildly subnormal adults in hospital, had received short-term care. The proportions were less, but the order was the same for those at home. Thirty-one per cent of the severely subnormal children at home, 14 per cent of the severely subnormal adults at home, but only 3 per cent of the mildly subnormal adults at home, had received short-term care.

Many of those at home did not need short-term care, but the files gave the impression of, and the visits confirmed, the need for readily available short-term care which was acceptable to the parents. A fair number of the parents did not want their child to go into a sub-normality hospital for short-term care. In view of the justified public concern about many of the subnormality hospitals, this is not sur-prising. In addition, the pressure on short-term beds is such that application for one has to be made months in advance. It is difficult to find a short-term bed at short notice to help cope with a crisis.

The frequency with which short-term care was received varied considerably. From time to time it would be a single occasion to deal with a crisis. More often it would be an annual event. Interestingly, it was the severely subnormal at home, both children and adults, who contained the largest proportion of those who had received short-term care at least three times. One extreme example was a very severely handicapped boy who received two spells of short-term care a year for five years until he was admitted at the age of ten. Without this help he would have had to be admitted much earlier. The files made it clear that the provision of regular, adequate and acceptable short-term care helped some families enormously. The visits under-lined its importance and it is discussed further in connection with the visits.

Support from social workers

The middle of the period covered by the survey was marked by the passing of the 1959 Mental Health Act, which came into force in November 1960. This had a considerable effect on social work in the Mental Health Service, comparable with the upheaval following the setting up of the mental health departments of local authorities in 1948. One result of this has been noted already, namely the steep reduction in the number of ESN school-leavers who were reported to the Mental Health Service. Another aspect which affected the way the social workers operated was the removal of the requirement that the mentally defective should be visited regularly unless they had been discharged from the register. As a result of the 1959 Act, both the register was abolished and the requirement to visit.

On balance, this more flexible and informal approach was an improvement. There were cases where visiting was quite obviously unnecessary and bitterly resented. In one distressing case the sub-normal's wife had no idea her husband was considered subnormal until she saw a postcard from the Mental Health Service suggesting that he be examined with a view to removal from the register. This played at least a part in the subsequent break-up of the marriage.

Before 1960 the files gave the impression that because visiting was officially required in certain cases, where there was no such obligation, informal visiting was carried out only rarely. This was in spite of encouragement from the Board of Control to carry on friendly visiting. The contrast between the attitudes of the two regimes was shown by two quotations. One of the 'old school' wrote: 'I pointed out that we were under no obligation to visit Jennifer and sort out her problems, as she had been discharged.' In another case a trained social worker wrote: 'I said that although Mavis had been discharged we were only to glad to give any help we could.' The old requirement to visit affected both parties. Not only did the inspectors tend not to visit when they did not have to, but also the fact of having to accept compulsory visits made the clients unwilling to accept voluntary ones.

This change in the pattern of visiting was reflected in the number of current and non-current cases. A non-current case was defined as one where there had been no contact for the previous twenty months, that is from 1 January 1967 to 1 September 1968. The practice of the mental health department was to go through the files at intervals, as a result of which some cases would be classified as non-current. Some of the cases shown as current may have been classified as non-current between 1 January 1967 and 1 September 1968. It is certain that many cases treated as non-current on the basis of the date of the last contact had not been specifically classified as such by the Mental Health Service. The yardstick used here is simply the date of the last visit.

Virtually all the children had been visited or had had contact with the Mental Health Service in the previous twenty months. The discussion therefore concentrates on the adults. In the case of both children and adults, if they were attending a training centre this was counted as contact with the Mental Health Service. The number of current and non-current adult cases is shown in table 10.7.

Table 10.7   Number of current and non-current cases among mildly subnormal and severely subnormal adults at home

	MSN No.	%	SSN No.	%
Current	228	31·2	250	55·6
Non-current	502	68·8	200	44·4
Total	730	100·0	450	100·0

It is no surprise that over two-thirds of the mildly subnormal adults were non-current. The proportion of non-current cases is almost the same as the proportion that were either in open employment or were housewives. It is, however, rather surprising, on the face of it, that over 44 per cent of the severely subnormal adults at home were non-current. Only 20 per cent of all the severely subnormal adults at home were either in open employment or were housewives, and by definition those who were attending training centre were counted as current cases. It would seem that there were about 100 severely subnormal adults at home who were not attending anything outside the home who had not been visited for at least the previous twenty months. Table 10.8 provides a useful commentary on these figures.

Table 10.8   Mean age reported, period of surveillance and age last contact of mildly subnormal and severely subnormal adults at home, by current and non-current cases

		MSN		SSN	
		Current	Non-current	Current	Non-current
Mean age		18·0	16·1	10·3	12·4
reported	SD	8·35 SD	3·83 SD	5·78 SD	4·05
Mean period of		22·4	14·0	21·0	16·7
surveillance	SD	11·85 SD	8·96 SD	11·37 SD	9·76
Mean age last		40·5	30·1	31·3	29·1
contact	SD	15·35 SD	9·81 SD	13·50 SD	9·79

SD = Standard deviation

This table shows that the severely subnormal adults who were still current cases were reported earlier than the non-current. The greater age at which the non-current cases tended to be reported would be the effect of a number of people on the borderline with mild subnormality who were at ESN school and were not reported until they left school. Such people are likely to be quite competent socially and in all likelihood the majority of them had been left alone quite rightly. It is difficult to accept, however, that this was true for all the severely subnormal adults who had not been visited for the previous twenty months. This reservation is strengthened by the fact that thirty-three of these adults have at least one major handicap (the major handicaps are those described in chapter 9). Of these:

17 had one handicap
8 had two handicaps

        2 had three handicaps
        4 had six handicaps
        1 had seven handicaps
        1 had eight handicaps.

Seventeen, it is true, only had one handicap. However, even if these seventeen are disregarded, there remain sixteen with at least two major handicaps who had not been visited for at least twenty months. It is possible that some of these people had become the responsibility of another welfare agency, but this was certainly not true of all the cases.

Where it was a matter of physical handicap and the family was coping perfectly well, the mental welfare officer may well have left a card and told the mother to get in touch if help was needed. There is also the perceptive point made by one of the mental welfare officers in the department, who said that where the subnormal was severely physically handicapped and he knew that he had no realistic help to offer to the family, he suspected that he let other more pressing cases prevent him visiting. This ties up closely with the question of adequate facilities, which has been discussed in the previous sections. If there is a glaring gap in provision, like the lack of day care for severely handicapped adults, it is putting the social worker in an impossible position to expect him to give 'casework support' to the family when what it needs desperately is practical help. The subnormal underline the absurdity of expecting the social worker to give the client the help he needs, if adequate facilities are not available.

This is one aspect of the social worker's work with subnormals and their families contending with a serious lack of facilities for the severely handicapped. At the other end of the scale one mental welfare officer began the record of his final visit to an elderly mildly subnormal woman: 'Miss Frith greeted me with the suavity born of thirty-four years manipulation of social workers.' In between there was a whole range of needs. Some needs were best met by the mental welfare officer leaving them alone; others by regular visits and spells of short-term care; for some others there was little the social worker was able to offer. Those who were visited most frequently were the severely subnormal in an institution. This occurred in the period immediately before they were admitted. These visits were connected with either the crisis leading to admission or the administrative arrangements for admission or both.

The people best qualified to comment on the help the social

workers gave are the recipients of the help, and so the matter will be discussed further in the light of the visits.

Other help

Sheffield Society for Mentally Handicapped Children   Sheffield has a thriving club for the mentally handicapped which caters for adults as well as children. In view of this a note was made where the sub-normal or his family had some contact with it. Very few of the files referred to this and an entry was made from the current membership list of the Sheffield Society for Mentally Handicapped Children. On the whole the club caters for the obviously retarded, and so most of the subnormals who are members of the club are severely subnormal. Many of the mildly subnormal would not want to have anything to do with a club which suggested that they were at all subnormal. Consequently, there were comparatively few mildly subnormal in the club, a total of only twenty-six. There were eighty-six severely sub-normal among the members. Thirty-nine were children at home (17 per cent of the total), forty-one were adults at home (9 per cent of the total). The remaining six were in hospital. Though the club only touches a comparatively small proportion of the total, for those that did go, it was an important social function. It was also a valuable meeting ground for parents facing similar problems. Many of those who attended also went to training centre. The club is unable to cater for the severely disabled. The files indicated that there were many other subnormals who might benefit from the informal social con-tacts of the club, if some means could be found of contacting them.

Support from relatives, friends or neighbours   The files did not give much information about this aspect of the subnormal's life. The number of unknowns was very high indeed, well over half the total, but the indications were that many more families where the sub-normal was at home were receiving a fair amount of support. Many more families where the subnormal was in hospital had not been receiving much support except for the mildly subnormal older institution group. This was most marked in the case of the severely subnormal children and the severely subnormal younger institution group. All this establishes is that there is an association between the amount of support that the family received and admission to hospital. But the direction of the difference is what one would expect and, more important, these figures do something to indicate the quality of life that the families experienced. The support given by friends, relations and neighbours was investigated in more depth in the visits, and this aspect of the care of the mentally handicapped is discussed more fully and with far sounder data in chapter 17.

Conclusions

The types of help that have been discussed in this chapter have been concerned with the ordinary routine of living. Going to school or going to a training centre became part of the family's routine. If the subnormal does not go to school or does not go to a training centre or any sort of employment or occupation outside the home, the family's routine will be different and it is very likely that the strains will be greater.

The cases where the family received some support from its relatives or friends were those cases where this help or support was given as a matter of course, as part of the family's daily or weekly routine. The provision or not of short-term care for the subnormal may have decided whether his family was able to go on holiday. The critical importance of provision in the role of the social worker was also pointed out.

The data are not such that hard conclusions can be drawn from lack of certain provision or help and admission to hospital, but here, as in other aspects covered, there is a consistent pattern. Where there was a lack of the sort of care and support which would enhance the life of the family, there was an association with admission to hospital. Quite apart from this association there is the question of the quality of life that these subnormals and their families enjoy and the part that the provision of certain basic facilities can play in improving it. There could hardly be a better illustration of this than the letter from Frances's mother, which was quoted at the beginning of this chapter.

11   Findings from the files – some conclusions

The pattern of admission to hospital

When the overall pattern of factors associated with hospital admission is considered, certain broad features stand out.

Among the mildly subnormal, leaving aside the small number of mildly subnormal children, there was a definite pattern of factors, mostly connected with behaviour and management, which marked off the younger from the older institution group and those at home. The families of the younger institution group were also distinguishable in some ways, for instance they were more likely to have unsatisfactory relationships within the family and the standard of housekeeping was more likely to be markedly low.

There is a singular lack of such distinctiveness in the older institution group. We can say that those in the older institution group were not among the most able; most of them were not employed outside the home, and they tended to need a certain amount of supervision. But there were many more of whom this was true who were still at home. The only difference of any substance between those at home and those in the older institution group was that those in an institution had no one else to look after them.

A similar distinction can be made in the case of the severely subnormal. The various factors which have been considered fall into three broad categories: first, the subnormal's behaviour; second, his physical incapacities; and third, his family's level of functioning.

The greatest concentration of problems in these three areas occurs among the children. The subnormal was likely to be admitted when his care subjected the family to considerable stress, by virtue of his behaviour or physical incapacity. Such stress throws a considerable strain on the family and any weakness in the family structure made the subnormal's admission more likely. Three important family factors were the mother being subnormal, unsettled family relationships and poor physical health of the mother. There was a strong indication that lack of outside family support was important as well. Cases where many of these factors were operative were urgent, and

167

they would be admitted almost invariably while the subnormal was a child.

The position with the younger institution group was almost the same as with the children, but to a lesser extent. The same sort of stresses were operative but the most serious cases had been admitted to hospital. The younger institution group shows the effect of various degrees of stress over a period of time. If the family functioning was very inefficient, the family simply did not manage to keep its difficult subnormal child at home until he was sixteen.

The effect of stress and time is made evident again by the older institution group. Very nearly all the subnormals whose behaviour presented problems had been admitted. Families which were not functioning reasonably effectively did not manage as long as this, but the mothers who had managed were getting old and ill and possibly suffering from the effects of caring for the subnormal. When the mothers were unable to care for the subnormals any longer, whether through death or illness, there were two physical factors which militated particularly strongly against a relative taking them on—namely, incontinence or such lack of basic social skills that they needed help with feeding.

Such was the broad pattern of hospital admission over the whole age range of the severely subnormal. The contrast between the younger and older institution groups is clear, as it was with the mildly subnormal. The main difference is that the older severely subnormal institution group was slightly more distinct from the home group on two counts which affected the physical care of those in it. It is worth considering that incontinence and difficulties in feeding can lead to normal old people being admitted to an institution. The sharp contrast between the children and the older institution group shows not only the effect of the death or admission to hospital of the more severely handicapped or disturbed, but also the different needs of these groups and the different provision which is required to meet those needs.

Some general points

The emphasis throughout the book so far has tended to be on reasons for which subnormals were admitted to hospital. The balance will be restored in the second half, which deals entirely with the care of fifty-four severely handicapped adults at home. This will deal only with those who were severely handicapped and so there are some points that arise from the files which can be considered most suitably at this point.

Possibly the most valuable aspect of reading the files was that it was possible to gather some idea of the subnormals' lives as a whole, not just a short snippet concerning a month or two, or a year or two, connected with some crisis. In many cases the contact with the Mental Health Service was short, but from the files as a whole it has been possible to obtain an overall picture of various patterns of 'career' that subnormals with various abilities or disabilities, various advantages or disadvantages can expect. The main exception to this is that once the subnormal was admitted to hospital he was not followed up unless he was discharged subsequently.

The picture that emerged from this varied from the depressing lack of provision and opportunity for the most severely disabled to the considerable number who were doing ordinary jobs or were married and bringing up families well and competently.

A follow-up study of 197 married mental defectives was carried out in Sheffield in 1958–9 by Shaw and Wright (1960). They found that while a rather large proportion of the children was attending an ESN school or had been reported as ineducable (the proportion was seventeen times higher than for the Sheffield school population as a whole), and while twenty-six families could be described as problem families, nevertheless forty families out of ninety (44 per cent) where the man was a defective and thirty-eight families out of eighty-seven (44 per cent) where the woman was a defective seemed to be living reasonably happy and normal lives. As the marriages listed for investigation in this study were only those recorded in the case notes, the actual number of marriages will be considerably higher. The less serious the case, the earlier he or she would be discharged or contact would be dropped, and thus the greater the chance that the marriage would not have been recorded in the case notes. In view of the greater competence of those with whom contact was only brief, it is fair to assume their marriages were on the whole likely to be more successful than those covered in Shaw and Wright's survey. There was a pleasing note on one of the enquiry forms for the survey. In the file the inspector had written about the wife, when she was younger, that she was epileptic, illiterate and of poor mentality. The note read: 'Husband well known to duly authorized officers who say that they were surprised that the wife is mentally defective. She is the mainstay of the family and actually brings her husband to the office when he is in need of treatment. She keeps the family together.'

The key figures which need to be born in mind are that virtually two-thirds of the mildly subnormal adults at home and one-fifth of the severely subnormal adults at home were either in open employment or were housewives.

One aspect, which has had to be left on one side, is what happened to those who had been in a subnormality hospital at some time in the past. The evidence suggests that many of the 124 mildly subnormal and forty-two severely subnormal who had spent some time in a subnormality hospital in the past made a good adjustment when they were discharged. Fifty-one of the mildly subnormal and fourteen of the severely subnormal had been in hospital for at least ten years. One such person was admitted in her early twenties after her mother died and she had created difficulties at home. When she was thirty-seven she was allowed out to do a job on licence from the hospital (this was during the war). She was discharged finally from hospital at the age of forty-eight, and after this went through a period when she was living by herself, unable to work and finding the time hanging heavily on her hands. At the last visit recorded in the file she was sixty-two years old and the mental welfare officer wrote:

> Bridget married seven years ago . . . she introduced me to her
> husband who seemed very sociable. Their flat is well furnished
> and clean. There is a warden who is available of whom Mr
> and Mrs Rogers spoke very highly. Bridget and her husband
> seem to enjoy a very comfortable relationship and there is no
> evidence of any financial hardship.

There were similar cases to this and also cases where the change in the person's behaviour was quite astonishing. One girl was expelled from a residential ESN school at the age of fourteen. The school reported on her:

> She must be recognized as being a danger in any community,
> and will in time have to be segregated in the interests of the
> community.

When she was seventeen she got married, and subsequently had four boys. Despite many rows with her husband, she and he settled down to a considerable extent when they got a house of their own. The final report when she was twenty-six read:

> Philippa has been into the office on two occasions, possibly just
> to let off steam about herself, the kids and her husband. She
> is as coarse as ever but nevertheless is honest and likeable.

There is no evidence that she had been in any trouble with the authorities since then.

One could not be so optimistic about all cases. East India Dock Road is not the most hopeful of discharge addresses for a rather unstable, mildly subnormal young woman.

Cases such as those of Bridget and Philippa, and there were others, show the need to take cognizance of the whole life-time of a person labelled as subnormal. The necessity to do this is underlined by the different characteristics associated with the admission of children, younger adults and the older adults admitted on the death or illness of a parent. This raises large questions about the role of the social worker and the sort of provision that is needed to help subnormals and their families at different stages in life. What has been lacking so far in the discussion is that while it has been possible to show that, for instance, incontinence was associated with admission to hospital for the older severely subnormal adults, it has not been possible to show how the families with an incontinent severely subnormal adult at home managed to cope. The picture is incomplete because there was a total of forty-six incontinent severely subnormal adults admitted to hospital, but there were fifty-three at home. In all the factors associated with the admission to hospital of adults, there were more at home with that characteristic than there were in hospital, with the exception of those presenting a serious behaviour problem or where there was clear evidence that the subnormal was mentally ill.

The extensive analysis of what factors were associated with admission not only decided which families it would be valuable to visit, but also showed aspects of caring for the subnormal at home which needed attention. It is the positive factors of how these families managed to cope and what help they needed in order to cope more easily that are explored in the visits described in Part II.

Part II

The visits

12   Introduction to the visits

When the coding of the files had been completed and the analysis was due to begin, the decision had to be taken about whom to visit. The key issue was which group of those at home would give the clearest insight into what community care means in practice. The general principle was clear. They should be a group whom one might have expected to be in hospital. But the answer needed to be more specific.

In the course of the analysis, the difference between the mildly and severely subnormal became more and more obvious. It was apparent, in view of this difference, that either one or the other had to be visited. Many of the questions which would be relevant to the mildly subnormal would not be relevant to the severely subnormal. Ultimately the decision was made to visit the severely subnormal. One of the chief reasons for this decision was that it appeared that the mildly subnormal who might be visited would often be families with social problems, and families who fell into this category would hardly be ideal for seeing how care by the community could work.

It was felt that it would be far more valuable to consider the severely subnormal. Their families are most often normal families with an extraordinary problem, and they would be able to give better clues about how care by the community did work or might work.

The basis on which the families were chosen was described at the end of chapter 9. Eleven major handicaps were identified. These were: a severe disability in walking, total inability to talk, serious incontinence, epilepsy weekly or more often, clear evidence of mental illness in the subnormal, inability to dress himself, inability to feed himself, needing considerable supervision, and being a serious behaviour problem at home, in his locality or at training centre. All those subnormals who had two or more of these major handicaps were chosen. The only exception was those who needed constant supervision. Even if the necessity for constant supervision was the only major handicap, cases requiring it were also included. Constant supervision was associated very strongly with admission to hospital and we were particularly interested in finding out how families managed to cope with this sort of pressure.

In the course of deciding how the major disability score should be made up, another important decision had to be taken. Many of these factors meant much less if the person was a child. Incontinence in a child of six is very different from incontinence in a man of twenty-six; many normal children of six cannot be left on their own for very long, but if someone of sixteen or over cannot be left for more than a few minutes, this is unusual and not something that parents expect. This means that the major disability score was only fully relevant for adults. The analysis in chapter 9, which showed the considerable difference between children and adults, makes this clear.

This led to the decision to limit the visiting to adults (i.e. people of sixteen or over). There was a variety of reasons for this. In the past, more attention has been paid to children than to adults—for example, K. S. Holt in his study on the effect of mentally retarded children on their sibs carried out in Sheffield in 1958, and Sheila Hewett in her study of cerebral palsied children (1970).

While the severely subnormal are children, it could be argued that the problems are likely to be the problems of ordinary children writ large, and that the difference is one of degree not of kind. Once the child reaches sixteen, the distinction will be more marked—this person is clearly different and is not going to be independent. A child is expected to be dependent; an adult is not.

Once a severely subnormal person reaches sixteen there is a change in provision. Anyone in the special care unit for the very severely handicapped is excluded at sixteen and there is no provision for him apart from a hospital bed. In taking the adults, those who had been excluded from the special care unit were visited and the effect of this lack of provision was seen.

The decision to concentrate on the adults meant also that the families visited were families who had been coping for a long time, and this raised one of the most critical aspects of community care—namely, that families often have to cope for many years. How they do so is a matter of great importance. Also, the sibs of these subnormals, if any, had often left home and the parents were older. How the family and community respond to this situation is critical.

Once the decision had been taken to visit severely subnormal adults living at home, with either two or more 'major handicaps' or needing constant supervision, it was possible to pick out the families to be visited. There were fifty-nine families. In five of them the subnormal only needed constant supervision.

There was a lapse of over eighteen months between the deadline date used for coding the information from the files, 1 September 1968, and the visits. The visits were carried out from May to September 1970. In order to increase the number of families eligible for visiting, those who were children on 1 September 1968 but had subsequently had their sixteenth birthday were examined to see if any had at least two major handicaps or needed constant supervision. This added seven cases, one of whom only needed constant supervision.

In preparation for the visits, all these cases were checked with the Mental Health Service. It was found that five had died, three had gone into permanent care in hospital, one had left Sheffield and one could not be traced. In one other case the man concerned had been a serious behaviour problem but had since married and there had been no contact with him for seven years. It was felt that it would be unwise to visit him and his wife, and so he was excluded. This left fifty-five cases.

Before the visits were carried out, sixteen pre-pilot visits were conducted with similar families in Nottingham. Two of the subnormals proved to be mildly, not severely, subnormal and, interestingly, in view of the decision to concentrate on the severely subnormal, they were very different from the rest, and the guided interview schedule which we were developing did not fit them at all. The fourteen remaining interviews were valuable, and by the end a schedule had been developed, designed to establish the capacities of the subnormal, how the family managed to cope with him, and the part that family, friends and neighbours played in looking after him. The schedule was based on one used by Dr Kushlick's team in Wessex.

The revised schedule was piloted in eight interviews in Sheffield with families with a multiply handicapped, severely subnormal at home, who lived in the new areas which had been excluded from the survey. A few minor modifications were made as a result of these visits. The guided interview schedule which was used in the main visits is shown in appendix D. During the pilot visits and the main visits a tape recorder was used whenever possible. Material from the pilot visits has been used in some places. Where this has been done it has been noted that it was from a pilot visit.

The first contact with each family was made by the mental welfare officer responsible. He or she told the family that they would be contacted by the research worker or his assistant, and gave them a brief idea of why we wanted to visit them. Once the Mental Health Service had let us know that a family had been told, the person who was going to undertake the visit[1] wrote to the family to arrange an interview, enclosing a stamped addressed postcard for them to reply. Out of the fifty-five families contacted, only one refused.

Successful interviews were carried out with all the remaining fifty-four families except one. This was an extremely interesting interview with the old mother of a middle-aged man whose behaviour presented considerable problems. His two 'major handicaps' were both behaviour problems. Otherwise, he was hardly handicapped at all. He was present throughout the interview and the interviewer found it quite impossible to go through the schedule. The interview turned into a slightly guided monologue from the mother with occasional remarks from the subnormal. The result was fascinating but totally uncodeable. This case has not been included in the tables, whose total is therefore fifty-three. In practice, this man's behaviour was far more characteristic of the mildly subnormal (his IQ was 48) than the multiply handicapped severely subnormal.

The chapters that follow are the result of these interviews, but before going on to consider the interviews it is worth giving thought once more as to what is the point at issue. Is it how can we stop people having to go into hospital? Or how can we decide who should go into hospital? Or is it what measures are needed to enable the subnormals and their families to get the sort of help they need to live lives that are worth living? In the early part of the century we went through a stage where institutional care was considered the answer. More recently we have been through a stage where it was felt that the subnormal should be kept at home at any cost. We are now at last *beginning* to break down the artificial *administrative* dichotomy between home and institution, and to consider the issue from the standpoint of the needs of the subnormal and his family and the reorganization that is needed in the light of these needs.

The selection of those with certain handicaps who were still living at home does not mean that these were the successes, compared with whom those families whose subnormal had been admitted were failures. Rather they were chosen as a critical group who could provide valuable clues to what does happen when such people are kept at home. This provides the necessary raw material for the next question about what measures are needed to enable subnormals and their families to get the help they need to lead lives that are worth living.

The aim of the visits was not to accumulate evidence of the need for more residential provision, but to find positive factors relating to care at home which would lead to a clearer knowledge of those aspects of it which would enable total provision for subnormals and their families to be planned. For many of the more able subnormals it was possible from the files to see a factor that helped towards satisfactory care at home, for instance, the ability to do an ordinary job, or the fact of having no severe disabilities, or attendance at a training centre. But where the subnormal was seriously handicapped it was less easy to see the positive factors. The files were only able to hint at the importance of factors, such as the relationships within the family, which made care at home possible. It was at these positive but elusive factors, which contribute to the quality of life, that the visits were directed. This meant attention to much mundane detail which makes up the business of living; but the underlying question was always, not home or hospital, but what contributes to the quality of life of this family, and what is needed to improve this quality of life?

13   The subnormal people who were visited

Fifty-four families with a severely subnormal member at home were visited, and in order to do justice to each subnormal and his family, fifty-four categories would be needed. It is, however, possible to suggest four categories which match the details to a reasonable extent.

The four categories can be described most easily by reference to figure 13. The principle employed in the top section on disabilities is the more disabilities, the more dots. One dot represents a mild disability, two dots a severe or total disability. In the case of 'temperament', if the subnormal's temperament was assessed as being livelier and more energetic than usual, this is shown by one dot, and if it was uncontrollably excitable, this is shown by two dots.

In figure 13 a reference number from 1 to 53[1] has been given to each family. The first refers to that with the greatest number of disabilities and problems in 'the daily grind', the fifty-third to that with the least. The four categories into which they can be divided are: the very severely disabled (1–14), the severely disabled (15–32), the moderately disabled (33–47) and the (comparatively) mildly disabled (48–53). Some cases might be moved up or down a category, but on the whole these divisions appear to fit the facts.

The disability of four of the very severely disabled was virtually total and they could do nothing for themselves. One of them was Angela who was in her early twenties and her parents' only child. When she was twenty-one months old she contracted tubercular meningitis and since then had been totally disabled. She suffered from epilepsy occasionally and was partially blind. She could not sit up by herself, let alone move about. She was quite unable to dress, feed or wash herself; she was totally incontinent and unable to talk at all. She needed everything doing for her, and her mother, who had a heart condition, had to lift her and turn her over. She remained in bed the whole time. She had never attended any day care centre nor had she ever been in hospital for short term care.

The least disabled end of the very severely disabled scale was Richard who was in his late teens and lived with his widowed mother in a house in an old industrial area. He could walk quite well but he was rather deaf. He could not dress or wash himself. All his food had to be cut up very finely for him. He could not chew and it took a very long time to feed him. He could not feed himself at all. He could not talk and he was completely incontinent. He had about three pairs of pants put on him and a pair of plastic pants, but this did not absorb the urine he produced and so he wetted his trousers as well as his pants regularly. His socks and shoes were also wetted and so the shoes rotted quickly. He wet the kitchen floor during the interview and started spreading it about the floor with his feet.

The division between the very severely disabled and the severely disabled is by no means distinct. Two of the severely disabled could, from the point of view of disabilities, be counted among the very severely disabled. They owe their position to the fact that they presented fewer problems. Both of them were comparatively young. More typical of this group was Jean who was in her early thirties and lived with her widowed mother in a council flat. Her main problem was severe epilepsy. She had fits every night. They were minor fits but she had had major fits which had left her paralysed for a while afterwards, and the use of her left hand was still not quite what it should be. Her walking was fair but she needed a hand. She was unable to dress or wash herself at all but, provided she was given some help, she could feed herself. Generally speaking she was continent, but when she had fits in bed at night she was likely to wet the bed. Her talking was fair and she was capable of carrying on a very simple conversation.

Jean's behaviour was very quiet. A very different case was Helen. Physically Helen was very fit but she was quite unable to wash or dress herself, although, given a bit of help, she could feed herself. She could only say a few words and had no bladder control. The main problem was her restless and unpredictable behaviour, which led to her temperament being coded as livelier and more energetic than most. What this meant can be gauged from her mother's reply to the question: Do you find that she has any habits or mannerisms that are difficult to live with?

'When she can't make you understand she has a paddy, and I'll tell you what she's got the habit of recently, she's pinching everlastingly, every time I go near her she is pinching. [The bruise marks from the pinches were clearly visible on her mother's arms.] She is at me all the time: . . . she's always on

the go, and now walking . . . she's pinching you all the time
she's walking, yet we've never been away without her for an
hour, holidays and the lot.'

The importance of any dot which appears in line eleven, temperament, will be appreciated.

The number of physical disabilities was considerably fewer among
the moderately disabled. Typical of them was Ruby who was in her
middle thirties and lived with her parents, both of whom were over
seventy. Her sight was poor and getting worse, but she could look at
magazines on a good day. She had a weak heart but she was not
handicapped at all in her walking, could dress herself and only
needed a bit of help with washing and feeding. She was fully continent. This gives only half the picture. During the interview she
tended to be rather restless and kept going to the lavatory and coming
back and making a great performance of taking her shoes off and
arranging herself cross-legged on her chair. This was apparently
typical behaviour. She appeared to have a capacity for getting the
household to revolve round her. She was never left alone in the house
and, 'she's not interested in going out; she will not go out; we can't
persuade her to go out.'

Philip, who also falls into this category of the moderately disabled, provides a marked contrast to Ruby. Although he was more
disabled, his care seemed to be felt as less of a burden. Philip was in
his early twenties and lived with his parents in a pleasant, modern
local authority house on the outskirts of Sheffield. Physically he was
healthy and capable but, 'the only thing with him is his nerves and
that affects him very much. Children's voices or anything with a
high pitch seems to upset him very much.' He needed a good deal of
help with both washing and dressing but he could feed himself.
During the day he was continent but he needed help. His mother
said: 'Well, before long he'll be fetching me. He seems to want me to
be there. He can undo his trousers and sit on the toilet but he always
wants me to be with him and then I have to fasten him up.' At night
time he was completely incontinent. His biggest handicap was his
complete inability to talk. His mother said that when he was upset,
'he makes a certain noise which I know [it was an extraordinary dog-
like whine], and if we are walking and we are in a nice quiet spot he
has a little lilt which I know is his happy sound'.

The mildly handicapped form a more separate group. It is questionable whether some of them fall into the category of multiply

handicapped at all but the selection of any group is bound to have marginal cases. In practice it was extremely useful to visit the families of some less severely handicapped people. One of these was Maisie who was in her middle forties and lived with her parents in a small terrace house in an old, well-established working-class area. She needed some help with dressing and washing but, except for her rather limited speech, these were her only handicaps apart from her mental retardation.

Her handicaps and the handicaps of the others in this mildly disabled group were mild indeed compared with those of the very severely disabled, but they remain a considerable burden to live with. Consider the answer of Maisie's mother to whether she could go out by herself at all: 'Well, I never let her, not trusted her, because if anything happened I'd blame myself. Knocked down or owt like that.' This may tell us as much about the attitude of Maisie's mother as it does about Maisie, but it also indicates something of the impact that Maisie had on her parents' life.

The illustrations of the four categories have given an idea of the range of disabilities. One effect that all the subnormals had on their families was the way they restricted the family's freedom of action, especially the mother's. Almost all the families were subject to the sort of restrictions which are associated with a pre-school child. In the case of those attending training centre, one could say that the restrictions were more like those imposed by a child at infant school. The hours they attend are very similar. But this state of affairs had not been a matter of a few years, just a stage through which the family passes, but had persisted for the subnormal's life-time, and the ages of those visited ranged from sixteen to seventy-one. (The mean was twenty-nine.)

The restrictions to which these families were subject provide the framework within which their lives were lived and their problems existed. Twenty-four out of the fifty-three were not left in the house on their own for more than five minutes, nineteen were not left for more than an hour and only ten were left for over an hour. Nine were not even left in a room on their own for more than five minutes.

Mothers were asked what their main problem was, and quite often this limitation was mentioned.

'The main problem is the tying down of oneself, that's the most irksome thing. I can't say, "Oh it's a lovely day today, let's go into the country." I can't. If I am going to do that arrangements have to be made.'

'We can't do as we like, we can't go out when we like, we can't take Andrew anywhere we like and we don't have any social life.'

This perpetual restriction affected many aspects of living, for instance shopping, going out or even making a phone call. The father of James, an over-active young man who could hardly be left at all, gave a good idea of what this restriction felt like. When asked if his son could be left alone in the house, he said:

'No, I could slip out into the garden for five minutes or so or something like that.' Mother: 'And I could hang out the washing or something like that.' Interviewer: But you wouldn't leave the garden? Father: 'No.' Interviewer: But being able to go out into the garden afforded some relief? Father: 'Yes, but in the past month [during which James had been in hospital] . . . only last night I went out into the garden and my wife came out and I said, "Good heavens, what are you doing here?" This feels like freedom, the fact that the two of you can do something together; and we're going out tonight. It was arranged on the spur of the moment last night and we didn't have to make any complicated arrangements.'

The same father described the period during which James had been in hospital as 'a second honeymoon'. The impact of this perpetual restriction on freedom of choice and movement was a recurring motif in many interviews. One widow with a very severely handicapped daughter said: 'Sometimes I feel these four walls are just like a prison.'

There was one factor of outstanding importance which affected the extent to which the mother in particular was tied. This was whether the subnormal attended a training centre or not. Seventeen out of the fifty-three did so. Figure 13 shows that it was the less handicapped who attended a training centre. (Attendance at training centre is shown by two dots on line 29 in figure 13.) The lack of day provision for the severely handicapped has been mentioned already in chapter 10 and will be mentioned again later on. Six of the others did receive day care at least once a week, either at a hospital, from the Spastics Society or at a centre for the physically handicapped shown by one dot on line 29).

Naturally those mothers whose subnormal attended a training

centre were tied considerably less than those whose subnormal did not. It is most unfortunate that those who were most disabled were those for whom there was least provision; but the extent of disability was not the only factor which prevented the subnormal attending training centre. Some who could go, and indeed had gone in the past, did not attend. A factor of pervasive importance in this and many other respects was the attitude of the mother, and to a lesser extent the father, to the subnormal. This colours so many aspects of the family's life that, some idea of the subnormal people themselves having been given, the attitude of the parents to the subnormal must be considered next.

14   The attitude of the parents

Different attitudes

The mother of Philip, the young man mentioned in the last chapter who could not talk at all and needed a lot of looking after, replied when asked if she felt having him had made her feel lonely and cut off from other people:

> 'Oh no, we'd been married nearly nine years when I had him, and I often think rather than not have one I would have Philip as he is. I think it's something fairly special actually, well I think it's brought something rather special into my life, I think my husband does as well. . . . I suppose . . . more contented I think, I don't know, I think they bring an added something into your life. It's hard work, and worrying at times, I think they also enrich your life quite a lot. I think you get your values right anyway. There's no false values attached to your life, with children like Philip you get things more into perspective.'

This was perhaps the most positive statement of the value of having a mentally handicapped child. More common on the positive side was a clear-minded and whole-hearted acceptance of their mentally handicapped child. The mother of Edna, a moderately handicapped girl of twenty-seven (pilot), said:

> 'The only thing I can say is that you've got to accept it. It's hard, isn't it, but you have to accept it. And really in my opinion they are your responsibility first and foremost . . . they belong to you, don't they, you see, and that's how I've always felt. You are much better if you've got a good husband, and if you've got good neighbours it's made a lot easier. And a lot haven't.'

By no means all the families and mothers felt like this. The mother of Diana, a twenty-year-old woman whose main handicap was very severe epilepsy, came from Poland. She was asked if she felt lonely:

'Well, what life have I got. . . . I came from Warsaw and you sit here and you wish you had never come. The only thing that holds me is I've got a good husband. It's not a good life.' The same woman, when asked if she had any plans for the future, said: 'No, there's nothing to look forward to.' Another mother, a widow, whose daughter was in her forties, moderately handicapped and would not talk, said, when asked if she belonged to any society or club or church: 'No, I don't belong to anything, I don't belong to any church because I'm bitter.'

Central to any understanding of the mother's and family's attitude was the parents' acceptance of the fact that the subnormal was handicapped. Sheila Hewett makes this point well in the final chapter of her book *The Family and the Handicapped Child* (1970, p. 207). She finishes by quoting the words of the mother of a severely mentally and physically handicapped child of six:

'You've just got to accept them for what they are and not keep wishing they were something else, not keep wishing they were normal. Well, you naturally *wish* they were normal, but it's no good to keep longing for them to do things you know they can't do. You've just got to accept them for what they can do.'

Mrs Hewett concludes: '"You naturally wish they were normal." This mother surely speaks not only for the mothers who contributed to this survey but for all mothers of handicapped children. She expresses precisely their first and final dilemma—the acceptance of the unacceptable.'

Time after time this point about acceptance was implied by what mothers said. Acceptance of their child is not all that has to be done but it is the essential first step without which nothing else is possible. Ruby's mother put it like this:

'I look at it like this, you couldn't believe it was right, you couldn't bring yourself to believe that for a long, long time, then when it gradually dawns on you, you feel a little gradual improvement, and you'd think "Oh this was it", but it wasn't you know. That was the worst thing, accepting, knowing, bringing yourself to terms with what you'd got in front of you, then it just comes.'

Edna's mother, who has already been quoted, was equally explicit: 'It's hard isn't it, but you have to accept it.' The mother of Bridget, a moderately disabled woman in her early twenties, put it more harshly: 'Well to tell you the truth, I've got what you call hardened to it. One lady said you've learned to accept it. I say I'm hardened to it.'

This acceptance of the fact of the handicap and at the same time of their child as a person, a handicapped person, demanded much of the parents, especially the mother. Above all it demanded self-knowledge. Acceptance of others *as they are* demands acceptance of oneself as one is. This can be detected in what Ruby's mother said: 'That was the worst thing . . . bringing *yourself* to terms with what you'd got in front of you, *then* it just comes.'

The way in which the subnormal came to be accepted varied. In some cases, though not many, it seems to have taken place quite naturally and easily. This was so for the unmarried sister who looked after Jennifer, who was the oldest subnormal visited. She was seventy-one and moderately handicapped. Her sister had been looking after her for twenty-seven years, ever since her mother had become incapacitated and subsequently died. Her sister was asked:

> You've lived with Jennifer all your life? She replied: 'Yes, she's always been here [Jennifer is seven years her senior]. That is why I look on Jennifer as a normal person. I think perhaps that's one of the things that people don't realize, Jennifer is a normal person to me because she's always been here you see.'

Acceptance of the subnormal was not always reached so easily. Lilian was a very severely disabled woman of thirty. The main problem was her constant activity and unreliable behaviour, for instance she was likely to try to snatch a potato out of boiling water and eat it. Her mother was asked whether she herself was keeping well. She replied:

> 'Yes, I didn't at one time. I went through a bad period at one time, but I was fortunate in realising that it wasn't so much my health as my mind. I used to pray for her to die because she was so bad, she used to cry all night, and I found that praying for her to die made her worse and it made me ill, until one night Phil was away working in Derbyshire, and I'd been from the top of the house to the bottom and it was sparkling, and she soiled bed, she didn't just soil bed but she ran about and wiped her hands all over bathroom floor and bathroom door and it smelled terrible and I was furious. I went through hell that

night, and that was the turning point, and I said to my sister
and anyone that came, "In future, no-one ever tells anybody
Lilian will never get better. In future everybody has got to say
Lilian is going to get better", and I found that with that positive
mind she did start getting better, and I stopped praying for her
to die and started praying for help for myself. I think if I
hadn't realised that it was all in my own mind, I would have
finished up in Middlewood [mental hospital]. You've got to get
used to things, accept them more or less, it's no use fighting
against conditions, you just make yourself ill doing it, you've
got to accept them and make the best of it.'

Olshansky (1965) makes a similar point when he talks about the
chronic sorrow of the parents of a mentally handicapped child and
how the process of coming to terms with the fact of the handicap is a
continual process which takes place over a long period.

Little mention has been made of the subnormal's father but the
attitude he takes is naturally important. Findings from the visits
about this were very indirect and the father's attitude was shown for
the most part in the extent to which he helped to look after the subnormal. This is discussed in chapter 17. In one case, however, the
mother was quite explicit about the help her husband had been:

'When I first had Henry, I used to cry for hours over him and
I used to think, oh why should it be me, everybody else has got
a normal baby but me, and my husband said, "Well, you can't
help him with crying, you'll just have to accept him, you'll find it
easier when you have accepted it."'

This suggests that in some cases the father may be the best person
for the professional helpers to talk to when trying to help the mother
to acceptance of the facts of the situation. Naturally this will depend
on the individual father, but the possibility is worth considering.

In just one case it appeared that even after nearly twenty years
the parents of one very severely disabled man had still not really
accepted the fact of their son's handicap. The interviewer (J.P.L.)
commented: 'They seem to have shut themselves off from family and
neighbours and live in a sad small world of their own, hoping desperately that one day a miracle might happen.'

There is an important difference between these families and the
families visited by Mrs Hewett. The oldest of the spastic children she
visited was eight years old. Among those visited in Sheffield the

youngest visited was sixteen. This means that the acceptance of the subnormal is something that happened some time ago and has become so much part of the family and part of the mother that they are hardly aware of it.

Furthermore, the different families have accepted their subnormals in different ways. One very simple way of describing this is on a negative/positive axis. At the extreme negative end there was the unrealistic hope and withdrawal into fantasy of the family with the very severely disabled man, mentioned above. Next, there appeared to be a very few families who were looking after the subnormal almost entirely from a sense of duty. The obvious instance of this was Shirley, a severely handicapped woman of forty-seven, who was looked after by her maiden aunt and unmarried uncle. She was not able to do very much for herself. The most wearying feature of caring for her was that she was totally incontinent and smeared herself with her faeces. Despite all their efforts the house smelt strongly as a result. The interviewer (J.P.L.) commented:

> Shirley is looked after by her maiden aunt and unmarried uncle who took over when Shirley's parents died because they felt some obligation, but they are both over sixty now and find the burden almost too much. Unfortunately the waiting list for permanent care is so long that they have been told that unless something happens to them there is no hope of getting her anywhere.

This was the one case where the family definitely wanted permanent care for their subnormal.

The next point on the line which the attitude of some families suggested, again not very many, about five, was one of resignation. Daniel's parents (pilot) provide an example of this. Daniel was in his early thirties and was very severely disabled. He could do almost nothing for himself and did not appear to be able to communicate at all.

His parents had received hardly any help in looking after him until he had received short-term care within the previous two years. The sheer 'grind' of caring for him seemed to have worn the mother down to a level of weary resignation. For instance, when she was asked if she thought that looking after Daniel had affected her health at all, she replied, 'I don't think so really. I mean he is my son and you've got to do it, you know what I mean, you feel as though you have got to do it. Sometimes it gets topside of you, doing for him, I am fifty-eight, fifty-nine next, as you get older you get tireder.' When she was asked what the main problem was in her case, she replied: 'Well nothing really, just that we should like to go out together more, that's what we've missed really. I mean we just take it for granted, he's thirty-two now and we've done it, you've got it to do. As for him going away, well, people keep saying, "Why don't you let him go?" but I've always said I'll do for him while I can.'

More common than this resigned attitude was a realistic accept-ance of the subnormal for what he or she was, and a recognition of the hard work involved. The majority of cases clustered round this point. This is only to be expected because otherwise many of them would have been in hospital. All those who were quoted earlier as examples of acceptance would come in at this point. However, there is a further stage discernible which is only reached after there has been a realistic acceptance of the subnormal. This is a positive enjoy-ment of the subnormal, who occupies a valued role in the family; in short, he is loved. This can be seen as the positive end of the nega-tive/positive axis. This appeared to be the stage that Philip's family had reached. Philip was mentioned at the beginning of this chapter. The same could be said of David's family. David was severely dis-abled, unable to do anything for himself, incontinent, non-ambulant and unable to talk, yet his mother said:

'It's amazing what satisfaction you get out of him having pleasure, as long as he is happy, you are happy. . . . Fortunately my husband and I are about the same temperament, we've lived with it that long. Twenty-two years you've got yourself into a way of life. You don't stop and think about it, it's there and you do it.'

This positive/negative axis is very crude and can only serve to give some indication of the attitudes of the families to their subnormal member. Five stages have been suggested. At the negative end there is withdrawal into fantasy, then sense of duty (withdrawal of affec-tion might be a more accurate description), resignation, acceptance and, finally, love. The different stages overlap; for instance, there is no suggestion that only those who may have reached the fifth stage loved their subnormal member. The stages are a simplified model.

Only when the reality of the subnormal's handicap has been accepted, is a further step possible. Indeed this step is almost as important as the initial acceptance, if the parents' attitude is not going to slump into one of submission and hopeless resignation. It is an attitude of realistic expectation, of accepting the subnormal's limitations, yet at the same time encouraging him to do as much as possible. A quite amazing example of this is what Judith's mother did. Judith was very severely disabled. She looked as though she could only sit in a wheelchair. Her mother was asked if she could move around herself and this was her answer:

'Well yes, but she's giddy because she is drugged that much. It's a big asset actually. Some days I can take her shoes off and she can walk round this house . . . she wasn't going to walk by the way, she were just going to sit. And in two years . . . because I went to an osteopath because I was just desperate. You burn and are not satisfied with the doctors, and he said to take her off drugs: there's no reason why she shouldn't walk, when he examined her legs—and that were enough for me, and I thought, well, she is not going to sit. In the first place you see she wouldn't get up, she just used to sit. Well I used to take her to the hospital for exercises . . . until I learned how to do them myself. [They taught her mother to help her to crawl like a baby. This took two years.] Well, my husband used to sit there and he'd say "for goodness' sake Doris stop it", because I got on his nerves. He loves her, but he would have been content to let her sit. It got on his nerves because she were crying all the time. I used to stand her there and *make* her take two steps. . . .

'She didn't know a door from a space when I started her walking. She knew that she went through this door, but I think she thought it were permanently open, but her brain didn't tell her it was closed and she used to go smash into it like a budgie out of a cage when it goes blind. We got four steps, we got marvellous right up to this door, and I knew she hadn't the sense to know it was a space. Anyway we started putting her hand on the handle and pushing it, and she used to cry, but we did it, week in and week out, she could open a door you know in six months.

'The same with coming downstairs. Up to her being ten years old I could carry her up and down if she was asleep, but she was putting weight on and I got so I couldn't carry her. Well, my husband were doing a bit of part-time job at night you know; she was just lounging in a chair; she'd perhaps be lounging in a chair all day; you didn't know what to do with her, she wouldn't lie on the settee, and I got to the stage I couldn't take her to bed, because she was too top heavy. She still is, that's only one thing I can't do, you see she always tries to do two steps instead of one step, and she overbalances me, and I've never tried since she was perhaps ten or eleven, but coming down I had the training to do with that you see. I knew I would be on my own all day. Mind you, she'd never been able to come downstairs without two so I thought, well, I'm going to be handicapped if John's at school, I've got to do something, so we started again, teaching her to hold the banister. She didn't want to hold it, terribly stupid you know these backward babies, so I used to put her hand on the banister and she'd pull it off, I'd put it on, slap it, so I thought well, we have to do it the hard way. I used to put her botty on the top step and pull her legs which weren't very nice, and slide her down you see, she'd cry. Right. So I said, "If you don't hold that banister we're both going to fall, and if your mummy falls I can't look after you." You know all these things I'd say to her, so she'd hold it again for so long, and eventually it registered you know, it registered that if she didn't hold that banister I were going to pull her legs, and it weren't very comfortable for a girl at that age, and of course she comes down now with me helping her. Now she gets to the top of them stairs and her hand's straight out to that banister, and she walks down.

'Nobody knows just what I've done, you can sit and talk about it, but you can't imagine how long it takes. You think it's never going to happen . . . and you see now, what would I have done? I would have to have carried her or have a wheelchair upstairs and take her to the toilet and bathroom. . . . Now he [her husband] wouldn't have had the patience with her, you see she cried all the time I was making her do these little jobs. She cried. . . . But I sort of persevered and I never knew what an asset it was going to be.'

A similar sort of attitude was evident in Joyce's mother. Joyce was even more disabled, yet her mother would encourage her to try to say words and take part in her own way in communication, even if it could hardly be called conversation. (What her mother said on this subject is related on page 199.) In different circumstances it would not be difficult to imagine Joyce being completely mute.

Whom the subnormal was living with

Not all of the subnormals were living with their parents or mothers, though the majority were. Table 14.1 gives the breakdown.

Table 14.1 Whom the subnormal was living with

Parents	32
Widowed mother	12
Divorced mother	1
Mother and stepfather	1
Widowed father	2
Father and mother's sister	1
Unmarried sister	2
Maiden aunt	1
Aunt and uncle	1
Total	53

In forty-six cases the mother was part of the household. The aunt at the bottom of the table had been looking after a totally disabled seventeen-year-old boy since he was three; she had lived in the same household as he since his birth, and in terms of relationships was effectively his mother. Two of the subnormals were living with their fathers. One of these was only very mildly handicapped. The household of the other subnormal man living with his father was run by a married sister who lived near by. It was this sister who was interviewed. In the one case where the subnormal was living with his father and his mother's sister, his care was undertaken exclusively by his aunt.

The mother figure was the mother in forty-six out of fifty-three cases, an aunt or sister in six cases. In one case, which was only marginally relevant, there was no mother figure at all. The man mentioned in chapter 12, who has not been included in the tables, was living with his mother.

The importance of whom the subnormal was living with can be appreciated better when the extent to which he could communicate has been considered.

The families were drawn from all social groups, and for such a small number the proportions were not markedly different from those for the whole of Sheffield. The figures appear in table 14.2.

Table 14.2   Socio-economic group of the families

Professional	4
Intermediate	6
Skilled	28
Semi-skilled	5
Unskilled	8
Undefinable	2
Total	53

The importance of the subnormal's ability to communicate

This section deals with the subnormal's ability to communicate, not simply his or her ability to talk. The two are by no means the same. Table 14.3 gives an idea of the capacities of the subnormals in communicating.

Table 14.3   Talking or communicating

Can join in general conversation	4
Simple conversation	12
Simple sentences	8
A few words	9
Gestures, grunts, noises	14
Not at all	6
Total	53

Some of the subnormals could talk quite well. In certain cases almost too well. The sister of June, an older subnormal woman (pilot), was asked if June had any mannerisms which were particularly difficult to live with. She replied: 'Well, cursing, wicked, violent language. God knows where she picked it up.' Her sister felt she could not leave her with other people because, 'She pulls this friend to pieces something cruel and when she [the friend] comes in and she's talking to me, she's knocking her all the time; she's shouting out and mocking her.'

Very few were able to take part in general conversation but Freda's mother said:

'Oh Freda gets on well with anybody. If we have gone into a cafe, I have tried to place her to be unobtrusive so she won't talk to anybody, but you can bet your life that she'll get somebody into conversation. She always does. She is very friendly.'

In one of the early pilot interviews, being carried out jointly by both the interviewers, Ann, the rather difficult epileptic subnormal woman, came in half-way through the interview and started interviewing the interviewers, enquiring whether we were married, how old we were and had we a lot of pound notes. Later on she announced that it was her birthday the next day and she was 'Sweet twenty-six and never been kissed.' Ability to communicate at this level was unusual. Those who could converse were generally able to do so with only one person at a time, and their conversation often had the rather irritating persistence and repetitiveness of small children. For instance, Freda's mother said of her: 'She keeps saying "ey, ey"; it just annoys you sometimes; she keeps saying "Mummy" to attract attention.' The parents of the more severely handicapped Patricia remarked on the same thing: 'There is so much repetition of the few things that she says. You know she'll ask the same questions time and time again every day.'

If the subnormal were able to talk in a fairly intelligent way, this made him far more of a companion to the mother. This was the case with Susan, who, although she was severely disabled, could talk quite well.

The problem was most acute when the subnormal could not speak at all. Where the subnormal's other disabilities were not too great, this did not appear to be so serious, but even so Hugh's mother said of his ability to make friends:

'He is so handicapped, not being able to communicate, but the other lads, they seem to be fond of him. When we picked him up from the bus from his holidays, we walked down town with another chap and he says: "I like your Hugh," he says. "We're pals, aren't we Hugh?" Of course Hugh could not answer.'

For some mothers their child's inability to talk hurt more than anything else. Christine was a very severely disabled woman in her late twenties. Her mother said: 'I would give anything if Christine could speak, but of course she can't.' In the case of the moderately disabled Nancy, one of the things which hurt her widowed mother most deeply was:

'She won't talk to me now you know. She hasn't talked since her dad died, that's fourteen year ago. There's no conversation, but if I say anything to her she'll answer me "yes" or "no", just answer me that's all. When she was younger she was a proper mimic, she'd make anybody laugh, and chatter away, but she won't speak now.'

The subnormals' inability to talk or make themselves understood affected their contact with, and care by, other people. Consider the case of Elizabeth. Elizabeth had been normal until about ten, then her condition deteriorated until she was able to do very little for herself. She was quite unable to talk. She had had an older brother Stephen who had died, to whom the same had happened.

Her mother was asked if she had ever contemplated letting Elizabeth go into short-term care for a while.

'No, we did that with Stephen. People kept saying, "you ought to have a holiday." Eventually . . . I said yes and the doctor arranged it. . . . It wasn't a bit of good, we went away and I had him on my mind all the time. When he came out he had bedsores and had lost half a stone in weight. You see, he had gone just like Elizabeth, he couldn't ask for anything, or speak, and it just wasn't worth it.' Interviewer: Would you say that one of the major things that stops you is the fact that Elizabeth can't speak? 'Yes, you see I can understand her, but nurses haven't the time to see to them. Poor Stephen, I discovered they'd had him sitting out, it was a nice day, but they'd put him a pair of glasses on which they'd found in his locker, but it was this old man's when it came to it. They got mixed up and Stephen was sitting in this chair with these little old man's glasses on, things like that, can you imagine it? He didn't wear glasses.'

Arthur could just manage a few very simple sentences but had also had an unhappy experience of short-term care ('He came back just like a frightened little animal.') and he couldn't tell his parents what the matter was and so, 'If we never go away again, he's not going there any more.'

It is clear that if the subnormal could not speak, not only was he very vulnerable, but also his parents were bound to feel much more protective about him—and not without justification. But of course the problems extended further than just contact with other people. The families and mothers of the subnormals also had difficulty in understanding, and this despite a life-time's experience. For instance,

Arthur's mother said: 'Occasionally we have difficulty getting the message across because he doesn't talk very clear. If he can't mime it or do it in a song it takes us ages, then he gets frustrated . . . he isn't violent, but he gets really annoyed when we don't understand.' James's father said: 'Of course the worst thing with these children is that you cannot reason with them. You cannot even bribe them. I don't know how much gets through to him really.'

The response that James's parents got from him was limited. There were cases where communication was even more limited. Lilian was a very severely disabled woman in her late twenties and could do nothing for herself, but she could walk and she was highly over-active. When her mother was asked if she could communicate at all, she said:

> 'Only way that I know she wants to go to the toilet is when she comes to me and pulls her dress up for me to take her pants off, but she doesn't tell me: and we know when she's frustrated because she'll blow her top off and this breathing heavy is only when she is annoyed, that is one way we found out when she was annoyed. When we went out anywhere and we wanted to go one way and she wanted to go the other she'd start breathing heavy then.'

The response from Angela was virtually zero. She was permanently in bed. Daniel, the very severely handicapped man (pilot) who was mentioned at the beginning of the chapter, responded hardly at all to his mother. She said:

> 'No, he can't tell you when he wants anything, he never does, it's just when he is mad. He can't make you understand anything really. I mean he can't speak, he can't say, that's how it is. He could have toothache or anything. We don't know.'

Contact in these last three cases was very limited. But there were subnormals who were equally disabled, or very nearly so, with whom there was far greater contact. Rupert was a very severely disabled boy of sixteen (pilot) who could do nothing for himself except, to a very limited extent, wheel himself around the house in his wheel-chair. But within familiar surroundings he was capable of responding. He enjoyed the movement on the television, he recognised hymns and used to hum them. Whenever there was strange company he would 'switch off' but with his parents he was capable of responding.

The same was true of the very severely disabled Judith. The interviewer had asked if she ever disturbed her parents' sleep.

'Oh yes, she does, some nights you know. She can go for three nights and never sleep.' Interviewer: And don't you sleep either? 'We do now, we can tell by the sound of her voice whether she is in pain or whether she just can't sleep and she is talking to herself.'

Joyce was also very severely disabled. She was permanently in bed and could not even sit up on her own, but she was capable of some communication. She could not really talk at all but she did communicate to some extent by noises. She made some attempt at words, but these were very indistinct. Her mother said:

'I can understand her a lot and relations can. She associates people with different things. Now the lady next door who comes to sit in, she once burped when she was here. Now, every time that lady comes in here, she [Joyce] makes that noise: she forces herself to do it because she connects her with that. We don't bother because it amuses her, and she gets a right whirl with it, and she does a lot of laughing. And different people like that she connects with different things.'

Violet was very severely disabled and could not talk, but her mother said: 'She'll look at me and I can sort of read her.' David could not talk at all either, but when his mother was asked if she ever felt cut off, she replied: 'I suppose you could say you are sometimes. I don't feel lonely because I've got Dave and I talk to him, and he in his particular way talks back, you know, and we chat together.'

Bernard was rather the same. He was very severely disabled, could do nothing for himself, could only walk with difficulty and could not talk at all, but the interviewer (J.P.L.) noted at the end of the interview schedule: 'Bernard is, however, quite a charmer with a twinkle in his eye and I imagine is very pleasant to live with.' His mother remarked that Bernard could sing quite tunefully and that he sometimes used words when he sang.

Enough has been said to indicate that even with some of the very severely subnormal and very severely disabled, some real communication was possible in quite a few cases. It will be equally obvious that the examples given are not simply about communication but fundamentally about relationships. Communication in these cases was only possible because there was a relationship. The way in which the very severely disabled Joyce managed to communicate is particularly interesting. The previous example of Judith was, strictly speaking, an example of the parents understanding Judith's noises, but this was just one part of the way in which communication between Judith and her parents was maintained. In the case of many of these severely disabled people, communication only took place through people with whom they had an extremely close relationship. The implications of this are important and are well illustrated by Nancy, who had refused to talk, except for yes and no, for the fourteen years since her father had died. If the subnormal's communication with the world depends entirely on one person, what is going to be the effect on the subnormal when the relationship with that one person is broken, for instance by the mother's death? This is a point of some significance, and is considered in more detail later on.

Now that the importance of speech and communication has been made clear, it is possible to consider the role that the subnormal occupied in the family.

The place of the subnormal in the family and the attitude of the parents

If a family is to cope with a subnormal at home for the length of time that these families had done, the family was bound to make certain adjustments in order to be able to cope. It is not normal for an adult to require, for his or her whole life, the care that a small child needs, and a family providing such care is bound to be different in some ways from the average.

This difference will be seen not just in terms of the care the subnormal needs, though this is a vital part of it, but also in the emotional attitude of the parents to the subnormal and the emotional position that the subnormal occupies in the family. The critical aspect was the extent to which the family was turned in on itself and emotionally bound up with the subnormal. At one end of the scale there was the family where the subnormal was the centre of his parents' lives to the exclusion of all else, and his parents were completely bound up with him. (This family was mentioned on page 189.)

The other end of the scale is much less easy to describe, because it is not so tidy. The subnormal is not the emotional centre of the family and the family is not totally bound up with him. Yet, at the same time, he is loved and valued. Such families generally had a good many contacts with family, friends and neighbours, and the subnormal appeared to be involved in the general commerce of living rather than hidden away in a little world of his own.

One of the best examples of this is Joyce, who was very severely disabled indeed. The interviewer was never quite able to work out the many relatives or friends who called in at various times, but this answer to a question about the mother's brothers and sisters gives some idea of how the family functioned. Mrs Fenton had two sisters and two brothers.

'The eldest lives quite close. She is the one whose caravan I go to stay in when I go on holiday. I see her every Tuesday and Friday. They come up, and when they come up, if ambulance hasn't come I hang on as long as I can, but if time's pushing up to half past ten they'll say, "Go on, and we'll stay while you come back if ambulance hasn't been", and while they're here my sister and sister-in-law, that helps to bath Joyce, they'll do my mother's ironing because she can't stand. This sister-in-law comes in on Monday, Tuesday and Friday. Monday she comes to help bath Joyce, on Tuesday she is here with my elder sister. Sister-in-law's husband, my brother, is on turns. When he is on nights he pops over before he goes to bed, and if he's over and Joyce is still in bed, he'll go up and carry her down.

'Then I've another brother, but we don't see much of him. He lives quite close. Then I've another sister who lives quite close, that's the one whose husband took us up into Yorkshire Dales, and it's their girl what sits in with Joyce, and boyfriend.' Interviewer: Is this mostly at weekends, that they sit in with her? 'Well Thursday, if her dad can't get up she'll get up in place of her dad, and then me and her mother have an hour at tombola.' Interviewer: So you see all members of the family quite frequently? 'Oh yes, we all sort of live in a circle.'

These two families indicate the two ends of the scale. It must be emphasized that the attempt to outline such a scale is only a tentative sketch of a complex situation, but if the general axis from an inward looking, subnormal-centred family to one which is not and has wider contacts with society can be accepted, at least provisionally, it is possible to fill in some of the ground in between the two extremes.

There was a number of families who concentrated almost entirely on the subnormal, with little contact with the world outside, though the isolation was not as extreme as that of the family of the very severely disabled young man already mentioned. One such family

was Diana's. The interviewer (J.P.L.) noted at the end of the interview; 'Diana is the centre of their existence. They never go out without her and as she is an only child they have no-one else to show their
affection to.'

A similar family was Hilda's. She was a moderately disabled
woman in her late twenties. The interviewer (J.P.L.) noted: 'She is
the centre of their lives. The parents appear to cling to Hilda as
someone who needs them.' The extent to which this was the case can
be gauged from her mother's answer to the question: Does the fact
that you do not leave Hilda with other people make things difficult
for you if you want to go out?

> 'Well, we're not people for going out you see, we're not that
> type of people, we're satisfied with our home and that's it you
> see. We never have gone out. We never left the others. I have
> two married. It's just our way, people are like that, some of
> them. We don't bother you see, we are quite satisfied at home.'

The needs of the subnormal, especially if he was very severely
handicapped, sometimes became quite explicitly the centre of the
mother's life. The mother of a very severely handicapped young man
replied, when asked if having him had made her feel lonely:

> 'No, he has made my life. He's made me feel happier. He's my
> god now. I think more about him than about my husband
> because I think he needs more looking after than my husband.
> My husband can walk and he can't. If he went away I should
> feel lonely because I've been used to looking after him.'

By comparison, in another family with an even more severely
handicapped young man, the subnormal managed to be the object
of the shared concern of the family, rather than the mother's emotional needs being in the forefront. This did not entail denying him
love. His mother said: 'You've got to shower a lot of love on them.
Keep going and giving him a kiss and he'll look forward to that.'

The relationship between the mother and the subnormal tended to
be specially close where there was no husband. In some cases the
subnormal was treated as a companion, to his, or more often her,
own gain and the comfort of the mother. The mother of Susan, a
moderately disabled woman in her middle forties, said:

> 'Well, she is a companion for me and I don't know what I
> would do without her. She was a very small baby . . . and when
> we took her home from hospital the doctor said, "You are

taking a great care home with you", and we never thought we would rear her. I think she has been sent for a purpose, I'd have been lonely on my own without her. You see you lose your husband just when you need him, when you are getting old.'

It is interesting that out of the sixteen cases where there was no father or father figure, the subnormal was a woman in twelve cases and a man in only four. Moreover, two of the men were not severely disabled.

The relationship between the subnormal and the mother is bound to be close. One would expect it to be closer if the father had died, but in some cases the exclusiveness and tightness of the bond between the two must be viewed with some reservations in the light of the point made at the end of the last section. If the mother is the subnormal's only link with the outside world, the only means of communication, what is going to happen when the mother dies or is too ill to carry on caring for her subnormal child? One example of this is what the mother of a very severely disabled woman, who could not talk at all, said when she was asked if she would like to go away for a holiday.

'Only if she were there. I really and truly couldn't leave her. She's more or less my world and I think I must be hers. I never leave her and I always take her wherever I go.' Later on she said: 'Ever since I've been on my own I've had her to bring up. I've been mother and father to her, and through me being on my own it's made me kind of cling more to her with her being in the condition she's in. Instead of mother and daughter, it's more like sister and little sister.'

In many ways this close and positive relationship is just what the subnormal needs, and it seems unfair to criticize when it is provided. Furthermore, it is difficult not to treat the subnormal as a dependent child when he acts just like one and demands the love and attention a dependent child demands. Sheila Hewett (1970, p. 142) made just this point:

For many mothers of handicapped children, an already intensified situation of interdependence is prolonged. A mother caring for a six-year-old who still behaves like a young baby in most respects, has no alternative but to go on mothering him as though he really were a baby, even though she can see the perils of this situation both for herself and the child, particularly when no day-care is offered.

Mrs Hewett returns to the same point a little further on in the same chapter (ibid., p. 148).

Mothers made the point that to be sent away from home is harder for the children when they have not been used to spending even the day-time with people other than their families, and this certainly makes it harder for the parents to adjust to their going. Once more, it seems that the more disadvantages a child sets out with, the more will accrue to him as time goes on, unless much greater efforts are made to reverse this trend than is the case at present.

Some of these families where the subnormal was very disabled and the mother or parents were very much bound up with their subnormal represent the result of lack of such help as day care not over six years but as many as sixty and 'the perils of this situation' to which Mrs Hewett referred were all too obvious. The situation is a difficult one because it represents an indefinable excess of something that basically is entirely commendable and right. The role of the social worker could be extremely important in this situation and will be mentioned in chapter 18. Here we are concerned with the attitude of the family and in particular with the role of the subnormal in the family.

It is quite impossible to draw a hard and fast line between the subnormal being given the love and care he needs and the mother or the parents allowing their own emotional need to love and care for someone who is dependent on them to become uppermost, to the detriment of the subnormal's long-term interests. It is equally impossible to say at what point the concentration of the family on the needs of the subnormal becomes a matter for concern and imperils the well-being of the family. Furthermore, it is necessary to state loud and clear that many of these parents had been left in a psychologically difficult, if not entirely hopeless, position in which they were simply not given the help they required.

Though it is not possible to indicate at what point giving the subnormal a valued role in the family topples into the subnormal becoming an object of the mother's emotional needs, it is possible to show some families where the role of the subnormal and the relationship within the family appeared more creative.

One aspect of such families appeared to be the ability to keep a certain emotional distance from the subnormal. Rejection was no part of this, rather could the attitude be described as loving exasperation with the subnormal instead of submissive acceptance. One father said: 'These people are pests in the nicest sense.' A similar viewpoint seemed evident from the severely disabled Patricia's father: 'Another thing we find frustrating is lack of speed, for instance coming downstairs. Well, it's sort of a choice between saying "come along sweetheart" or "get a move on" and you've got to make it work out to be "come along sweetheart".'

In two families in particular the presence of a younger daughter, in both cases still under sixteen, appeared to be a considerable help. In one of these, the daughter was nine years younger than Henry, the very severely disabled subnormal. The mother remarked:

'You know, if I could have had my time again I'd have had a family I think. When we had Henry it kind of put us off. He was nine when my daughter was born. She is such good company, and she brings such a lot of good company in that I wish I had a bigger family. For her sake, for my daughter's rather than Henry's. We try and keep things as normal as possible for my daughter. She has always had to come second . . . but she's never grumbled over it, never.'

The family of Joyce shows the difficulty of illustrating the well-integrated attitude to the subnormal, because this is linked so closely with the relationships with the wider family and the neighbourhood. A brief description of the relationships of Joyce and her mother with their wider family and friends was given on page 201, as an example of a family which was not turned in on itself and the subnormal. The point is closely akin to the one made about communication. Communication with the very severely disabled was only possible in terms of relationships: so the attitude of the family, where the family had refused to turn in on itself, can only be expressed properly in terms of the family's relationship with the wider family, neighbours and friends. For this reason a proper consideration of this must be left until these relationships are discussed in chapter 17.

Where the subnormal had become the centre of the family to the exclusion of all else, it has been possible to define his or her role. Where this has not happened, the subnormal's role can only be described in terms of the wider relationships. There was one characteristic which was common to the better-integrated families. It took many different forms. This could be described as an openness which contrasts with the closed attitude of families at the other end of the scale. Elizabeth Bott, in an extra chapter called 'Reconsiderations' in the second edition of her book *Family and Social Network* (1971, p. 248), quotes C. C. Harris's comment on her original book. Harris says: 'Perhaps the really lasting significance of Bott's study is that she has made impossible the proliferation of studies of the internal structure of the family which takes no account of its social environment.' It is the 'social environment' of the more 'open' families which has to be considered to make sense of the role the subnormal had in the family.

There are two additional points to be made. First, the primacy of the mother's or parent's attitude was very obvious. The more closed families tended to have severely limited contacts with family or neighbours. To discuss these limited contacts without considering the parents' attitude is meaningless. The second point is connected closely. Sometimes the family of the subnormal feels stigmatized by the subnormal's defect and withdraws from society. This too is best considered in the wider context of the general attitudes of society and relations with neighbours, and will be referred to in chapter 17.

With one partial exception all these families were looking after their subnormal because they wanted to. The difficulties that all of them had encountered to some extent, and with which they had coped in differing ways, were essentially the perils of loving a person, but in their case the already considerable perils of loving someone were compounded by the fact that that person was severely subnormal and often multiply handicapped. To end this section here is the splendid assertion of the mother of Amy, a severely handicapped woman of fifty-nine. The mother had looked after Amy all her life and was ninety-one years old at the time of the interview. She was asked if she ever left Amy alone in a room, but she evidently thought the question was about leaving Amy for good, and she retorted: 'No, and I never will while I live and I never have done and I never shall do and I like a drink of beer, I've always had a drink and I shall always have it while I live . . . it's that as keeps me going.'

The long-term effect on the family

A clear distinction must be made between the family being completely bound up in the subnormal and the family being organized to cope with the needs of the subnormal. The two are very different. Good organization and attitudes from the other members of the family can mean that the family is not so turned in on the subnormal. For instance, David's mother said about mealtimes: 'We have a system and everybody falls in with that system.' The families had been living with their subnormal for so long that their system for coping had become part of their lives. 'We've just organized things, we've lived together until we just blend.'

This definition needs to be set against the rest of the chapter. It was evident in families where the attitudes of the parents seemed rather strange, as well as in families where the attitudes seemed very sound, that they had lived together until they had blended. Whatever research workers or social workers might think about their attitudes and the awful things they were doing to the subnormal's psyche, the state of affairs had persisted so long that they had generally reached a way of life which they found tolerable. As David's mother put it: 'Twenty-two years you've got yourself into a way of life, you don't stop and think about it, it's there and you do it.'

15 The daily grind

When the mother wakes up in the morning what prospect does she face? What is she going to have to do before she goes to bed in the evening? What are the problems of everyday living with which she has to contend?

The daily routine

Sleep First of all, how much sleep have the subnormal and she and her husband had? In half the families (twenty-six) the subnormal did not disturb the family's sleep at all. Of the rest, seventeen found this was a lesser problem, and ten a marked problem.

In the case of Trevor, a moderately handicapped man in his middle twenties, he did not disturb their sleep very much: 'Well, sometimes he has a little nightmare and jumps out of bed. It doesn't happen very often, but he's scared of sleeping on his own.' This problem has been solved, but at a price.

'He won't stop in bed, he is in and out of bed all night, so he's been sleeping with my husband, and I sleep in his bed. It's no good us all being disturbed. We let him do that. It's better like that.' Interviewer: Does this mean that when your husband sleeps with him you do get a decent night's sleep? 'Yes.' Interviewer: But if he doesn't sleep with him you don't. 'No.'

Quite a few families dealt with problems of sleep by the subnormal sleeping in the same room, and occasionally in the same bed, as the mother. Twenty-three of the subnormals shared a bedroom, but in some cases it was with a brother or sister. The widowed mother of one very severely disabled girl shared a bed with her daughter.

'With me waking up when she used to have fits, I've never got into habit [of sleeping]. I can't go to bed and wake up next thing and it's morning. Sometimes she gets a bit of cramp and I have to rub her leg.'

The mother of another very severely disabled girl adopted a similar strategy, though she did not actually sleep in the same bed. She too was a widow.

All these cases were considered to be lesser problems, but the first one was considered a resolved problem because his parents no longer lost much sleep. The latter two were considered unresolved problems because the mother's sleep was still broken. The distinction is not always very clear but it is one which is worth trying to make. The problem seemed clearly resolved in the case of the severely handicapped Jennifer.

'She used to disturb my sleep when she had fits. I went through a terrible time with her. But now she goes to the toilet, I've lost my hearing a little and I couldn't always hear her. The difficulty is that when she gets into bed sometimes, she wouldn't cover herself up properly, so I had a buzzer made so that, when I turn it on in my bedroom, when she opens the bathroom door the buzzer goes off by my head, then I can go and attend to her.' Interviewer: Are you buzzed quite often at night? 'She always gets up at night.' Interviewer: So your sleep is always disturbed at least once? 'Yes, but I'm quite used to it, so I wouldn't say my sleep is disturbed unduly.'

The distinction between a resolved and an unresolved problem is made on figure 13 by an oblique line across the one or two crosses representing a lesser or marked problem. A single cross by itself indicates a lesser unresolved problem; with a line through it it represents a lesser resolved problem. Sleep is line 12 on the diagram, in the section on 'The Daily Grind'. Eight of the lesser problems were resolved and nine unresolved.

If the problem was a marked one it was much less likely to be resolved. In only one case out of the ten where sleep was a marked problem could it be described as resolved. It could be a serious problem, as the following examples show. In both cases the question was: Does he or she disturb the sleep of the family?

Lilian was a very severely disabled woman in her late twenties:

'Mind you she is wonderful now, you should have come a few years ago. She used to go three days and nights without sleep, sleep a couple of hours, and then go another three days and nights without sleep, she never stopped crying from morning to night. She didn't cry with tears, it was just one continual noise, she does sleep better at night than what she used to do.' Interviewer: What is her sleep like now? 'She takes a long time to settle down, and she soon wakes up.' [At this point Lilian made a horrible noise, a sort of howl and yell.] Interviewer: Do you get a lot of that noise at night? Father: 'Last night when I went up to bed, she went to bed just before me, and she started off like that.' Interviewer: And how long can that go on for? 'Oh it can go on for two or three hours.' Interviewer: So she does disturb your sleep quite a bit? 'Well, I'm used to it so it doesn't bother me. There's another thing, you can't turn over in bed, you can't blow your nose, you can't sneeze, or straight away she is doing this [making a noise and getting out of bed]. We've got used to it so we don't notice it. There are lots of things that you just accept, whether anybody else could accept it I don't know.'

Judith was a very severely disabled woman in her twenties:

'Oh yes, she does, some nights you know; she can go for three nights and never sleep.' Interviewer: Does she have fits in the night? 'Yes, well, we jump up, you can't do anything but she could vomit, and she may be lying face down and could suffocate. She always wakes us up when she has a fit. She very rarely has small fits now, they're nearly always the big, terrible ones, and this is when she interferes with our sleep.' Interviewer: How often does she have these fits? 'About one a week, sometimes three or four times a week, and it changes her whole personality, you know, and she can sit up all night and all day and all night and all day again, it's unbelievable the sleep she can do without, and I just don't know what to do. I give her anadins and indigestion medicine, it worries you, you don't sleep as content.'

Judith's parents had been helped considerably by the provision of a cot bed:

'She has a hospital bed now. Before she had a hospital bed she had a divan, she could get out of that divan herself, straight to the door, and that great thing I taught her of opening a door, she could open her own bedroom door. Years ago, before we had this hospital bed, I don't think we had three nights' sleep a week through the night, because she used to get out of the divan when she was fed-up and she used to go to the gate (at the top of the stairs) and rattle it, and she wanted to go to the toilet, not to wet, and about three years since something went to my brain and it said "why don't you get her a bed with sides on?", she was sending us barmy you know, and I wrote to the welfare officer and asked if I could have a bed, and they came to see me and that was the time that I got these papers [incontinence pads]. It dawned on me that we might get a good night's sleep because it used to look as though a bomb had dropped on her bedroom. Perhaps she'd have wet on the carpet as she got out and all like that, anything could happen. It was through me enquiring about the bed that I got these papers, I'd never heard about them, it's wonderful Sheffield, the Health Department, I've not asked for a lot but what I have asked for, you know, a chair, I've been quite satisfied.'

The value of such help as a cot bed and incontinence pads was immense. Incontinence pads were mentioned as a great blessing by several parents.

Getting the subnormal up.   However the mother had slept, she still had to get the subnormal up. Judith's mother found this very trying:

'That is my worst part of the day, that's my biggest problem. If I could just walk down and get my breakfast ready, but there's Judith. Usually she's wet and I can't come downstairs without changing her. That is my biggest problem, because I feel washed out, if I could just walk downstairs and have a cup of tea, that is my biggest problem, because I do have to do little bits at night when they go to bed. I do like to keep things a bit tidy, so if I can't do things in the day with Judith, when she's upset, I do them at night, and lots of times I don't get to bed while about twelve o'clock, I'm soft really then I'm absolutely jiggered in the morning.'

This was considered a marked unresolved problem. Problems in getting the subnormal up are shown on line 13 of figure 13. The figures are shown in table 15.1.

Table 15.1   Getting up

No problem	28
Lesser resolved problem	11
Lesser unresolved problem	4
Marked resolved problem	5
Marked unresolved problem	5
Total	53

In quite a few cases the mother left the subnormal in bed in order to have a bit of time to herself. The mother of the moderately handicapped Philip said:

> 'He does like his sleep out. I do find it's better to let him have
> it because he is more relaxed. He can become a bit tiresome
> if he is tired.' Interviewer: Do you sometimes leave him in bed
> in the morning? 'Yes, I do, and I get on with my work and then
> get him up. He likes a good ten hours' sleep.'

There was no problem there.

Nor was there any problem with Norman, a moderately handicapped man in his fifties. His aunt said: 'He doesn't get up while about half past ten because doctor said it would always do him good to have plenty of rest. Well, that gives me a chance to get biggest part of my work done.'

Slowness was one of the problems. 'We don't rush her,' said the mother of Norma, a severely handicapped woman in her late twenties, 'she is slow and she is put about if we hurry her, she is soon upset, kind of thing, she works up you see, she is soon very upset.' This problem was often solved by simply letting the subnormal get up or getting him up in slow time.

If the subnormal was attending training centre, however, it could be a source of difficulty. The mother of a moderately handicapped young man who attended training centre said: 'Oh, I do have difficulties, yes. If his dad has forgotten to tell him the time before he goes out of the house it's a tremendous job. You can sit on his bed for quarter of an hour trying to get him up.' This was considered a lesser unresolved problem. Such problems are not peculiar to the mentally subnormal but their handicap, even with the less severely disabled, did add another dimension. This was apparent with Trevor:

> Interviewer: On an ordinary weekday morning, is the problem
> simply that it is very difficult to get him out of bed? 'Yes.'
> Interviewer: What do you do about this? 'Well, I have to
> threaten to get the belt on, but you see, he can set about me
> now, he's a man and he's quite strong, and he has set about
> me.' Interviewer: Recently? 'Yes, he gets hold of me and squeezes
> me, I get terrible bruises. The other week he got hold of my
> hands and he was biting me, and I had to hit him in the face
> to make him stop. After that, when he comes round, he's all

right, it's just like a brain storm.' Interviewer: Does it happen almost every morning? 'Well, twice up to now this week, and Tuesday morning I had a job getting him off the toilet. He was on from half past seven while eight o'clock, and I said, "Oh, come on Trevor, you'll have to get up." Ten past eight and I reckon I'd fetch belt and set about him, but I can't you see, there's not much room in the bathroom, you've no room to get out of the way, so I don't really dare say much to him. Anyway, he got up.'

This was coded a marked unresolved problem. In at least three cases, one of them in the pilot, the subnormal had stopped attending training centre because of the difficulty of getting him or her up in the morning.

Among the more severely disabled the problem was a more physical one of lifting, holding, washing and dressing an adult who could do very little for himself. This was the case with Judith, who was mentioned at the beginning of this section.

In the case of the totally disabled Terence, although everything had to be done for him, there were really no problems:

'My sister next door comes in and gives him a good bed bath, he is stripped and washed all over, that's her job for him. She is finished then and I feed him and give him his tablets. She's always in and out you know.' Interviewer: How do you get him downstairs? 'We carry him down, I don't think he'd be above two and a half stone.'

But lifting and stairs were often a problem. The very severely disabled Henry's mother said:

'Well, I get him up in the morning because his dad goes just gone seven.' Interviewer: Is this quite a strain? 'Well he has to be lifted downstairs. I can manage it, well I've managed it up to now.' Interviewer: Does he help you at all? 'No, I just carry him. I'm always glad when we get to the bottom of the stairs.'

The mother of the severely disabled Amy admitted:

'Well, I have to take my own time to tell you the truth. I have to wash and dress her. I like a good hour. If I have my own time I am not breathless. I am getting a bit short of breath now you see.'

This was hardly surprising because the mother, whose forthright views have been quoted already (on page 206), was ninety-one. Interviewer: But don't you find this a problem? 'No, no, it's just routine.' In spite of the calmness with which Amy's mother coped with the situation, old age and increasing feebleness were often a source of anxiety and physical strain.

The process of getting the subnormal up was a part of the routine which threw a heavy strain on the parents, in particular the older ones, and especially if the subnormal was severely disabled. One aspect of this which was often mentioned was the difficulty of carrying the subnormal up and down stairs. The efforts that Judith's mother was prepared to make to train her to come downstairs have been mentioned already. In two pilot visits the problem had been solved in one case by leaving the subnormal upstairs, where she was rather isolated, and in the other by her sleeping in the sitting room, where her parents could never get away from her. In this second instance the mother's back had been affected by lifting her daughter and she had to wear a surgical corset.

The help of the father could be important in this respect. In one case in the pilot study, the father had got a job where he was permanently on the night shift so that he was always available to do all the lifting involved in getting up and putting to bed his almost totally disabled son. But getting the subnormal up in the morning was a job which generally fell to the mother. In only three cases did the father get the subnormal up; in one instance it was a joint operation, in two further cases some other relative got the subnormal up and in thirty-three cases it was the mother's job. Fourteen of the subnormals got themselves up.

Putting the subnormal to bed   The problems were very similar to those of getting up. It was sometimes a little more difficult because the subnormal generally had to be taken upstairs. In the case of Judith, her mother could get her downstairs but she needed her husband's help to get her upstairs. This was often the case.

> 'If his dad wasn't here I don't know what I should do. He [his father] goes out once a fortnight at night with a friend; Henry was asleep on the hearthrug and I was tired, but I couldn't go to bed until his dad came in for getting him upstairs.'

The help of the father was often essential for getting the subnormal upstairs to bed. It was frequently a combined operation. 'No, her dad helps me with getting her upstairs.' 'Only my wife and I can manage her upstairs.'

Where there was no father, a friend or relative occasionally came in to help. In one case it was a friend, in another a son (if he did not come, the seventy-one-year-old mother carried her daughter into the bedroom herself) and in another a brother-in-law.

In one case handrails had made the difference. 'We don't have any difficulty now. We used to have, what with pushing him up the stairs. Climbing with one handrail he couldn't manage. Now we've got two handrails, he's up in no time.'

There were also some problems where the subnormal would not go to bed. One or two would not go to bed until the television programmes finished completely. Indeed the period that one severely disabled young man was up appeared to be related not to the sun but to the television programmes. It was quite common for the subnormal to go to bed at the same time as his parents. One very severely disabled young woman insisted on her mother doing so.

Bathing   Bathing presented similar problems to those encountered in getting up and putting to bed, and they were almost entirely with the severely disabled. If the mother was on her own, bathing was often a difficult operation. 'It takes me three-quarters of an hour. I generally wash her hair and sponge her legs, and then about once a month I give her a full leg bath, it is a problem that.' In one case it was the father's job.

'I've bathed her for years. Some little time ago I was finding it difficult lifting her from the bath . . . then one morning I tried a new technique of getting her out of the bath, I simply drag her up the side of the bath, in other words the bath is taking part of the weight. You see she is no help at all.'

The father was seventy-five years old.

Where the subnormal was as disabled as this, the mother generally had help with lifting, from the father or occasionally a relative or friend. It is not difficult to see why this was necessary with the very disabled James.

'This is a two-person job. He doesn't get bathed all that regularly, he'll get washed down stood up, but to go and sit in a bath requires two of us and he's very awkward to get out. He is scared very easily. If his foot slips it will take him ten minutes to get into the mood again to get out. He is a big lad, he must weigh thirteen stone.'

Three cases are of particular interest. The first is Joyce. She was difficult to bath.

'We were once bathing her and she twisted, and water went in her mouth, well if we hadn't been there she would have drowned. She hadn't the sense just to turn her head and put her head up, and there were two adults in bathroom with her. After that we bought one of them bathmats with suction pads at the bottom, which does stop that slipping about.'

Her mother had the help of her sister-in-law once a week but, even with the two of them, carrying Joyce through to the bathroom was difficult and her mother considered this her main problem.

'Well it's that bath. Myself I think if there were a home help, even if it were only once a week, to come to see to those main things. . . . I mean you can bed-bath them but it is not the same as them laying in a bath. . . . You know what these ambulance men use, a chair on wheels, well she's got an ordinary wheelchair, but we were saying if we got one of them, two would be able to carry her downstairs [to the bathroom which was downstairs] on one of them. Mrs next door would come in perhaps, or sister-in-law; at the moment one has to get hold of her legs and the other of her arms sort of thing. With that we'd be able to put bathtowel straight on chair and wheel her straight to bath, and it would save a lot of heavy lifting and it would be more comfortable for Joyce, but I haven't heard anything. Social welfare woman at hospital did her utmost to try and get me one. She said, well it had finished with her now and it rested with Mr Grinton [the mental welfare officer], and from there it went to somebody else, but we still didn't get it.'

Judith's mother had had some help with bathing but it had not been very successful so she was back to relying on her husband.

'Oh, that's a problem these last two years, just that getting older business. I did have a nurse to help me periodically, but the nurse could never keep a proper time, or perhaps I'd have the nurse come in the morning which was all right, but it got that nurse came afternoons. Well it were harder work waiting for the

nurse than me bathing her, so we had to squash it.'
Interviewer: So you bath her? 'Yes, I bath her, but what I do,
I always bath her when it's nearly time for her dad to come
home from work. I can put her in all right, I can bath her and
wash her hair, it's getting her out, drying her. She is fighting
you, you see, she's struggling, she's a big girl, she is about
eight stone, she doesn't stand still for you to wipe her, so we
work it now that she either gets bathed on a Sunday when he is
at home—she only gets bathed once a week now—or Friday
night, as the car draws up she is all ready to come out, and he
helps me. Because I haven't the energy to go back and wash
bath out, I used to be so exhausted, he washes bath out, so we
work it like that now.'

However in the case of Christine a bath attendant came once a
fortnight and this was much appreciated.

'Oh yes, she loves to get bathed, she loves the water, but we
have to lift her in and out you see, it's hard work, and we got a
high bath as well.' Interviewer: You have to lift her in and out?
'Yes, me and the bath attendant, she comes once a fortnight,
we have to manage the other week.' Interviewer: How do you
manage? 'Well, it's not fair to Christine I think, I give her a
good wash down, and I get her feet in water, and wash her
legs and feet well, we've got to manage like that. It's not the
same as having a nice bath, is it? The bath attendant is a
very capable lady.'

A little later on she said: 'If she likes people she'll give them something of hers. She's got to know Mrs Middleton, the bath attendant.
She'll give something to Mrs Middleton. She sort of got trust in her
now.'
Joyce's mother had never heard of a bath attendant. It was clear
that help of this kind would have been much valued by several families.

Housework Three specific questions were asked about this—whether
the mother had any difficulty with cooking meals, cleaning the house,
or doing the washing. The only one which posed problems to many
families was cooking meals, and even here only ten reported any
problems, and six of these were considered lesser resolved problems.
   In only one instance was the problem serious. The very severely
disabled Lilian's mother said:

'It's a fight when you want to bake, it's a fight to keep a lid on a saucepan, if you didn't watch it she'd try to grab things out of saucepan, she can't resist saucepans.' Interviewer: How do do you deal with this? 'We have to keep our eye on her the whole time. If I want to go upstairs and left anything on stove, I put that latch on [a latch high up on the door].'

For most of the other mothers the problem was the one common to mothers of small children of having them in the kitchen and under their feet while they were cooking, but they were not small children, they were large adults. The problems arose generally from the subnormal wanting to be in his mother's company. 'I just have to put her in a chair and put a strap round her, you know, in case she gets up quickly. Occasionally we do a lot of baking with her like this, holding my arm, because she likes to watch you see.' And similarly: 'It's a little difficult sometimes. It's only a small kitchen you know; she overpowers you a little bit because she likes to be there.' In both cases this was considered a lesser resolved problem.

The effect of the undramatic but persistent fact of the subnormal's presence was obvious in the case of one mildly disabled but rather awkward young man. The question was: Do you find that having him around makes cooking difficult?

'Oh yes, because he never stops talking, never ever. He even goes to bed talking, he goes to sleep talking to himself.' Interviewer: Does that mean you do most of the cooking when he isn't there? 'No, but it means I have to persevere and keep on saying, "go and look at the television", or I have to bring him up and sit him down. But I have to persevere with him and do it in between, you have to have patience, sometimes it runs out but there it is.' Interviewer: It is quite a problem then? 'It is a big problem, yes.'

Here the problem was considered lesser but unresolved. In three cases the subnormal actually helped with the cooking. Betty was only mildly disabled. She was in the pilot group.

'She will lay the table, and when we've done, or just before we've done, she is clearing the table. Tell her what to do and she'll help. She is very good help for that.'

Cleaning the house presented hardly any difficulties. This was often because the mother had got things organized, like Violet's

mother. 'Well I have a method you see. If I don't get it all done at
night-time, I leave her in bed until I have done the remainder, and
then I get her up and she can have all my attention.' But it is worth
noting that, in this and other cases, the lack of problems was bought
at a price, namely that of having to do the housework in the evenings.
Christine's mother lost part of her one valuable free day when
Christine attended a day centre. 'Well, I have a struggle with the
bedrooms because I have to come back on Wednesdays and tidy her
bedroom up, because I can't leave her you see. She doesn't like
stopping in here [the sitting room] without me long.' Julian's mother
gave the bedrooms a good clean when he was in short-term care
because he made cleaning awkward when he was at home.

Some mothers also had unusual problems to contend with, for
instance, having to watch that the subnormal did not bite the flex of
the Hoover. But generally this was not a problem and nine of the
subnormals helped with the cleaning. Naturally those who helped
were the least handicapped.

The amount of washing to be done depended very largely on
whether the subnormal was incontinent or not. Thirty of the fifty-
three were continent, though seven did need help; ten either wet their
beds or had occasional accidents; three had no bladder control and
ten were totally incontinent. The most important help here was
naturally a washing machine. Table 15.2 divides the problems
according to whether the family had a washing machine or not.

Table 15.2   Problems with washing

	Washing machine	No washing machine
No problems	25	2
Lesser resolved	11	4
Lesser unresolved	1	0
Marked resolved	6	2
Marked unresolved	0	2
Total	43	10

As might be expected, the only major unresolved problems with
washing were where there was no washing machine. The answers to
this question illustrated graphically the way these mothers just got
on with the job, and the way they had organized their lives in order
to cope.

Bernard was totally incontinent:

'Well, I have to wash every day for him.' Interviewer: Do you find there is any problem doing it? 'Well, some days I get real fed up with doing it. But I try to tackle it and think, it's a job that's got to be done, so don't moan about it.'

Richard was also totally incontinent and his mother had a lot of washing to do as a result. She had no washing machine and no running hot water. The gas geyser was broken and she could not afford to have it mended. She took the sheets and large things to the launderette once a week, but this cost her fifty pence, which was quite a proportion of her weekly income (£8.90). However, she appeared to take these problems in her stride.

The attitude of the mothers to this time-consuming and rather disagreeable chore was well summed up by one mother in the pilot survey: 'I have a washing machine; it's no trouble, I don't let it bother me.'

Meals   There were two aspects to meals. First, there was the actual process of feeding the subnormal. Sometimes this was difficult and took up a lot of the mother's time. Second, there was the subnormal's behaviour at meals. One important feature of this was whether it affected the possibility of his parents taking him out for meals. At the moment it is the first aspect with which we are concerned. The second will be considered later.

This first aspect was important mainly for the fifteen who could not feed themselves at all. The business of feeding the subnormal added to the jobs to be done and the time taken in caring for the subnormal, even if it presented no real problems. This was evident in the case of David.

'Oh no, we have a system, and everybody falls in with that system. We three, my husband, Pamela [David's younger sister] and I, have ours first, and David's is kept on a warm plate. When we have finished everybody else gets on with what they're doing and I give David his, and he is happy with this situation. You see it takes a little bit longer for David to eat his, so therefore I think I might as well get on with mine while it's hot because he can't eat his as hot as we do, so there's time to get the temperature right. No, we don't have any problems at mealtimes.'

Later on, David's father said how nice it was for his wife when David was away in short-term care, and she did not have to spend quarter of an hour to twenty minutes after every meal feeding him.

Slowness in feeding was sometimes a problem and in a few cases the subnormal was thoroughly awkward, like the very severely handicapped Sybil.

'She is very fussy. If you go to give her something she'll lift her hand up and push you away with her hand, and if you've got rice pudding or Weetabix you've got it all down you before you know where you are, she'll only have what she thinks she'll have.'

Problems of feeding the subnormal were generally absorbed into the routine of the household. Some of the answers told one a good deal about the way the household was organized. One mother, when asked if her daughter's behaviour at mealtimes presented difficulties, said: 'Well, it doesn't, because I am used to it. To me with her being like that, she always comes first. I always feed her. I should say the house revolves around her.' The more serious effect of the way the subnormal behaved at meals on the social life of the family is discussed later on.

Shopping 'You're forced to have food, aren't you?' as one of the mothers said. This was a potential problem for every family. Where the subnormal was mildly handicapped it was much less of a problem, and two of them could actually help with the shopping if they were sent with a list to a shop where they were known.

For the rest, there were various ways in which the shopping was managed. If the subnormal went to training centre this generally solved the problem. Seventeen did so, but they were the less handicapped, and therefore these were the families which were least likely to have problems with shopping anyhow.

A further six received some form of care one or two days a week. All of these subnormals were quite seriously handicapped, and this assistance gave the mothers their main or only opportunity for shopping during the week.

All these mothers had long enough to do both local day-to-day shopping and also more major shopping in the centre of town, though the irregularity of the time at which the ambulance returned sometimes meant a scramble to get back for it. For the other families these two different types of shopping demanded different tactics. Day-to-day shopping was most often done by slipping out of the house for up to half an hour and leaving the subnormal alone, often in bed. The distance from the shops was important. In this respect the mother of the very severely disabled Richard was lucky. She did not take him shopping because he would not go inside the shops and the road was busy. But the shops were only about twenty-five yards away and she could slip out and leave him for five minutes, or if he was in the yard the neighbours would keep an eye on him for the few minutes she was out.

Richard's mother was a widow. So was Gerard's (pilot), who said: 'Well, I only shop at the stores across the road, and I lock Gerard in the house.' Christine's widowed mother had found herself in some difficulty after Christine had been in hospital for a spell of short-term care.

'I used to get up about eight o'clock and leave Christine in bed until about half past nine, and dash off to the shops. They're only just here at the corner. I used to just dash there and back and get her up, but now she is awake, she's sat up and waiting to get up at half past six, so it's a bit of a problem now.'

It was widows especially who tended to have difficulty over shopping. Susan's mother was seventy-one and she had to rely entirely on her daughters and friends.

'There are no shops near. I have to depend on other people.' Interviewer: And you can't go out by yourself at all? How do you manage? 'My daughter has been this morning, she brought me some bits. My friend, she is bringing me some, I have another daughter that comes this evening, she'll bring me bits in. Otherwise I can't get to the shops. You see, wherever I go it's a hill.'

If the father was alive the family was in a much better position, especially if they had a car as well.

'No, my husband and I co-operate between the two of us. He does the weekend shopping Saturdays, and I fiddle about during the week sort of thing, popping out for short periods while David stays at home. Pamela [her young daughter] did the shopping today. The shops are very close, and I do most of the day-to-day shopping in the immediate vicinity, that's the normal

weekly routine. If I go to Cockaynes [a department store in the
city centre], it is usually a Saturday afternoon, and I go to the
market while I am in town. My husband is at home, you see,
on Saturday afternoon, so there is really no problem.'

'Well I go before he gets up, luckily he'll stay in bed you see.
I've got a bolt on the bedroom door and I lock him in the
bedroom. I go out as soon as the shops open about nine o'clock,
and the main shopping I do on Saturday when my husband is
at home.'

Shopping was often quite an elaborate arrangement, which had
been working for some years.

'I catch the ten minutes to two bus on Tuesdays, and I'm back
for ten minutes to three. Well, with my husband running around
he usually pops home at half past two to see if he is all right.
Then I don't go shopping any more until Friday morning.
Well, his father takes him. He comes at ten o'clock and takes
him Friday morning. It's quite all right with the firm, they know
that he takes him whilst I go and do the weekend shopping.
He's done that for years. That's the only day when my
husband comes home to lunch. So I can stay out from ten
o'clock until half past two. . . . I shop from Friday up to
Tuesday, and then from Tuesday up to Friday.'

Husbands, daughters, sons, neighbours, all helped. Most commonly it was the husband who had a very definite role in getting
the shopping done. In three cases where the father was either retired
or off sick for a long period, he was largely responsible for the
shopping, and there was no problem. Amy's mother, the ninety-one-
year-old, managed with her home help (nine hours a week) and
tradesmen calling. 'She [home help] goes to shops for me. And they
all come to door—breadman, coalman, 'taterman, milkman. They
all come and Amy knows 'em all 'cause she points through
winder.'

However, where the subnormal was severely disabled, just popping
out to the shops for the day-to-day shopping was often difficult, and
leaving him or her a source of some anxiety. A refrigerator helped
in some cases, but this could only reduce the problem, not solve it.
Judith's mother shows the problems and difficulties that can attend
even such an apparently simple aspect of living as 'popping out to
the shops'.

'Well I have to go when she's in bed . . . usually I only go twice a week, you're forced to organize it, especially when Judith's got her off days and she may have a fit. It's a major operations going just to the shops some days.'

Keeping the subnormal occupied　This was not a major problem in many cases. Thirty-nine of the fifty-three reported no problem. In some cases the subnormal was incapable of doing very much. He was occupied or kept himself occupied in a variety of ways.

The mother of the very severely disabled Violet did not find this a problem.

'No, because I talk to her and she'll listen. And also I can kind of read her, you know I can read the expression in her eyes.' Interviewer: What does she do? 'Well she'll generally just sit in chair, and she watches whatever you're doing until time comes for the television or we'll have music from wireless. When it's nice I'll take her outside and give her a walk outdoors round the garden and watch flowers and everything. She's quite content.'

The sister of the almost as severely disabled Jennifer also found keeping her occupied no problem.

'That is her occupation, having the book. I buy her a book every week, and she has a packet of envelopes and she loves to put these scribbles into envelopes and call those her letters. That's her delight. Also she looks at books and of course television occupies her all evening. She keeps herself happy, I wouldn't say occupied because she does so very little, but she is quite happy.'

For the more active subnormals a garden, especially a confined one in which they could be allowed out alone, was a great help. It was with Helen, who was always on the go. 'She amuses herself. She just wanders round the garden all day. The neighbour at the bottom is very good to her and they all know her you see.'

Some of the mildly disabled were capable of doing a good deal more. Ernest is one example of this.

'He seems to occupy himself a lot. He goes out, and he might make a run for his tortoise. He used to have rabbits, he always used to be busy messing about making rabbit hutches or knocking things together. Now he's got his dog, and he takes him for a walk. He seems well occupied. He has a crayoning book and jigsaw puzzles. He seems pretty contented.'

A very few of these more able subnormals presented a problem if they went out by themselves. Ernest was one of these.

'He doesn't get into trouble, but we do get these children on the road that call after him which makes it very difficult for him really, because if he says anything to the children they go home and tell their mothers, and then they're down at my dad's to see what he's been shouting for. They never think their own children will call them.'

Julian's main handicap was his epilepsy. He could go out by himself, and this had been a source of difficulty.

'Well, he only goes a little bit round about, round the block or so, and he can go to his cousin's about five minutes' walk away.' Interviewer: Does he ever get into trouble when he goes out by himself? 'No, not really, unless he gets mixed up with these youths. Luckily it was only once this year that we had a little bit of trouble.' Interviewer: What happens? Do they bait him? 'You see, they get the girls with them, and they teach him all this he shouldn't know—well I'm not saying he shouldn't know—but everything's on you know. They are sitting back thinking of being entertained, and the old lady put me wise. Round the back of the pub it's pretty dark, and you see Julian will do anything for anybody as long as they'll be friends . . . and so they egg him on to do things, it's very rare he is out after dark. You see if he got with them and. . . . Well I'd look such a fool you know going round there. He'll say, "I'm not coming, and that's that" and they all grin and so forth. So I ask him two or three times, and then father has to go, and I say, "Oh well, I'm sending your dad", and probably by the time he's got round one way they've egged him on to go home the other way, so they won't get caught, but we've a good idea who they are. It's just catching them red-handed. At one period he would say they were taking his money off him.'

But this only affected a small minority of the families. There were two instances of marked unresolved problems and three of lesser unresolved problems (such as the two examples given). Most of the subnormals were unable to go out by themselves. For many of them the problem was not what they did do but what they did not do. The mother of the moderately disabled Bridget said:

'Well, that is a problem love, trying to keep her occupied. She likes to do something and she knows she can't. I take her upstairs with me sometimes to dust, but she's sometimes not interested and she'll lay on the bed. That's the main thing though . . . you don't know what's in their mind or what's coming over them. But one thing that helps is that she goes and plays cards with an old lady across road every Monday afternoon.'

This was considered a lesser unresolved problem. There were three cases of this but there were eight cases where the problem was marked and unresolved. The problem was sometimes one of sheer boredom. The very severely disabled Henry's mother said:

'Yes, I feel for him, I think, "Oh he must be getting bored."' Interviewer: How does he occupy his time? 'He can't do anything. He looks at my club book, apart from that he's nothing he can do really, he can't use his hands enough; he'll look at the television and enjoy it. Even when he went to the day nursery he didn't do anything.'

With the very over-active Lilian the problem was more pressing.

'She won't take any notice or anything.' Interviewer: How does she occupy her time? 'Just by being a nuisance to herself. Sometimes she'll pull her hair out, gripping her neck.' Interviewer: Does she like playing with water? 'If I'm washing she likes them suds and that.' Interviewer: Will this keep her occupied for any length of time? 'Oh no, just a moment, that's all. When my daughter is home we have teddybears and dolls and all sorts out, but she is not interested. For the most part she occupies herself sitting down and wandering around. She is always looking for something to eat like, she'll go and pinch dog's dinner if you don't watch her. I have seen her pinch bone off dog.'

Those who were over-active and demanding were particularly difficult to live with. James was in short-term care at the time of the interview, which is why his father is talking of the past.

'He wanted your full-time attention.' Interviewer: So whatever
you're doing . . . 'He'd want to be there. He didn't want to join
in, he wanted you to take notice of him and do what he wanted.
He would bring you things. He had some tins which he played
with, he would thrust these at you and collect them round you,
and you'd find that if you were sat here reading, by the time
you had finished you were surrounded by things which he had
brought.' Interviewer: And he wouldn't do anything by himself?
'Nothing at all.'

Julian presented a rather similar problem.

'Yes, he likes a change often, he'll have a good play with his
records, but I've got to be part of this: "Listen to me and my
records." He likes looking at books and motorcar books, he's
piles and piles of these motorcar journals, but then "Read what
it tells me about it." He always likes to be near me, to be in
conversation with me. He's always at the back of me, whatever
you're doing you turn round and . . . but if you're feeling a bit
low yourself and every time you turn round you bump into
somebody, it gets you all tense.'

Destructiveness was related, but only ten families felt this was a
problem, and it appeared to be resolved in five cases.

Those who were over-active and created the sort of difficulty
which has been illustrated were a small minority—there were only
eight cases where it was a serious problem. The larger problem is the
one of the subnormal being utterly bored and just vegetating. This
gives the subnormal little chance to develop what potential he has.
The role of training centres or day care is clearly critical here. Not
only does it make things much easier for the mother, but it is much
better for the subnormal. There were two cases of very severely disabled older subnormals who seemed quite intelligent, but they had
nothing to do and spent their days doing their best to annoy those
who were looking after them.

For the mother, too, a break is essential or the day can seem very
long. Christine's mother said: 'It's a very long day if you get up early.'
Stanley's mother said how, during the weekends, 'he sends me up
the wall'. Richard was very severely disabled. He had attended the
special care unit up to the age of sixteen, then he had had to leave. A
friend of his mother's called in near the end of the interview. She
summed up the position pretty accurately. 'Main problem is boredom

for Richard and monotony for her [his widowed mother]. You know it's never going to alter.'

A structure for coping

One of the problems in the interviews was that the parents had organized their lives round looking after their subnormal for so long that they were in many cases unaware of what they had done. In the description of the daily grind such phrases as, 'we've learnt to live with it after so many years' kept on recurring.

The way in which they coped was by evolving a routine. Sometimes that routine was very rigid, because this was the way the mother could cope best, or it was what the subnormal had come to expect, like the mildly handicapped Anthony (pilot).

> 'He is a creature of habit. Eight o'clock is his time in the
> evening for orange juice. He is not so fussy about breakfast
> time . . . but anything else, lunchtime, at the weekend, has to
> be at the right time. And his cup of tea and ginger biscuits—
> it has to be a ginger biscuit. And on Sundays he'll condescend
> to eat a piece of cake. Otherwise it's ginger biscuits, and on
> Wednesday morning he has a Kit Kat. That's because I used to
> go to the Post Office on Tuesday morning and I always brought
> him back a Kit Kat, that's from right when he was a tiny boy.
> And that was always on a Tuesday and he ate it on a
> Wednesday morning.'

On the other hand there were families which had evolved no less of a routine, but the keynote of it was its flexibility. The mother of the very severely disabled Ursula (pilot) kept on saying during the interview, 'We [Ursula and herself] please ourselves', and so they got up and had meals when they wanted to.

But whichever way it was the families had created a structure within which the family could cope with its subnormal member. His care was only possible within that structure, in the same way that the care of a baby or a small child is only really possible within a structure of routine. The description of 'the daily grind' of these families has shown some of the detailed ways in which these families dealt with the unavoidable tasks of everyday living.

If the subnormal can be seen as being cared for within a structure, it makes it easier to pick out the various forms of help which combined to create the structure within which the subnormal lived. This structure was generally based on continuing care by one person, normally the mother, though in a few cases this first-line care was shared completely by the parents; in one case the father was virtually in charge of the household.

On the base of the continuing care by this person it is possible to pick out three further elements from which this structure was made up. First, there were various devices employed by the family, such as putting a lock on the bedroom door; or having a padlock on the garden gate; or a particular technique for getting the subnormal out of the bath; or a way of getting the subnormal downstairs.

Second, and closely linked with this, were routines which involved the help of another person, often the husband. Many examples of such routines have been given, such as the father lifting the subnormal out of bed before he went to work; husbands or friends who carried the subnormal upstairs; sisters who helped with getting the subnormal up or bathing him; husbands, relatives or friends who helped with shopping.

Third, there was official help, ranging from the provision of incontinence pads to help with bathing, day care once or twice a week, or attendance at training centre.

The emphasis here is on structural help which relates to the daily or weekly routine. Because it is structural help it needs to be help which fits in with that structure. That means that it must be regular, reliable and punctual. The provision of incontinence pads, for instance, met this requirement, so did the training centres, but the help that Judith's mother was given with bathing did not (see page 216), while that which Christine's mother received did (page 217). The twice-weekly day care in hospital provided for Joyce did help, but its usefulness was reduced because the transport was not punctual. Help from neighbours often did not reach the level of structural help, for instance the neighbour who 'sometimes helps with shopping but not regular that you could rely on'. But a distinction needs to be made between neighbourly help, which is simply not structural, and official help, which is designed to be structural help but is provided in such a way that the families find it difficult to fit it into their routine.

Structural help must fit the routine of the families who are being helped. It is not the only type of help that is needed, but if adequate help, whatever its source, is not given at this level the family is unlikely to be able to cope and the subnormal will be admitted to hospital, or, in the likely event of no bed being available, the family's standard of living and quality of life suffers, sometimes seriously and irreparably.

The cost of keeping the structure intact

Financial   Lilian's parents had been given a car by their son, but could hardly afford the petrol to run it. There was no question of taking Lilian on a bus. Richard's mother could not afford to have her gas geyser repaired, even though this was her only source of running hot water.

Virtually all the families suffered to some extent financially, either because of the actual expense of looking after the subnormal or because of the fact that the mother could not work. No attempt was made to assess the families' financial position. They were simply asked: 'Do you feel you have suffered financially from keeping N at home?' Twenty-seven of the fifty-three reckoned that they had no financial problems, but this reflects *not* their financial position but what the mothers *felt* about it. One mother said: 'Well, I've never thought about it. I don't think we look at it quite like that.'

All the help that most of the families received (in summer 1970) was £4·90 supplementary benefit and, where they had enough money, £150 income tax relief for a dependent person. The expense could be considerable. Christine's mother was entirely dependent on social security payments.

> 'We just manage, we've got to be careful. Fuel is my big worry in winter because Christine feels the cold very much with having coeliac disease. I don't know how much it is now but they used to give us half a crown a week for fuel in winter.'

The brother-in-law of one of the people in the pilot study made the same point about fuel. 'There is an extra bedroom in use. Extra heating is needed. Two hundredweight of coke a week goes on the sitting room fire especially if she is ill.' In addition, his wife, the subnormal's sister, had had to give up her job in order to look after her.

The expense of clothes was often mentioned. Leonard's father mentioned this.

> 'Well, yes, they are heavy on clothes, they are heavy on shoes, they don't lift their feet up.'

Daniel's mother (pilot) made the same point. He was very severely disabled.

'Well, yes, with him creeping on floor, I'm forever buying him jeans, he doesn't wear them out only at the knees; you can see his shoe toes . . . they're good underneath, when he wears them out I just have to throw them away, that's all, I can't have them mended.'

The clothes themselves were sometimes more expensive. Helen's mother found this was the case.

'I pay more for her than I pay for my own, because I can't dress her in these silly teenagers' things. Being backward, she'd look silly, so I've got to go and pick the clothes and pay whatever price they say.'

In the case of Harold, a moderately handicapped young man, it was not just clothes.

'He is very heavy on clothes, shoes and that. I can't keep pace with him, and he eats a lot. He always wants biggest meal there is put out, he'll get through eight pounds of potatoes a day.'

Washing and the expense of incontinence was another problem. The provision of incontinence pads helped both practically and financially.

The expense could be more far-reaching than this. One father had had to refuse promotion because this would have meant having to move. A sister who was working had had to give up her car because of the expense of paying someone to look after her subnormal sister at home. Holidays tended to be more expensive. A few families had to hire a car because the subnormal could not travel in a train or coach. Helen's parents found they had to hire a large caravan.

When these families had so much to contend with, it seems unnecessary that they should have had to contend with the sort of thing that Christine's mother did.

'They only give me £4 18s. 0d. a week for her, and she is on a special diet. I've had to write to the Manager. I've only just had the book for this week, otherwise I only had £7 8s. 0d. I brought it to his notice that when she is in hospital suppose I was visiting her, what can I do with my £7 8s. 0d. and nearly £3 rent out of it. It's going to leave me on a very tight string. Well, anyway, he has sent it to me. I've got a cheque for £1 10s. 0d. But if I hadn't drawn it to his attention they wouldn't have sent anything.'

The Chronically Sick and Disabled Persons Act 1970 gives the local authority the chance to do more for these families than has been done in the past. It is to be hoped that full advantage will be taken of it.

The parents   The wear and tear on the parents, especially the mothers, was much more important. Two of them were ninety-one and one mother of seventy-one was still carrying her daughter to and from the bedroom quite regularly. One of the ninety-one-year-old mothers had had a heart attack recently but the only thing that really troubled her was that she could no longer see well enough to thread a needle.

The health of the mothers tended to be poor. Seventeen of the fifty-three reported no trouble, eight something which was not an active problem (that is a lesser resolved problem), twenty-one a lesser unresolved problem and five a marked unresolved problem. In two cases there was no mother or mother figure. In many cases it seemed as though the mother simply did not let herself be ill. The question was: 'Are you keeping fairly well at the moment?'

Both the following two cases were considered lesser resolved problems.

'I have duodenal ulcers at the moment. I am on a milk diet.'
Interviewer: So this affects how much you can do, does it?
'Yes, I've got to watch how much I do and how much I leave for tomorrow.' Interviewer: But you manage all right, do you?
'Oh yes.'

Ken's mother had had a pain in her side, which had been X-rayed. It was thought that this was due to her carrying Ken upstairs. This had been solved for the moment by the husband and son carrying Ken upstairs.

The mother's health was considered a lesser unresolved problem in twenty-one cases. The following examples give some idea of what is meant by this.

'I have this Bell's palsy. It was two years ago now, and it took me overnight. But apart from this I'm quite well. Anaemia has been my worst trouble.'

'Some days I have bouts and do's like that. I'm having tablets but it's not touching it at all, and sometimes I feel all swollen

out, my body is all swollen out, and I feel really ill some
days, but I've had to stop taking the tablets this last fortnight
because I've had a pain in my kidneys.'

No distinction was made between mental and physical health.
This was partly because both the interviewers felt unqualified to
make an adequate assessment of mental health and also because a
question about general health might be more revealing. One mother
who had a nice sense of humour was well aware of the connection
between mental and physical health. She asked the interviewer:
'What do you call that long word when you think there is something
and there isn't?' Interviewer: Psychosomatic? 'That's it, I am having
that just now.'

There was no doubt that the strain had told on some mothers,
and several had had nervous breakdowns and more had received
treatment 'for their nerves' at times: 'I am on librium you know.'
'There's times when I have to take them black and green capsules
for my nerves you know.' A neighbour said of one mother: 'Well, it
has affected her nerves, I can tell you that. Mostly I think it's her
not going out anywhere.' The mother said: 'I think you get depressed
at times, you know. Things get on top of you at times, and then it
sort of passes off.'

In five cases the mother's health was considered a marked unresolved problem. In these cases the mother's health was quite
seriously affected.

'I have my ups and downs actually depending on Evelyn.
One day I feel fairly well and another day, when Evelyn has
been showing off, my nerves get topside of me.' Father: 'In fact
in the last twenty years you've had two nervous breakdowns,
haven't you?' Mother: 'Yes, once I tried to commit suicide.'
Interviewer: So you would say that looking after Evelyn has
affected your health? 'Oh yes, definitely I would.'

One mother was confined to a chair and required regular hospital
care. The house was run by the husband.

The health of the father did not appear to have been affected by
the subnormal to the same extent. Nineteen of the thirty-seven
fathers had no health problems, eight some lesser resolved problem,
seven a lesser unresolved problem and three a marked unresolved
health problem. One father, who played a large part in the care of
his daughter, said cheerfully:

'I'm all right, I'm not a healthy man really, I've got arthritis and a curved spine, and blood pressure and skin trouble, but apart from that I am fairly well.'

A factor which affected the health of some of the mothers was whether they had reached the menopause. This was most in evidence in the early pilot visits. This may well have been because a larger proportion of these visits was undertaken by a married woman (J.P.L.), whereas the majority of the visits in the main study was undertaken by a man (M.J.B.). In a few cases this was a factor of some importance, and this could be a period when the mother needs special help.

Any policy of community care must face the fact that with the services in their present state, and very possibly even if the services were improved substantially, the cost in terms of the health, both mental and physical, of the people looking after the subnormal is often high. It is for the parents themselves to decide if the cost is too high, but high it remains.

The break-up of the structure

The most likely cause of the break-up of the structure within which the subnormal is cared for is the death or illness of the mother or person looking after him. There is little that can be done about this except provide good residential care, though in some cases other relatives do take on even very severely disabled relatives. In six of the fifty-four families visited, the family had continued to look after the subnormal at home after the death of the mother.

The structure alters as the family alters. As the other children leave home, a source of help departs. When they have children themselves it is likely that the amount of help they will be able to offer will be still less. There is also the constant ageing of the parents, but one factor which may ease the situation temporarily is the retirement of the father. In two cases (one pilot) this had lightened the load on the mother considerably and possibly given the subnormal another decade at home.

The signs of the potential break-up of the structure may well be evident in advance, and it may be possible to provide the necessary structural help. For instance, one mother depended very heavily and almost exclusively on her mother, who was becoming very frail. This was making the family very vulnerable and they needed some structural help before the grandmother became unable to help any further. On the other hand there was evidence in another family that the care of the subnormal might jump the generations and the subnormal's contemporaries might take on the care of the subnormal, because they were a willing part of the present structure of caring for the subnormal.

Conclusion

The emphasis in this chapter has been on the sheer physical grind of looking after the subnormal. If the subnormal was in hospital, as most of the very severely disabled were, society would provide twenty-four-hour care for a life-time. The needs of these people at home should be considered in the same sort of way. A day at home is just as long as a day in hospital.

16   The quality of life

One of the mothers who was ninety-one declared of her drink of beer, 'It's that as keeps me going.' For others it was bingo, the annual holiday or going out on summer evenings with their husband. This chapter considers those wider aspects of living which contribute to the quality of life. If the last chapter was about the bread and butter of daily routine, this chapter is about the jam or even the cake. It recognizes the importance of the rights of the parents and the other members of the family, as well as those of the subnormal.

But it would be a mistake to think of these various forms of relaxation and recreation simply as compensation for the intolerable and wholly unpleasant job of looking after the subnormal. As was pointed out in chapter 14, this was not the case. Most of the mothers derived positive satisfaction from looking after their subnormal and were spending the vast majority of their waking hours doing so because they wished to. (It is true that even if they had wanted institutional care for their subnormal they would probably have had a long wait, but only one family wanted their subnormal admitted as soon as possible.) The strains imposed have been described and should not be underestimated, but looking after the subnormal was not the same as a prison sentence. Judith's mother expressed the important aspect of positive satisfaction experienced in caring for the subnormal. She had been talking to the interviewer about how she had taught Judith to walk and open doors and come downstairs (see pp. 192–3), how, 'She wets and wets and wets', and how she disturbed their sleep, when she broke off, saying, 'I must get her and show you all these things because I'm proud of her.' Later on when she was talking about short-term care, she said: 'It's terrible to leave her, I hate it. And when we come home, first thing I know I've another pleasure in store. I know it's for another fifty weeks but it's my pleasure to fetch her home. Oh, it's lovely.'

The restrictions on the parents

However, having made this point, the complementary one that the parents also needed a break does not need labouring. The life of the

236

parents was a life of restriction. They had none of the freedom of action that parents with adult children would expect normally. The extent of this was considered in chapter 13 (pp. 183–5).

The restriction was more than simply the length of time the subnormal could be left. Another aspect of it was the way he or she behaved when taken out, and the difficulties attendant upon having a meal out, for instance. For the very severely disabled this was often a 'non-starter', but for many this was at least possible in theory. In practice there were difficulties.

Interviewer: Can you take her out to a meal? 'No, because she wouldn't sit on a chair at the table, she sits on the floor. At Bridlington we took her out one day to a cafe, but she wouldn't sit down, she sat on the floor. Well, it makes you feel, you know . . . you're embarrassed, people watch her you see, and people they watch you, and I set about them many a time.'

'The thing which is disturbing, is we would have liked that she had been better at table so that we could have had an occasional meal out.' Interviewer: You can't manage this? 'No, frankly mealtimes are a messy job.'

The consequences of difficulties with feeding or the way in which the subnormal behaved at meals is all too clear. The extra freedom gained by those families who were able to take their subnormal out to a meal was valuable, even if there were only a few other households to which they could take him.

Interviewer: Does behaviour at mealtimes present difficulties? 'No, Martin doesn't get on with his meal, that's all. He's a slow eater.' Interviewer: Can you take him out to meals? 'Yes, mind you, I only take him to my own family, them that knows him sort of thing. I wouldn't take him to a complete stranger, but to old neighbours and friends I could take him.'

'When she has been away at the hotel she's behaved quite all right. When we are out with her she sometimes can't eat something, and she is inclined to panic a bit so you have to have lots of big paper handkerchiefs and just hold it to her mouth, and she can spit it out, and we get on all right like that, so we can take her out.'

The first subnormal mentioned above was moderately disabled and the second severely disabled. The next two were very severely disabled.

'We take him in cafes and he is going to Butlins for his holidays. I find they are very good with invalids there. We go out every Sunday somewhere, his daddy is very keen on fishing, and we take him, and if we go to the seaside we go in a cafe. He's usually good.'

'We can take her out. My husband's boss's wife, she is very kind, she fetches us to lunch, she lives in a beautiful house at Totley, and they are very genuine people. They take an interest in her even though my husband has been dead six years. She takes us up, I like it and all up there, we see how the other half live, it's lovely up there. But it's not just a bit of snobbishness on my part, it's the goodness of this lady, to think about us, that touches me, but it's a beautiful house and garden, it's very nice to go there even if it's only for one day. No, she sits at Mrs Clumber's table and she is very good.'

The additional freedom that these parents enjoyed was valuable, and the quotations show the extent to which this could widen the family's horizons. This was not the only aspect of the subnormal's behaviour which was likely to clip the family's wings. The naivety with which the subnormal behaved was sometimes a matter of acute embarrassment.

Stanley was only mildly handicapped but his behaviour made life rather difficult for his parents. His mother was bringing him back from the centre of town on the bus.

'Coming home on the bus he saw a man who unfortunately had his trousers undone, and his immediate reaction was at the top of his very loud voice to say, "Mother, that man has got his trousers undone, he's very rude." He realized what my boy was saying, he looked down and he saw his zip, and he pulled it up, and he said, "Ow" and Stanley immediately said, "Have you hurt your Peter Leicester" at the top of his voice. The man had to get off the bus, I was going to get off, but the man got off you see. He wouldn't let the matter rest, he kept on shouting across, "Have you hurt your Peter Leicester?" and of course I was so embarrassed, I daren't take him on a bus I'll be quite frank with you.'

Unfortunately the result of this incident is that Stanley's mother *never* takes him on a bus and this restricts their freedom of movement seriously.

Arthur's behaviour was difficult in this sort of way. His parents were talking about going on holiday.

'You see, if Arthur goes anywhere he plants himself on other folks.' Father: 'If we go to a place like the seaside, we've got to go to fringe of crowd so that we're on us own. If we went in to a crowd as soon as he saw anybody playing with a ball or that, it doesn't matter how far away it was, he'd go for that ball, but now he's twenty-three, we can't let him go into a crowd like we used to do. When he was small people used to accept him, but now, they look on him and think, "Oh". Until they see that he is a backward lad, they are amazed, because he isn't that type to look at. He has a normal face. He has to do these little tricks before people realize that he is backward. Naturally a normal young man wouldn't go and kick somebody else's ball, and then you get that uncomfortable feeling until people know. Up to the point that you know that people have accepted him for what he is, it's a bit dodgy.'

The over-active Lilian, who was very severely disabled, was also likely to embarrass her parents in this sort of way.

'I have to hold on to her, and it's hard work holding on to her. I couldn't take her into a park and sit down. If I took her to the seaside on sands, and somebody rattled a piece of paper she's there, and she is not very polite you know when she goes, and she'd drag a bag off people to see what was inside, so she is a nuisance to other people.'

In the examples just given, the subnormal interfered actively: the attitude of people to a passive aspect of the subnormal's behaviour, for instance slavering or grimacing, is slightly different, but the effect is often much the same.

The mother of the very severely disabled Judith said:

'She slavers terrible. If people didn't stare I'd push her to the end of the world. Ordinarily she sits like a normal little girl and I'm just proud that she looks like a normal little girl to a certain degree, but it's just this slavering you see, it's terrible. We took her to Bridlington last week and we put her in the chair to walk round the front you know, but people just stared, for all this on T.V. about these babies . . . it's not because you're ashamed of them. Quite honestly we're not ashamed, parents aren't, but it's just that they embarrass you with staring at them—adults, not children. So that habit of slavering just stops me from feeling quite happy taking her out, and we have to take her in the car and find a quiet country lane and a field where there's nobody can stare at her. And we're happy because nobody can stare at her.'

It is difficult to know whether other people's responses were really so curious or insensitive as the parents reported. It is hard to say to what extent the parents who were embarrassed projected on to other people their own feelings towards the subnormal. For the ordinary member of the general public it is not easy to know what to do. If one does look at the subnormal in the way one might look at any person, the criticism may be, 'people stare': if one avoids looking, the criticism may be, 'no one will look at my John'.

It is a difficult and complex situation and one with which parents may need help. There appear to be three aspects to be considered. First, there is the attitude of other people; second, there is the parents' personal attitude and feelings towards the child and themselves, which affect their awareness of the *actual* feelings of others; third, there is the parents' capacity to cope with their own feelings and/or the subnormal's behaviour or physical appearance in situations involving embarrassment, external insensitivity or hostility. This capacity to cope will be related to both internal factors (like 'damaging' experiences on buses) and external factors, like the presence and support of a husband or friend.

The attitude of the general public is considered in a slightly different context at the beginning of the next chapter.

Many factors combined to decide the extent to which the family's activities were curtailed by the subnormal being what and who he was—the parents' attitude, friends' and relatives' attitude, the public's attitude and the actual characteristics of the subnormal himself. The effect is that the family was not limited simply by how long the subnormal could be left, but also by these other less obvious factors.

Other factors affecting parents' outside activities

It is very easy to assume that all the parents wanted to go out sometimes, but not all of them did. There seemed to be two factors affecting this, which were often connected. The first was cultural, whether it was usual in that family's social milieu for husband and wife to go out together, and, more generally, whether the mother expected anything but hard work from life. The second was the extent to which the parents, or the mother, felt able to leave the subnormal. This is closely related to the extent to which the family's life was centred on the subnormal to the exclusion of all else. If the family's life was totally centred on the subnormal and in consequence everything else was totally excluded, naturally the parents hardly went out at all, and, granted that this was the way they wanted to live their lives, they did not wish to go out. Both these factors were evident in varying degrees.

Ruby's parents hardly ever went out together, and this appeared to be because they did not really expect to.

'We don't go out together, we haven't done for years, well of course you just take that in your stride because Harold [her husband] is always busy with his shopping; well, I used to go to the Happy Circle, it's only this last year I've got arthritis very bad and I never seem to have got rid of it, and I can't walk. So there's the pair of us, Ruby doesn't want and I can't, so we're all right, aren't we.'

It was difficult to disentangle this cultural aspect from reluctance to leave the subnormal. In addition, the real difficulties these families often faced before they could go out meant that they had become so accustomed to staying in that in some cases they had stopped thinking about going out. The aunt of the totally disabled Terence just did not want to leave him (but this is not a family that could be described as turned in exclusively on the subnormal).

'No, I don't (go out), me husband does, he likes to go for a drink, but I don't go out, I'd sooner stop in and watch telly, I'm not worried, I'm not bothered about going. I think that's the point of having these children, to keep them at home you've got to throw all your love on them, and stop in and look after them. I don't think it's any good if you're going to be leaving them to go off enjoying yourselves, I couldn't go and sit in a public house drinking knowing as he was in the house. If there was someone with him I couldn't.'

It would be interesting to analyse more precisely the impact of severe handicap on families from different social backgrounds. There certainly was a difference in ways the families responded to the pressures. Possibly the greatest contrast to Terence's aunt was

Henry's more middle-class parents, who had a highly organized social life which they clearly found very valuable (see p. 251). One point of particular importance was the expectation of the parents, especially the mother. The mother of a severely disabled man in a pit village on the outskirts of Sheffield was prepared to tolerate an apparently joyless life of undiluted 'slog' in a way few, if any, mothers from a professional background would.

These two aspects, cultural and conditional, interacting with personal attitudes and feelings, had an impact on the outside activities of the parents. It is impossible to say precisely what that impact was, but these points need to be borne in mind in the discussion.

Evenings and weekends

Evenings   Two questions were asked about this. First, whether the parents went out together, and then, if they ever went out separately. Table 16.1 shows the answers to the first.

Table 16.1   Parents going out together

Regularly	9
Occasionally	9
Never but would like to	5
Never but don't want to	11
Not applicable	19
Total	53

This question was naturally not applicable where there was no husband, or wife, with whom to go out. If the parents went out at least once a fortnight, this was considered regular. 'Occasionally' covered going out as rarely as once in six months.

The amount the parents went out depended first of all on the parents themselves, whether they were the sort of people who liked to go out and whether they came from a social background where it was usual to go out. This has just been discussed. Quite apart from this, it depended on whether anyone was available to look after the subnormal while they went out. If no one was available and this had been the situation for a long time, it was evident in some cases that the will to go out weakened.

In every case, except one,[1] where the parents went out together, either there was someone who would look after the subnormal, or the subnormal was able to be left on his own. Where there was no relative readily available to look after the subnormal, it generally meant considerable organization and effort for the parents to get out together. The sheer effort involved, superimposed on an already demanding daily routine, was often a crucial factor in limiting the parents' social activities.

The reactions of the parents to going out or not going out reflected once again the length of time they had been living with the state of affairs and the way they had accustomed themselves to it. Those who went out regularly liked it, those who went out occasionally quite liked it and the rest were not bothered. This can be seen in the examples.

In the following two cases the parents went out together regularly.

'That is when we get out together, every other Wednesday.' Interviewer: What sort of things do you do? 'We go to bingo. Or if we are celebrating we perhaps go to a show or have a drink and then have supper, I love to be waited on.'

'We'll go out for perhaps an hour or two when it's my night off and Pat [the subnormal's sister] will look after him. We've had to take the plunge and go out for an hour. Friday night I usually go out for an hour.' Interviewer: Do you find this a valuable break? 'Oh yes, little things you want to talk about that you don't want to talk about in front of Julian you can discuss at these times.'

Others who went out regularly went to a pub, old-time dancing or a working men's club. The pub was the most popular.

Those who only went out together occasionally tended to go to some special event.

Father: 'We keep saying we'll have more of these occasions when we go out. I've got the Philharmonic programme and I've been looking through, and I'll say we'll have some more Friday nights out, but . . .' Mother: 'It is more difficult with your sister, isn't it, and there isn't anyone else we can call on. You see, I've got two sisters but they are both at business and they've both got very full lives.' Father: 'When Patricia was younger we did have a day or two's holiday without her because then we could leave Patricia with my older sister, but then they are not able at all now, they are older than we are. My brother-in-law is over eighty and blind, and my sister is seventy-seven.'

'It's very rare. He fetches his mum and dad to sit, but they're getting on, they're in their seventies, we've been out three times since Christmas [i.e. in six months]. It's about four times a year, we go to his [her husband's] dinner and dance at the works, we go to the Parent Teacher Association dance twice a year, and the pictures once, so it's four times a year, and that will be our lot. If anything happened to his mum and dad we wouldn't be able to go really, because these functions, they're late you know, and you can't really ask your neighbours.'

More never went out together, and did not want to, than went out regularly. The case quoted below shows how this can come about by default.

Father: 'We're not bothered, that's grown on us, you know.' Mother: 'Yes, we would like to go out more but you don't realize that you creep within yourselves, the only thing we can do now is spend money on the house.' Father: 'I'd like to go out for a day's racing, or have a night at the dogs, or have a pint, but as the years have gone by I just don't bother, and I'm not worried.' Interviewer: Do you or your husband ever go out separately? 'No, we've said we were going to do, but we've never got on with it.' Interviewer: So this is a way of life that having Arthur has made you grow into? Mother: 'Yes, definitely, we're not that type of person. Had Arthur been normal like the others we wouldn't be like this. So for comfort we've built it round ourselves in our own four walls.'

The picture is slightly more complex when the fact of the parents going out separately is considered. This can be seen in table 16.2.

Table 16.2   Parents going out separately

	Father	Mother	Widowed (or single) Mother (figure)	Widowed father
Regularly	15	9	4	2
Occasionally	8	6	3	0
Never	11	19	10	0
Total	34	34	17	2

The men went out considerably more than the women. In some cases this indicates a certain indifference on the part of the husband, 'Oh yes, he's always going out, he likes his drink', but in others it reflects what was expected in that social milieu: 'My husband goes out. He is ready for a pint after a week's work. He goes out Friday, Saturday, Sunday.'

The women went out less often by themselves but there were six cases where both husband and wife went out by themselves regularly: 'I go to bingo once a week, and he goes for a drink on Friday.' More common (eight instances) was the father going out regularly and the mother never. 'He likes to go for a drink, but I don't go out. I'd sooner stop in and watch telly.' There was only one instance of the mother going out regularly (to bingo) and the father never going out.

In all this it is hard to separate social convention from social handicap as a result of having the subnormal living at home. David's father used to go out regularly but his mother never did, and her reply indicates the sort of pressures that can bring this about. The father's job put him in the intermediate social class (i.e. between the professional and skilled classes).

'I think it is very difficult for a woman to go out on her own and again, it is very difficult to have people to call us friends with these kiddies, because you are never sure from one week to another what you are going to be doing. I mean with people that we have known for a long, long time, probably since before we were married, if I wanted to I could 'phone them up and say, "Are you coming out tonight", but I couldn't make it a regular sort of thing. I think to myself, well, unless it's absolutely vital I can't. . . . I don't feel as though it bothers me not to go out, because once these have gone to bed that is me finished. I sit down, it doesn't matter what else needs to be done, I sit down and I watch television, and nothing, you know. . . . Even if there were mountains of washing in the back kitchen, I wouldn't do it once they'd gone to bed.'

The problems of going out were far more acute for the widows. For the few who did manage to get out, it seemed a great help. The fondness of one of the mothers who was ninety-one for her drink of beer has been mentioned already. There was another mother who was ninety-one and she also liked her pint of beer. She went out two evenings a week to the local pub while one of Elsie's many sisters came in to look after her. Another widow went out once a week with her sister-in-law to play tombola.

'It makes you forget things, not just the tombola, people what we know, what we sit with, we get talking and it passes right . . . it's only across at St Joseph's and it's laughs and what you get with people and comical expressions what comes in.'

Christine's mother depended on her daughter coming.

'Well if my daughter comes in decent time I'm going to see a lady I met at this convalescent home, because she is very badly in need of someone, her husband committed suicide, and she found him. It's knocked her sideways because she hasn't got any children. The first Saturday I came home from my time at the convalescent home I told my family I must go and see this lady because I promised. I went to see her last Saturday, and she enjoyed it very much, she said, "I hope you come again, you've cheered me up no end." It was nice for me as well.'

But in the majority of cases the mother never got out. 'I've got accustomed to it. It's my problem isn't it?' 'I've got so it doesn't bother me. I never go out but I'm not bothered. Me and Richard, we just go for a little walk round.' 'Oh no, I've never left her, I've never left her of an evening, never. I've never gone out at night, never.'

Weekends   Roughly two out of five of the families went out at the weekends with some regularity. Twenty-two families did, thirty-one did not. If the subnormal was severely disabled going out was only possible if the family had a car. In five cases where the families without a car did get out at weekends, the subnormal was not severely disabled physically. In the sixth case the severely disabled Elsie was taken out in her chair to the local park and her family reckoned that this was 'getting out at the weekend'.

For some families this seemed to be an important break.

'Yes, we go out every weekend, whether it's wet or fine. We go for a drive, and if it's nice we take the invalid chair and we pick a spot where it is nice and flat. We have certain roads that we know are flat, we give him a walk on there. But otherwise we park him where he can watch the traffic, and we just go for a little walk. We usually go with a crowd. There's my two sisters and my brother and another brother and sister, not ours, and another friend. There's a whole crowd of us, and they are very, very good and help us with him. We've gone with them for twenty-odd years.'

Helen's mother made the same point about a flat spot.

'She is a proper one for outdoor and, if my husband isn't working on a Sunday, when it's fine we're never in. We go to Chatsworth and all over. But I like it where it's flat, so we can let her walk on her own, where it's safe you see. It's got to be flat.'

But the problem mentioned in the first section about the naive behaviour of some of the subnormal cropped up.

'We get out if it's fine weather, out and away from people. We don't take Stanley where there's other people because if they are sat eating anything Stanley goes and asks them for some, or he shouts at them, "Can I have a bit". With the increasing number of cars on the road it is getting more and more difficult to find private places.'

But for some, weekends were a difficult time.

'No, I never go nowhere. I'm handicapped at weekends, nobody wants me at weekends. I've got nobody but these two backward boys. I can't go nowhere at weekends. You haven't got no husband to take you out in the car or anything like that. I don't know what it is comes over me on a Sunday, it's just same as if somebody come and took all that mattered to me out of my life and there's nothing left.'

Arthur's family found weekends rather difficult because he got thoroughly bored. Two other families reported the same problem. Arthur was moderately handicapped. The problem of the weekends seemed to epitomize the problem of living with and looking after Arthur.

'The thing is we just don't get any life, it's just the same thing over and over again, year in and year out. He is bored; it's become more boring as we've got older. I'm not capable of taking him and kicking a ball about with him. I tell you what we do, I fly a kite for him on Ringinglow Moors if it's been a nice breeze. He'll sit down, listen to his wireless, look at his comics, watch his kite, and I can have a read, that's me, happy.' Mother: 'But if there isn't a breeze you can't make him understand his kite won't go up, then he goes mad. But had his dad still been able to kick a ball we wouldn't have had any problems.' Father: 'As the years have gone by and he's got stronger as I've got weaker,

I've had to find a place on a hill where Arthur had to kick it
up and I could just tap it down. But I just can't manage that
now. We could do with the youth club coming and taking him
out, just to knock his energy out of him.'

Arthur's parents state the central issue. What matters is not
whether the family conformed to a middle-class model of social
intercourse but whether the members had 'any life' or whether it was
'just the same thing over and over again, year in and year out'.

Where the father or the husband of the woman looking after the
subnormal was alive, there were only four families out of thirty-
seven where the parents did not go out at all in the evenings, nor did
the mother go out by herself, nor did the family go out at weekends.[2]
In two of these families the family set-up was rather curious anyhow;
in the third the female relative looking after the subnormal was
really best considered as a solo mother (and has been treated as such
in table 16.2), and only in the fourth case was it a 'normal' family
which had centred its life almost exclusively on the subnormal.

But where there was no father or husband of the woman looking
after the subnormal, the mother did not go out at all in nine out of
sixteen cases. These women suffered from an accumulation of disadvantages. They could not go out with their husband, either because
he had died or because they had never had one; because there was
no one else in the house (in every case where there was no man of
the house, the household consisted of just the subnormal and the
woman looking after him), they were not able to go out by themselves
unless somebody else came in to look after the subnormal; and
where there was no man in the house the person looking after the
subnormal never owned a car.[3] This meant that it was often impossible for the subnormal and his mother to get out at all at the weekends.

This group shows more obviously than any other the extent to
which it was possible for these families to become cut off from the
mainstream of living, from the general intercourse of everyday life.
In these circumstances it is hardly surprising that the very close bond
between the subnormal and his mother, described in chapter 14,
developed in a number of cases.

A structure of living

In the previous chapter it was shown that the families had created a
structure for coping with the everyday needs of the subnormal. A

rather similar concept is useful here. A helpful question to ask is, 'Has the family developed a structure for the total business of living which keeps it within the general commerce of life?' The structure for coping may itself have this effect if, for instance, other members of the family are involved regularly in the daily or weekly care of the subnormal. A good example of this was Joyce. Some indication of the involvement of members of her family was given on page 201.

However, although the structure for living and the structure of coping must overlap, the former can be considered by itself. Instances of both isolation and good contacts with what is going on have been given. These indicate whether the structure of living of the family is such that the family is either a part of society or an isolated unit within society. The emphasis again is on structure. If the family has to make gigantic efforts in order to remain in touch, the effort required is likely to lead to gradual loss of contact. It is a question of what is taken for granted and what happens as a matter of routine.

Paid work for some mothers   There was a variety of ways in which the family kept in touch with the outside world. One of the most important of these was where the mother had a part-time job. In one case the sister looking after the subnormal did a full-time job, and found this a help in many ways. She was due to retire in the fairly near future and was concerned about this.

> 'I have rather a fear what's going to happen when I retire, it's getting near. I am rather dreading that, because money will be cut down to half, I shan't have the companionship of my work and the people at work, it is rather looming up to me.' Interviewer: Do you see any way through this? 'Well I hope I will be able to afford to have someone to do half a day's job, and I'll have to go out when they come in. I will not be able to afford Mrs Rastall like I do now. At work one can get away from it, and it is quite a different interest as well.' Interviewer: Would you say your job has made a big difference? 'Oh definitely, financially for one thing, and the company, for instance I never eat alone, here I'm alone with Jennifer, there it's company. I don't see my friends as much as I would like perhaps, but I wouldn't say that I feel lonely.'

But generally it was only possible for the mother to work part-time. This was very important for the mother of one rather trying young man.

'He's never turned on me. He's turned on his father more than once, but there again that was jealousy. At that period he seemed so attached to me he resented anyone having any conversation with me. He would sulk when they came to see me, he wanted me for himself, and I did have a bit of a nervous breakdown and I lost some weight, and I knew I'd got to do something. So I plucked up courage: I'd got to find something I could do at night for a few hours, so I went to be a barmaid, it's a very nice place, and oh it has done me good. I get very, very tired, but I've got back now that I can speak to people. I found out that my brain hasn't gone.'

Later on in the interview, the mother mentioned this again.

'The doctor said to me, "Whatever you do, keep going to work as long as you can, it will do you more good than all the pills I can give you", but this doesn't suit my husband really. He's a little bit fed up, "Oh but leave at the weekend, leave at the weekend", he says, but I can see myself now if I leave at the weekend; I can see him coming home tired and thinking oh, he'll have half an hour, and he'll be asleep in that chair for an hour or so, and I should be back in my old routine. I've no conversation, no adult conversation. Well I got to the stage where even with the neighbour that I said I could approach, if she was hanging washing out I would wait to go and hang mine out because I felt that I didn't want to talk, and I'd cross the the road if I saw anyone coming, I'd think, oh I don't want to talk.' Interviewer: How often do you go out to work? 'Five days, I have Tuesday and Friday off, and it gave me such a boost to think that my brain hadn't got dormant, that I could reckon up right and get a big order in, and in no time you know . . . it boosted my morale. It was a terrible ordeal the first week, but I knew that I'd got to do something and I really enjoy it. Though it's very tiring, I enjoy it.'

Another mother worked part-time in a pub: 'I mean it gets you out, doesn't it. It's a break for her as well. Oh, I look forward to company.' It was a break for her daughter because a neighbour, of whom the girl was very fond, came in to look after her while the mother was at the pub. Her husband worked on the night shift and there was a gap between him going to work and her mother getting back from the pub. The neighbour looked after her during that gap.

One other mother, a widow, after saying how necessary it was for her to work simply for the money, said in reply to the question, Do you enjoy working?:

'Oh yes, I think it takes the misery from having one like he is. When you've had other three wonderful children and you get one like this, it's heart-breaking, and to have a laugh and that amongst yourselves, you forget it. You forget your troubles.'

The mother of Richard, a very severely disabled young man, had had to give up work when he was sixteen and could no longer attend the special care unit. She missed her job very much.

Other social contacts   For some of the less severely disabled it made a big difference both to the parents and to the subnormal if they could take him or her into a pub. Four families mentioned how important this was. Sometimes Julian's parents went by themselves to the pub, which they valued, but,

'Other times we take him with us. He loves to go and have a pint of shandy, he thinks, "I am one of the grown-ups now." Of course the people know him and he really enjoys that.'

Douglas's mother also thought it did him good.

'When nice weather is on we get out. Sometimes we call in a new public and have a drink, Douglas will have a shandy and he is getting to meet people you see, because that seems to make him getting better in himself.'

Freda's parents were wondering about it.

'Some folks don't like to go out, do they? But I am afraid I am one that does. Now she is eighteen you begin to wonder if you could take her into a pub or anything, because we like to go for a drink.'

These are only minor instances of ways in which families kept in touch with life, but for these families it was important. A few families had things very highly organized, as in the case of Henry's parents.

'We take it in turns, my husband goes out one Thursday, and I go out alternate Thursday, then we go out every Sunday. We have about twelve ladies, we have a supper arrangement, my neighbours and I, and every fortnight we go to one of us for supper. Then about twice or three times a year we all go out to a dinner. It's been going on for about four years, and I discover this just breaks my monotony, and we have a good gossip. On the alternate Thursday he [her husband] goes out with a friend.'

However it was organized, where families had created a structure of living which kept them in touch with the world, the mothers did appear more buoyant. The amount the parents went out was only one aspect of the extent to which the family was kept in the mainstream of life. The structure of living depended heavily on family, friends and neighbours. The vital part they played is discussed further in the next chapter. Before that there are three other aspects to be considered.

Holidays

Hewett (1970, p. 125):

> The family holiday . . . although it is historically a recent phenomenon for the majority of the working population, is already very much taken for granted in many families. Perhaps the presence of a handicapped child seriously interferes with this activity.

Sheila Hewett asked families with a young spastic child about holidays and found that 71 per cent of her sample had been on holiday at least once since the birth of the handicapped child. Among the families we visited, almost exactly two-thirds (thirty-six out of fifty-three) had had a holiday at least once in the previous five years. The breakdown of this is given in table 16.3.

Table 16.3 Holidays

With subnormal regularly	17
With subnormal occasionally	6
Without subnormal regularly	10
Without subnormal occasionally	3
Never	17
Total	53

If a holiday were taken every year or almost every year it was considered regular, but if it was less often it was considered occasional, provided the family had been on holiday at least once in the previous five years.

Seventeen families had not been on a holiday at all during that period. In a few cases the problem was money. One such instance was the widowed mother of Richard, who would have liked to go on holiday but could not afford it. The difficulties of widows in getting out and about was mentioned on p. 248, where it was seen that in nine out of sixteen cases where there was no father (or father figure), the mother never went out in the ordinary course of events. Of these nine, five never had a holiday either. One old couple who used to go away regularly said: 'Well, we have been doing, but we can't now with being on pension. We have been going away, but we can't now.'

A strong reluctance to leave the subnormal was often a factor in not going on holiday. 'No, I shouldn't rest now, I've got into that routine. I wouldn't be happy to leave her behind.' The combination of this and the difficulty of looking after the subnormal away from home appeared to be decisive in quite a few cases. The real problems the parents faced in leaving their subnormal were well illustrated, even if in rather an extreme form, by what happened when the totally disabled Terence's aunt left him for a week.

'It's six years since we went away for a holiday, I went to Bridlington with my husband and my son, and my sister had him again for a week, and I rang up every night to see how he was getting on, and she kept saying, "He's all right, he's all right", and then when I came home we had to rush him off to hospital. He'd been poorly all week and she wouldn't tell me because she thought I would have come home, so we haven't been away since then because you see she's frightened.'

Twenty-three of the families avoided the problem by taking the subnormal with them on holiday; but this also meant that they were taking some problems with them. The two sisters who helped the ninety-one-year-old mother to look after the severely disabled Elsie explained:

'We have to take those two chairs, a chair what folds up and a seat to fit on it.' [When they go out she goes out in her wheelchair and they have to put a rubber on it in case she wets. They cannot take her into a public lavatory. They have a lot of washing to do when on holiday, and do it every day.] 'For instance, when we go down on to the sand we've got that washing to do. She's no control you see. That is the worst problem.' Mother: 'She's very good though.' Sister: 'Yes, she is good.

We don't know we have her, just that wetting and lifting up and down.'

The parents of the over-active Lilian faced more acute problems. The way she would drag a bag off people to see what was inside was mentioned on page 239. If they had a flat it had to be one on the ground floor, otherwise she would annoy other people with her walking around and shouting.

The mother of the moderately handicapped Nancy also had problems.

'She won't sit at the table and she sits on the floor, people stop and watch you, it hurts me, because children stand and watch you see, they stand on the sands and watch us.'

Martin's mother was a widow. He was only moderately handicapped and she would have quite liked to take him on holiday with her.

'If I had a husband I would take him with me, I wouldn't let him go away. I'm so afraid of the toilet part of it you see, I mean there's these hooligans, and I am so afraid of them taking advantage of him that I really wouldn't take him on a holiday on my own.'

But provided they could find suitable accommodation, this generally meant a cottage, a caravan or staying with relatives, a holiday was valued.

'Well, we usually get a cottage. Last two years we've had a very nice one with about two and a half acres of ground to it, and that's when he'll walk out and leave us because of all this ground, and he'll walk round or fetch me the milk from the bottom of the drive; it is in a little hole in the wall and he'd go and fetch that for me. Here, he wouldn't. There, with it being quiet, he would trot round the grounds. We all get a really good holiday, we relax because he's relaxed.'

An isolated cottage or caravan in a corner of a field was the most common solution families found, but in at least two cases the family was able to take the subnormal to a hotel. Butlins had a favourable mention as a place 'where they don't refuse to take people with a handicap . . . they provide ramps to everything for wheelchairs'. The same mother did mention that boarding houses and people letting flats were always likely to discover suddenly that they were full. This was not mentioned often, probably because the situation was avoided.

Rather fewer, only thirteen, went on holiday without their subnormal, and three of them only went occasionally. In such cases the subnormal almost invariably had to go into short-term care. For most of the mothers this was clearly valuable. 'We've been on holiday three times without Joe and it's sort of wonderful really' (pilot). However, where it was for the first time, the parents, especially the mother, sometimes fretted and did not enjoy it. This is tied up closely with short-term care.

Short-term care

Only one-third of the families had used short-term care at least once in the previous five years. Thirty-five had not used it at all in that period, nine had once or twice, nine had used it regularly. In a few cases this was because a relative or friend looked after the subnormal while the parents or mother went away. In other cases it was either the very strong reluctance of the parents to leave the subnormal, an unfortunate experience of short-term care in the past, or dislike of what was offered.

The reluctance to leave the subnormal has been mentioned already. It was often felt very strongly. 'No, I wouldn't want it. I would feel I'd done something wrong. I don't think it would be good for me.' Another mother said simply: 'No, I've never cast him off.'

Regrettably in some cases it was the result of unfortunate experiences in the past. Anthony was mildly handicapped (pilot).

'Only once and that was a disaster. That was to enable me to have a rest. We didn't see him for the full month and then when I collected him it was a poor pathetic creature we collected.'

Nancy was a moderately disabled woman in her forties.

'She went away for a fortnight in one of these homes at . . . and when she came home she was bruised all here, all here [on her thighs]. Her mouth was swollen up, and I don't think she really knew me. She just went away for one fortnight. See with her sitting on the floor I expect the children would kick her as they passed her, you can't blame those responsible for her really, you know what children are like, if they saw someone on the

floor they would give them a kick, wouldn't they. I had her in
bed a week, that's what I know about a home. That was when
she was going to school [i.e. at least twenty years ago]. So I said
she'd never go no more.'

Arthur was also moderately disabled.

'Well the thing is he once went to . . . and he came back just
like a little frightened animal. God knows what they'd done to
him.' Father: 'He'd lost two stone in weight.' Mother: 'He was
terrified, everything we asked him to do he did for us for a few
days, until he got the run of the house again, but something had
frightened him. He could have gone there again this year, but
we wouldn't let him.' Interviewer: And he couldn't tell you,
could he? 'This is the point you see, and whether it was one of
the inmates or too much discipline, we just don't know, but
they'd cut nearly all his hair off, in fact when we got home we
said, "If we never go away again, he's not going there any more."'

Another family refused even to consider short-term care in a subnormality hospital. This was the only choice they were offered. 'I
once saw a programme of places like . . . and I said to my husband,
"I would die if my son went there."'

However, for some the experience was just the opposite. The
young man who had returned from one hospital like a 'little frightened
animal' returned from another, 'and said he'd been on his holidays.
He had had a good time.'

Another young man had enjoyed his spell at another hospital.
'He'd only three complaints, the bread was too thick, the tea was
too weak and the bathroom floor was dirty. Otherwise he's
played at bingo, he had a lot of things stolen, his money, his
best shirt and things like that you know.' [But this didn't seem
to worry his mother very much.]

The new local authority hostel was very popular but this now has
only one place available for short-term care for each sex.

Short-term care was important to give parents a holiday, or at least
a break from looking after their subnormal. It was also important to
prepare the subnormal for eventual separation from his parents. The
point was well put by the mother of an older subnormal for whom
there had been no short-term care when her daughter had been
younger. When she was asked if she had ever made use of it, she
explained:

'No, that's the one thing that I say that I'd advise any mother take up whilst they are young. That break early on, I mean you see it afterwards, you think, "Oh, I don't want to go and leave her and that, and I don't want her to leave me", but if that was taken as a routine it would have made all that difference, because they accept it and you would accept it, but not when they are older, when they are set in their habits. But I would for any young mother or anybody just for that holiday period now and again.'

One family were quite explicit about the value of short-term care in preparing the subnormal for when they died.

'We have had his name down to be put in hostel for permanent care, but that will maybe take years. I've had it down five years, you know so that I can have him at weekends, I wouldn't have him taken altogether, I love him too much for that. This is something we're always thinking about because it's got to happen eventually, because when either of us finish our lives there is no-one to take over. I think it would be too hard as well for him, for us to die and then him to be taken in, cold turkey sort of thing. I'd far prefer him to go in whilst we are still alive and able to take him out and get him used to the idea. It's bound to happen eventually.'

One family with a very severely disabled young man had accepted short-term care for their son after refusing it for years. Both the parents felt that it had been an important step to realize that he could manage without them.

The provision of good and acceptable short-term care does sometimes, and could frequently, play a critical role in helping a family to learn how to live with its subnormal member, and to prepare him for his parents' eventual death. This was something which was uppermost in many parents' minds—the future.

The future

'Well, I worry constantly about what's going to happen to Christine when I'm gone, and that's at the back of all these throats I get.'

A number of the parents were getting quite old and what would happen to their subnormal was naturally a matter of some concern.

Eight of the mothers (or mother figures) were seventy or more, eleven were in their sixties, fifteen in their fifties and seventeen were under fifty. In two cases there was no mother or mother figure. There were only four fathers over seventy, eight in their sixties, fourteen in their fifties and eleven under fifty. In the remaining cases there was no father or father figure.

A major preoccupation it may have been, but the number of parents who had any clear ideas about what would happen to their subnormal when they could not look after him was very limited. This can be seen in table 16.4.

Table 16.4   Plans for the future

None	34
On waiting list for permanent care	3
Expect permanent care will be necessary	12
Expect relatives will take over	1
Hope relatives will take over	1
Don't think about it	2
Total	53

One very clear-minded mother whose subnormal was very severely handicapped said: 'Only definite plan I have, it sounds terrible but I do have it, if I came to be ill and I knew I was really ill and I knew I couldn't get better, I'd give him a bottle of tablets.'

A rather similar though less drastic attitude was, 'Only hope is that they go before you', but this was more evasion than plan, which one mother admitted implicitly when she said, 'I just pray that she goes before us'; and another said explicitly: 'I think perhaps I'm a bit of a coward, keep on putting it into the background, suppose have to some day . . . sort of . . .'

But as a mother in the pilot survey said: 'Well, what [plans] can you have? That's what you miss. No plans, you just live from day to day.' And this is what many of the families did. It is important to recognize that this could be a positive attitude and in view of the *present* provision it is also realistic.

'We just live from day to day, you know, and don't look too far into the future. One year is much like another year.'
Father: 'I think if with something like this you were to look too much to the future, and dwell on it too much, then I think you would get despondent.'

Lilian's mother expressed similar views.

'No, you can't think of the future, or you're punishing yourself.
As far as I am concerned, we've got faith in God and I've had
help. If we started worrying about what was going to happen to
Lilian, we'd worry ourselves stiff.'

In a rather similar vein there was the determination to go on doing
what was possible, while it was possible:

'Well, my plans for Violet for the future are while I've got the
health and strength to look after her I will do, and I give her
as much pleasure and happiness as I can possibly give her.
That comes within my reach, but apart from that I don't see any.'

Helen's parents expressed the same sort of attitude: 'We are giving
her a life while we are alive . . . while you can look after her you are
going to, aren't you?'

But for all this the subject of the future was a matter of deep-
rooted concern. Lilian's father revealed how impossible it was to
avoid thinking about it in some way. He went on after what was
quoted above:

'We think something will happen to make things right. I wouldn't
like to think of her going into an institution and I wouldn't
like to think of anybody else looking after her.'

This clearly did not solve the problem. The most common outcome
envisaged was an acknowledgment, generally reluctant, that care in
an institution would be necessary. 'I always think what is going to
happen to her when I've gone. See, she'll have to go in a home.'

Along with this acknowledgment there often went a positive desire
that the subnormal's brothers or sisters should not be 'landed' with
looking after the subnormal. Only two expected or hoped that relatives would take over the care of the subnormal. It was clear from
what the mothers said that this was a painful subject (and so the
interviewers did *no* probing on the subject).

'Well no, I suppose there is only one answer, isn't there?
If anything happens to us. I couldn't. . . . I don't think my
daughter-in-law would have him. Though she is very good.
I wouldn't expect them to, they're only young. I wouldn't dream
of asking them to. I think it is too much of a responsibility
and she's not grown up with it like we have.'

'When anything happens to me then of course he'll be put in a home. I wouldn't place the burden on my Phil or my daughter.'

Naturally the parents were very concerned about where their subnormal would go and whether he would be looked after properly.

'Well, I'm just wondering if, when I die, there'll be anyone who will take an interest in her, or whether she will just be one of many, sort of a number, that worries me. I know she is happy at . . . [a subnormality hospital] oh, it would be a break for me if she could go there, I'd be really happy about it, because they keep to her diet, they look after her, and she seems to be happy there.'

There was considerable anxiety about the ordinary subnormality hospitals.

'I tell you what I would like to know, is there any centre without him going into . . . [a big subnormality hospital]? We're getting older and wondering what is going to happen to him, that's my one dread, if something decent turned up like a Cheshire Home it would break my heart but I would let him go. It's come home to me this year what will happen to Henry when we get older, because I think now if anything happened to us suddenly it would have to be . . . [the same big subnormality hospital].'

Patricia's father made a similar point, but notice that he, unlike most parents, spoke about what he thought it would be like for *her*, rather than how *they*, the parents, would feel about it.

'Subnormality hospitals with sixty or more beds in a ward, you don't need me to point out to you that after the life she's had it would be pretty grim for her.'

A few of the parents had tried to save some money to help with the care of their subnormal when they died, but the great hope for those who knew about it was the new local authority hostel.

'He is depending on my life. I am only living for him. I'd never part with him while I take my last breath. No, never. I'm sticking my boy while my last, and I'm only praying he is for hostel.'

'We've made a will in his favour and Mr Pratt took us up to see that hostel and having seen that we felt more settled. It

was a nice place that. We were told that was the sort of place
he would go to.'

Dennis's parents had just joined the Sheffield Society for Mentally
Handicapped Children, which they found a help.

'You get to know more news and details about these homes that
are being made for these children. I want to go and visit that
one on Fulwood Road [the new local authority hostel] this week,
because I think for every mother it's a big thing, what happens
when I can't do, that is the biggest worry I think. We have told
Victor, if anything happens to us, not to keep him at home
because he has his own life to make, but to see that he gets
into a good home, not just pushed anywhere, and that they
will help him at the Mental Welfare Department.'

Anxiety about the future pervaded the life of most if not all of
these families. If they could be given the sure knowledge that their
subnormal would be looked after in a way that would satisfy them,
a great load would be lifted from them, and they and probably the
subnormal as well, would be much happier. As one mother said
when she was asked what her main problem was:

'We always wonder like whatever happens if she has to go away,
or anything happens to us. We've always that at the back of
our minds. I'd really like to know she was somewhere safe and
comfortable, that is one worry with us.'

Conclusion

This chapter has considered those wider aspects of the families'
lives which contribute to the quality of life. It has looked at such
aspects of the weekly routine as whether the parents ever got out in
the evenings or at weekends. In connection with this the concept of
the structure of living was introduced. The chapter went on to consider holidays and the use of short-term care. Finally, the long-term
question of the subnormals' future and the importance of this to the
families' well-being was discussed.

This completes the picture of the problems the families were up
against, the ways they met them and the general routine of their
lives. The next chapters consider the part that various sections of the
community played in helping and supporting these families.

17 Family, friends and neighbours

In the course of describing the way in which the families dealt with the daily grind of caring for their handicapped member and the ways in which they managed to obtain some relief, frequent mention has been made in passing of the part played by other members of the subnormal's family, friends and neighbours.

In chapter 15 the need for structural help was emphasized. It was seen that the key characteristics of such help were reliability, regularity and punctuality, that is, help which related to the structure of coping which the family had evolved. In chapter 16 the critical aspect of the various forms of social activity discussed was seen to be the extent to which they kept the parents and family within the general commerce of living. The importance of such a 'structure of living' was emphasized and its close relationship to the 'structure of coping'.

This chapter considers first the general tolerance, intolerance and understanding, or lack of it, in society at large, then the help given by the siblings, relatives and neighbours. After this the different levels at which help was given are outlined. Finally, some features, which either make it easier for the family to accept help, or make it more difficult for them to do so, are considered.

The tolerance and intolerance of society

The parents' interpretation of society's attitude to them and to their subnormal was related closely to their attitude to social activities in general. This was discussed at the beginning of the last chapter. However, the attitude of society, or the parents' interpretation of that attitude, was not only reflected in the subtle ways mentioned there but also more directly. A case in point was whether the father worked for an understanding firm. Bernard's father did. He took Bernard round with him in his car on Friday mornings while his wife did the shopping. 'It's quite all right with the firm, they know that he takes him whilst I go and do the weekend shopping.' The firm for which the father of one of the subnormals in the pilot study worked was very understanding and helpful. If his son had a serious attack of epilepsy, the firm would let him have time off.

Travel was another place where public attitudes were important. The problem of people staring has been mentioned more than once. There were more practical difficulties, such as the problems of folding chairs. These chairs can be taken on some buses but not on others. One mother in the pilot study said that it was very difficult with one-man operated buses. Some drivers were more helpful than others and, on buses where there was a conductor, the same was true of conductors. She said that coloured conductors generally helped. Ordinary members of the public did not help very often, in her experience.

More directly relevant to the lives of the families than the general tolerance and understanding, or lack of it, of society at large was the support and acceptance of the neighbourhood. There were four families visited, one in the pilot survey, where the subnormal and his family seemed to have the unthinking acceptance of the neighbourhood. These were all in areas of nineteenth-century working-class housing. In none of these instances did the neighbours actually do much for the family; indeed, in one case they had even got up a petition 'to have him put away'. Yet in each of these neighbourhoods there was an attitude of casual tolerance towards the subnormal.

On the other hand one family faced considerable problems in their present house because of unsympathetic neighbours. Stanley's parents were asked whether he could go out by himself at all.

'Yes, but I wouldn't allow him, because as I explained there's a wall just here and it only needs someone to turn and say to him, "jump it Stan, it won't hurt", and he would turn and jump it, he would take the word of what the person was saying.'
Interviewer: Is it the children? 'The parents are afraid, that's the top and bottom of it, they're afraid to let their children mix with him, and Stanley is inclined to go to them and ask, "can I play with you" and then their parents have told them no, they're not to go with him. They just can't accept the fact that he is mentally retarded and he is harmless.'

The tolerance of the neighbours could be very important. One mother in the pilot study told how her son was particularly fond of throwing heavy objects through windows. He still tended to throw things, especially if frustrated, but his mother said that now he opened the window first. Neighbours had been very understanding about finding strange objects in their gardens.

These neighbours did not give much active help, but such tolerance would have been valued highly by one family who had a neighbour whose behaviour appeared to be little short of vindictive and included such behaviour as banging on the wall to keep them all awake. Sometimes the neighbours appeared to be frightened. 'Everybody somehow seems frightened that you are going to ask them to do something. . . . I broke my arm but nobody helped.'

Contacts with neighbours will naturally be determined to a large extent by the attitude of the parents, especially that of the mother. The importance of this was well shown in the pilot survey. Two families lived in the same road not more than 300 yards apart. One family had contact with only one neighbour, the other seemed to know half the neighbourhood.

But there were neighbourhoods which did more than just tolerate the subnormal. The clearest example of this was the old industrial area that Arthur used to live in.

Father: 'He was born there, and born into their way of life;
they treat every child the same, they accepted them.'
Mother: 'If he'd been born up here it might have been different.
Among a lot of strange people it's terrible, it's terrible to move
with a child like that. To come up here it took me two years
to get over it. Neighbours used to come and say, "Your boy has
done this, your boy has done that", but the thing is he was used
to doing that in the old place, and they didn't mind. One
family used to have bread and dripping on the table for him,
and when he used to go in, they'd give him a slice of bread and
dripping, and he was happy. Another person would sit him to a
meal. Well you see, he expected it when we came up here.
Up here they didn't understand, down there they used to laugh,
they'd bring him back to me and say, "He's had his tea Joan",
or, "He's had a bit of dinner so if he doesn't eat much you
know what's wrong", but to move with a child like that is
murder.'

Arthur's mother mentioned the problem of moving. Two other mothers, one of whom also lived in an area of old industrial housing, the other in a more middle-class area, had decided against moving for just this reason.

Help and support from various sources

The help and support of the father   Table 17.1 shows how much help the father gave.

The seventeen not applicable were families where the father had died, except for one case where the subnormal was looked after by his father and a coding here seemed inappropriate. In the other case, where the subnormal lived with his widowed father, the household was run by a sister who lived in another house, but the father did give some help and in this case a coding of 'adequate help' was given. In two families the father figure was not the father but the stepfather in one case and an uncle in the other.

Table 17.1   Father's help

Much	14
Average	17
Very little	3
None	2
Not applicable	17
Total	53

In the five cases where the father gave either very little or no help, the family situation was rather curious in four cases, and only in one instance was the family comparatively normal. In the large majority of cases the father gave a fair amount of help. The help was considered average if the father took a regular part in the care of the subnormal, even if that part was small. If the father was working full time, which twenty-nine of them were, the amount in which he could help was limited. By these criteria the following instance was considered 'average' help. The mother is speaking:

'It's done me a bit of good to go to work at night. His dad looks after him at night you see, when I'm not here, and that has kind of brought him back to his father a little bit with being away from me, but apart from that he has no time.'

The help that the father of the moderately disabled Trevor gave was also considered average.

'If Trevor is a bit late coming home on his bus and my husband's come home before we are back, he starts getting Trevor's tea ready, and he'll get mine ready, so he's not bad at

that, and when he is not working Saturday and Sunday, he'll
wash me the pots.'

The help that Philip's father gave verged on 'much', and illustrates
the top end of help that was considered 'average'. He used to look
after Philip one afternoon a week while his wife went into town and:

'Sunday after dinner he'll take over where the food is concerned,
he'll bring in tray for us, and get us any drinks we want.'
Interviewer: Does he spend any time with Philip? 'He'll spend a
bit of time with him, trying to get him interested in things, and
try and get him in the garden.'

The fourteen fathers who gave much help were an integral part of
'the structure of coping' with the subnormal, and their help meant a
great deal.

'Oh, he is extremely good, he'll even wash nappies.'
Interviewer: What particular ways does he help? 'Well he'll take
him to bed for instance. He always takes him to bed, and he'll
undress him, and things like that. He can do all the things just
like I can, apart from feeding him. He can feed him, but he has
to do it separate, he can't do it and eat his own at the same
time like I can.'

'Yes, he does help me, he bathes him, he undresses him every
night, he helps me get him up in the morning.'

'Oh yes, he's not here in the day but he takes these little
things off you, you know, no I couldn't do without him, love, I
just couldn't manage. He sits like an old sheep, content, when
he comes in you know, and for all we've had her all these years
he asks a lot of daft questions. . . . But I couldn't do without
his help, and as I say, when he comes home at teatime he just
takes over and I can go in the kitchen and please myself what
I do . . . and he'll sit his-self down, she will sit with him, and
he's content you know. And if I'm preparing a meal at weekends
he'll jump up and give it her and take over like. You know,
little simple things . . . and he loves her just like I love her, and
well, I mean what dad would go to her at five-thirty in the
morning, see she were wet, and change her.'

It made a big difference in some cases when the father retired.
One such father said:

'We work as a team. Since I've retired I've done the best I can
because I know how tired my wife got, while I was out working.'

It was evident in some cases where the father gave this amount of
help that without it the subnormal would not be able to remain at
home. It underlines the disadvantages under which the widows
laboured.

The help of the fathers was in a different category from help from
other sources, because it was help within the family unit. The very
considerable help given by the fathers is a reflection of the fact that
the decision to keep so handicapped a member of the family at home
for so long was, almost invariably, a joint decision. In many of these
cases the subnormal would have been in hospital if such help had not
been forthcoming.

The help of the fathers provides part of the background against
which other help needs to be set. Now that we have seen the extent
and range of help that they did give, it is possible to look at the
other sources of support and help given to the family.

Help and support of siblings A distinction must be made here
between siblings living in the same household and those who had
left home. A total of nineteen subnormals had siblings living in
the same household. In one case the subnormal's two sisters were
looking after her and had virtually assumed the position of the mother.
In four cases the brother or sister was also subnormal and, in one
other instance, there was an unmarried adult son living at home.

In all the remaining cases the other siblings were children or young
adults, and generally played a very small part in the care of the subnormal. This was often the deliberate policy of the parents, who
expressed reluctance to encumber their other children with looking
after their subnormal sibling.

'We can leave him with him for a short time, but I think
James has had an effect on him. When they're young I think the
normal one sees the subnormal one having attention lavished
upon him. Raymond used to say, "Oh for goodness' sake shut
up, lad", but now he's saying, "When do you think he will come
home?" Almost a love-hate relationship. He treats him quite
sympathetically. I don't think it's fair to ask him to do much.
We only do it when there's no alternative.'

There were sometimes other reasons for not asking the other
children to help.

'The other boy has suffered with our not being able to get about, because of Andrew. He has been neglected, in fact he's been put upon to cover spaces like this week. He looks after him the hour between five and six o'clock, from when I go off to when my wife comes home from her job. We don't like to leave them too long, or they start scrapping.'

This was all that parents generally asked of their other children. Relationships between the subnormal, when the subnormal was not severely disabled, and the other children tended to be much like those between normal children. There were one or two instances where a sibling did a little more. 'We all more or less work together. Thelma will feed him, brings him downstairs. She's a very good help. If I can't go up to him she'll go and chat to him. We sort of all help one another.'

In one case the younger sister, a young teenager, was a considerable help. Her mother said: 'I go to the hairdressers' on a Tuesday. My daughter will sit with him until my husband gets back. . . . She's very good with him. It is a shame really, she is old before her time.'

This study did not set out to discover the effect of the subnormal on siblings, but most parents thought that they did have some adverse effect, and sought to reduce it to a minimum. This is one reason why siblings living in the same household were not a very important source of help. Only one gave much help and eight average help.

The subnormals' brothers or sisters who had left home were older than those living in the same household and they gave more help. The figures can be seen in table 17.2.

Table 17.2   Help of siblings not living in the same household

Much	10
Average	11
Very little	6
None	1
Not applicable	25
Total	53

In a very few cases the other children's lack of concern for their parents and their subnormal sibling was a cause of pain to the mother.

Interviewer: Are they any help to you? 'No, none whatsoever, they are not very nice to her either, she's a lovely girl too.'

But this was the exception. Distance prevented some of them from giving much help. Three-quarters gave considerable help. The help they gave varied. The very severely handicapped Judith's mother said:

'Every other week my son and his wife stay overnight and have her, yes, every other Wednesday. Yes, I've got a grand son, he's lovely. I say he's lovely, he is my son I know, but he is thoughtful.'

This was considered average help. So was the support that Trevor's mother was given.

Interviewer: You see your son almost every week? 'Yes, and we telephone almost every day. Sometimes he doesn't manage to get over every weekend because he is away working, but he does generally manage to get on a Sunday if he can.'

Note the importance of the telephone. Naturally the help brothers and sisters could give was limited when they had their own families. This was generally recognized by the mothers, as we have seen already when considering the parents' attitude to the future. For instance, one mother said of her married daughter:

'Oh, she's all right with her. Mind her love's for her own children which is right isn't it? But she is pretty fair with her and I don't think she'd like to see her away. But I won't burden her with her because she's had a bit of a rough do with her own little life, and I want her to have a bit of comfort with her own children. Because they are hard work, aren't they?'

Martin's brothers and sisters were all married and each of them had at least one child. They gave their mother much support. Recognition of the importance of looking after their own families ran through the mother's account, as the following quotation shows. She was a widow.

[The eldest sister was married with two small children.] Interviewer: Do you see quite a bit of her? 'She comes every weekend.' Interviewer: Do they get on well with Martin? 'Well, as I said, they've got their own lives to live; they've got enough to do; they've their own home to run; they both work; they come and see him, and they love him, but as for trailing him about with them, you just can't expect them to do it, and I don't.'

When the mother was a widow, the support of her other children was likely to be very important. Susan's widowed mother depended completely on her other two daughters for her shopping. Christine's widowed mother was visited every week by her daughter and grand-daughter. As for her son, 'He came last night. He comes once a fortnight. . . . He does many odd jobs for me.' The widowed mother of the severely disabled epileptic Jean had two sons.

> 'I've got the one son who is single, and who I send for if I
> think she's not going to be very well . . . he's on phone . . . so
> I can just get on phone and ring up and tell him to come.
> He'll come and stop because he is on hand then. Phone
> downstairs [in a tower block of flats] is never working, so we've
> got to go to phone on road. Well you can't leave them you've
> got to have somebody at hand.'

In the case of Elsie, whose mother was a widow of ninety-one, her brothers and sisters were almost entirely responsible for her, though she actually lived with her mother.

However, not all the parents had other children, and where the children were younger and still living in the same house, we have seen that the help that was given and expected was very little. For such families the help of other relatives was likely to be important.

Help and support of relatives   Only three of the families had no relatives at all. Relatives were the source of a good deal of support. This can be seen in table 17.3. 'Relatives' covers all relatives, including the grandparents, if any, and excludes only the subnormal's siblings.

Table 17.3   Help and support from relatives

Much	16
Average	19
Very little	7
None	8
Not applicable	3
Total	53

Some of the relatives were little or no help, because they were old or infirm or living a long way away. In some cases the fact that they were little help, even though there was no obvious reason why they should not help, was borne with equanimity. One mother had six brothers and sisters living in Sheffield, but there was very little contact. When she was asked, 'Do you feel you could ask them for help if you needed it, for instance if you were ill?', she replied, 'I don't think so, only one who might.' She went on to comment: 'We haven't fallen out with them at all, it's just one of those things that's happened with not going out.'

More often there was an undercurrent of bitterness in such phrases as, 'I don't get any help at all', 'None whatsoever', 'Oh no, they never bother, not a bit of help, no.' In one or two instances there was concern to excuse, explain and try to understand this lack of support.

'No, never. It's not because they don't love her. I know my youngest brother really loves her . . . but in this day and age nobody has time, but we were only saying the other night, "It's funny, nobody has ever offered to have her." They come, but they never say, "You go out". . . . . My nephew did once or twice but he started courting.'

In all these cases the help given by relatives was reckoned to be none. One step up was where the help was considered to be very little. This generally indicated goodwill but little else.

Interviewer: Could you ask your sister for help? 'Well I could but she's not so understanding with her. My sister has never had children to deal with, whereas my daughter has been brought up with her and that makes a difference.'

This was the coding given if the parents kept in touch with their own brothers and sisters but that was the extent of the contact. It also seemed to fit where help *was* available but the help was not given in the ordinary course of events; that is, it was not part of 'the structure for coping' or 'the structure of living'.

Interviewer: It sounds as though they help quite a lot? 'No, you have to ask. You never had to ask my parents [the mother's, now dead], but to be fair they will help, if you ask, they will do it, but not without asking.'

In fact they only asked about twice a year. There was a similar situation where the mother said of a relative: 'She really has enough of her own troubles without helping us, but if it came to an emergency I could always call on her like.'

If the contact with other members of the family was more regular than this, the relatives' help was considered 'average'. Ruby's mother, Mrs Franks, had two sisters surviving. One lived an easy bus ride away, 'That's the sister I go to see every week.' And the other sister lived at Barnsley, 'We go visiting; I went about two months ago. I got a letter from her this morning.' Regular contact rather than help was the distinctive feature of average help. 'My sister's daughters and two nieces, they come every Friday and bring children. I always have a houseful on Friday.'

Mrs Jacobs had three sisters and four brothers. They all lived in and around Sheffield. She lived very close to her mother and saw her brothers and sisters when they came to see her mother. The critical point here is what will happen when Jean's grandmother dies. It would seem very likely that her mother will become very isolated if the family reacts in the way that many did in Young and Willmott's Bethnal Green study.[1] She was a widow and lived in a modern block of council flats. Harold's parents lived in an old industrial area, and there was not the same sort of danger because they lived in the midst of a large extended family. The parents had nineteen brothers and sisters between them. Many lived near by and all except one in Sheffield. The mother was asked how much help her relatives gave. 'They pop in, they live round the corner most of them, he [Harold] goes and sits with his grandma.' Could you ask them for help if you needed it? 'Yes, I could ask.'

Having a relative who could be asked easily made a big difference. Philip's mother found this was the case.

'I've got a niece that comes quite regularly, that's my sister's daughter. She lives quite close, she comes up regularly to see me, perhaps once a month. She understands him very well, she knows him. He seems to take notice of her. There's got to be that feeling with Philip between people, he can sense a genuine kind person, and he reacts to that feeling. She is very good to him.' Interviewer: Do you feel you could ask for help if you needed it? 'Oh yes, if there is anything I wanted I could send down and Annette [her niece] would be here. She is the type that would say, "All right. I'll have a day off, auntie." I know that she would come.' Interviewer: Have you ever had to ask her for help? 'Only if it's shopping which I have not been able to do on Thursday. I've been able to go, and with my mind quite at ease.' Interviewer: She is easy to ask? 'Oh yes.'

Sometimes help was available but was not used. One mother had relatives willing and able to help. 'I think some of them you know are cross that I don't [ask them more often]. I do really, they'll say,

"It's no good offering help to you." Different times, years ago, they'd offer to do things but I'd never take them up on it, and I really think they got a bit cross.'

Help was occasionally available from relatives even if they lived further away. One mother and her daughter used to go and spend their annual holidays with a married brother at Cleethorpes, and the previous Christmas, when the mother had been ill. 'They came across, and the sister-in-law stopped. She is very good like that you see.'

Much help and support indicates that it had become a regular part of the family's routine. 'Well, his [the father's] sister, she's very good. That's his second home. She usually goes on holiday with us and it's nice because it's one more and she knows his little ways.'

James tended to be rather unsettled when he went out to other people's houses so, most frequently, his grandparents used to come and look after him at home.

'Yes, they might come up and look after him so that I could go out in the garden. They come up on a Saturday, my parents that is. This used to be a fairly regular routine, my wife would go down town, my mother would keep her eye on James, and my father and I would go out in the garden.'

Where a relative was much help and involved in the daily routine, this has often been mentioned in the course of describing the daily grind that the families faced. Terence was a good example of this. His care was the concern of many members of the family. The basic care was shared by his aunt and another aunt next door, but the help given by the family was much wider than this. There was an unmarried uncle who lived quite close and, 'If Terence is in hospital he helps me with the bus fares.' This uncle lived with a great-aunt who came down every day. Mrs Stokes, the aunt who looked after Terence, had two other sisters. One lived near by and her husband had a car,

'and she comes down every day without fail, and she will sit with him if my sister and I wanted to go up to the village, or wanted to go to town together. It's very rare we ask her, but she would do.' [She might actually come and sit a couple of times a year.] 'And her husband, he is good now, if he is poorly in night and I ring the hospital and they tell me to get him in as quick as I can, my son will run over to their house and he'll come with car. It doesn't matter what time of night it is, and take him, and he fetches him home from hospital, so we don't have to wait for an ambulance for him. They are a big help, and she comes every day to see how he is.' Interviewer: And what about your sister at Norton, do you see much of her? 'She comes on average once a week.' Interviewer: And how is she with Terence? 'Well there again we've never asked because she works, I've never asked her to come at all. Probably if we had asked she'd have come and stayed with him, she isn't frightened of him or anything like that.'

There was only one other instance of the wider family helping to this extent, and this was Joyce's family. This was mentioned on page 201.

More commonly, there would be one relative, almost always a woman, who was a particular help. Sometimes it was the subnormal's grandmother. 'Mother is a big help. She does more for Dennis than anybody. She can also interfere a bit.'

Sometimes it was a sister. 'Oh she is always here, she's just been round . . . she lost her husband and we are more close than ever now.'

Sometimes it was a sister-in-law. 'My brother and sister-in-law live next door but one . . . and they idolize her and do as much with her as I can. Really I don't think I could have coped if it hadn't been for her.'

Sometimes it was some other relative. A niece was mentioned by two mothers. One of them said, 'Oh yes, she's always round . . . Sylvia [the subnormal] likes her to come in.'

A striking feature of these families was the regular contact and the fact that the family relationships were in good working order. The knowledge that their family was behind them contrasted sharply with the 'none whatsoever' of those who did not have this support. A typical instance of the assurance this gave was the very severely disabled Tom's mother, whose sister used to come and look after him for an hour or so every weekend.

Interviewer: Is there anything else she does? 'No, but I know she would do, I know that she is there you know. If I did need her she would do.'

Help and support of neighbours

'Oh there's a real 'un here, she is a right 'tato, that one.
She is a frump and she is a gossip, and she knows it all, you

know what I mean, and a tittle-tattle, and all that. Her, she says that when she dies, she's taking her purse with her.'

Fortunately most of the families' experience of their neighbours was rather happier than this. This family did not appear to receive any help or support. It can be seen from table 17.4 that there were only two other families in this position.

Table 17.4 Help and support of neighbours

Much	14
Average	25
Very little	11
None	3
Total	53

Everybody had neighbours, and neighbours, by definition, are near. It required less effort for them to give at least a little support than it did for relatives who did not live near by. Most of those whose support was rated 'very little' accepted the subnormal, for which the parents were grateful, but did very little actually to help. The mother of the very severely handicapped Judith was grateful for such acceptance.

'Now the two boys next door, they came here some years ago. Now we were wheeling Judith in the sun yesterday afternoon, you know, in the garden, and acting daft really—now her eighteen-year-old came up the drive and he said, "Hello Judith", and now him saying, "Hello Judith" is grand.'

But Judith's mother was well aware of the limitations of what they could be asked to do.

'As I mentioned to you I've got a nice neighbour. She accepts Judith, speaks to her, passes me bits over you know, she's passed me bits of bedding. I couldn't say to her, "Would you look after Judith for an hour" because she's got a husband that's on nights regular so he is in during the day. I am not very often ill, but I was at Christmas, and I had nobody to have Judith, and my welfare officer didn't know. My husband were coming home in the middle of the morning and the lunchtime to see to us. He were bringing flasks upstairs, Judith had it for five days, but I was really ill. It made me realize then I had nobody.'

Where there was a large family supporting the subnormal and his family, there was not the same need for help from neighbours. For instance Elsie was accepted and greeted whenever she was taken out but, 'We've never needed anything. It's with her [Elsie] having a big family you see, you don't need any help.'

Otherwise in these families where the neighbours gave very little support, when the question was asked, 'Do you have any problems with your neighbours?' typical answers were, 'No, because we don't see them.' 'Oh no, we don't see much of them living up here' [in a maisonette on the first and second floor of the block]. 'We don't see much of them to tell you the truth.'

In some cases the subnormal's behaviour had a lot to do with it. 'Well, a lot have volunteered but we've never taken it up because we know what a handful he is. They wouldn't understand him.' 'She [an old lady] likes Hugh but he doesn't understand that he's got to be gentle with her, because she's a bit feeble now.' But it was also probably a reflection of the type of person the mother was. This is the same mother speaking as in the last quotation: 'To tell you the truth although we've lived here eight years I couldn't tell you the names of them. You see, they are all out at work or whatnot.' Another of these mothers said: 'I'm a little bit independent that way. It would have to be desperate if I went for anybody.'

Freda's mother made this point about herself.

'I am afraid I don't neighbour very much, I'm a bit stuck up.
I think it's having Freda, I'm on edge all the time wondering if they are going to accept her, because she is different.'

However, Freda's mother did have one neighbour with whom she got on well and whom she would be prepared to ask for help. This just took her into the average group. This was by far the largest group. These families seemed to have easier and more positive relations with their neighbours.

Mrs. Thompson said of herself: 'I can get on with anybody, as you might put it. I'm that friendly nature what people can get on with.' Interviewer: Are there any neighbours that are a help? 'Well, any of them would give me a hand. Say I'd forgotten a thing, I'd ask, "Are you going up the road for such a thing, would you mind bringing me that", and they would do. Or say I was full of cold and they'd say, "Will you want anything bringing, I'll bring it you, seeing you're not very well." Well that's when they have brought me things.' [But she has never asked any of the neighbours to sit in with Violet or anything like that.]

Their neighbours' tolerance of the subnormal in respect of the average group tended to go rather further than that of those who helped less.

'I've got two nice neighbours, the little girl next door is always in and out, and is used to him, and little lad, and he can shout to them, shouts their names; they come in and they are quite used to him. None of them seems to be afraid of him. One or two were when we first came up, but I used to say, "He'll not hurt you love." They accept him and are used to him.'

Most of Arthur's neighbours also showed considerable tolerance.

'Mind you, he's gone and done some tricks, gone in their outhouses, walked in their houses, gone and played the piano and all sorts. He'd walk through their house, not knowingly, he thinks everybody else's things are his, he'll just walk into people's houses and some don't like it. But he doesn't do that now.'

In some cases it was the neighbours who needed the help as much as the reverse.

'Oh, they're all friendly, but they need help, that's the thing. Now there is the old lady upstairs, she is stone deaf; she is eighty-six: and there's the new people, he is an ambulance man, they seem very nice people, and they've told me they'll help me any time if they can be of any assistance: and there's the old lady come back from hospital, she needs help: but this old lady she'll sit with Christine while I go to the chemist, I can safely leave her for an hour, she is getting on. But before that there was another old lady, she was nearly ninety, so I couldn't ask her for anything. I used to run errands for her.'

In the case of Diana's mother, her isolation was reduced by the fact that she could do something for her neighbours.

'They're very very good. But some are old age pensioners, others working you see, so there's not really anybody that. . . . They all come in for a cup of tea, pop in here. They are very good. If she has a birthday, I don't think anybody round here would not know. She has twenty odd cards, and they all bring little presents. They are all very good, because they've seen her grow up you see.' Interviewer: Do you feel you can ask them for help? 'If she is bad, anybody would help, but otherwise I am very independent. I've grown up that way, and I don't ask anybody for anything. I like to manage myself, and I couldn't ask—only for emergencies.'

Naturally some neighbours were more helpful than others, and one or two were sometimes particularly helpful. Three mothers mentioned what a blow it was when such a neighbour moved. Julian's mother had one particular friend about fifteen minutes' walk away.

'She used to live just across the road for many years, and if Julian's dad was at work and he got out of hand I could send for her husband and he'd come, they've got a way with him somehow and he loves them. It was a very big wrench when they moved away, but she comes to see him once a week without fail.' Interviewer: Can you ask her for help? 'Oh yes, she's real dependable.' Interviewer: Apart from these two is there anybody else you can ask for help? 'Well I suppose the people that I've known for years that live right close, if I was ever in such a dire situation I feel sure that they would help.'

The support that Julian's mother received was considered average because her close friend now only came once a week and support from other neighbours was limited. However, it was this sort of relationship that sometimes characterized those families which had much neighbourly support. One example of this was Philip's mother.

'For the most they are quite nice people, but as I say, there's the one just up there where we are friends, not just neighbours. We came together [to the estate when it was first built fifteen years ago].' Interviewer: And you could ask her for help? 'Oh yes.' Interviewer: Have you in fact done so? 'Oh yes, anything I needed or want, and it isn't very often I get depressed, but I can go up to Phyllis and we can cry on each other's shoulders sort of thing. It's the fact that I know I can go, and know that help will be genuinely given with a lot of feeling. It's quite a deep friendship really, one that I know no matter what I wanted she would be there to help.' Interviewer: Do you see quite a lot of one another in the course of the day? 'She'll put the flag up for coffee, and if she thought Philip wasn't well or anything she'd come down and have a little talk and sit with us sort of thing. She is a very nice person.' Interviewer: It must make a very big difference? 'Oh it does, it does really.'

In these families that received much support from neighbours, there were often references to the neighbourhood as well as individual neighbours. Richard was very severely disabled. He and his mother lived in an old industrial area. 'They're very friendly, they don't shun Richard. Everybody knows Richard and they are good to you. They are very good. I wouldn't like to go on an estate.' The neighbours appeared to give a lot of support and do things like fetching a bit of shopping or keeping an eye on Richard for a moment, without thinking about it.

Heather's mother expressed a similar reluctance to leave her present neighbourhood.

'Oh, they are very good. Well, they've been here all the time you see. That's one thing, I wouldn't like to leave here, you know, we're friends all round, and with her being born here it does make a difference.' Interviewer: Is there any particular way in which they have been helpful? 'Well, I mean in keeping her company and talking to her. Now, if she'd been home today she would have been sat outside in her wheelchair you see, and they'd sit on that little wall and shout to her, you know, and they have all pet names for her, she answers them back. They are very good that way.'

Friendliness and helpfulness were not limited to the old industrial areas. The severely disabled Alex lived with his parents on a pleasant, modern council estate. For the previous two years they had had a very friendly couple living in the maisonette above them. They went up there at least once a week. Mrs Davison was obviously pleasantly surprised by the way in which this older couple got on with Alex. They appeared to have 'the touch' for looking after him. There was also an old-age pensioner who lived in one of the two pensioners' flats which are included in these blocks of maisonettes, and they went in to have tea with her, or she came in to them, three or four times a week.

One widowed mother who lived in a big block of flats received a lot of help from the caretaker. The mother of the very severely disabled Joyce received much help from her family. She also received a great deal from neighbours. If she wanted to go round to somebody else's house she could summon her next-door neighbour.

'I get this ashtray, and we go I-tiddely-I-ty-pom-pom with the ashtray, and she'll know what it's for and she'll come round. When Mrs Farris lived across road I had a pink jug, she used to say, "If you need me stick jug in window", and I used to put jug inside window and even if any others used to chance to see jug in window, they knew what I'd put it in for.'

Mrs Farris, the particularly close friend of Joyce's mother, had moved from the immediate district, but she was still in touch with the family. She had had the totally disabled Joyce to stay for a fortnight the previous year while her mother went on holiday. A policy of community care cannot expect help like this as a norm, but it is impressive when it happens. Possibly the nicest example of neighbourly support, but also one which cannot be expected with much frequency, was when a delightful old widower who lived near by married the widowed mother of one of the subnormals.

Help and support from all sources

One indication of the extent of support is the number of other people with whom the subnormal could be left. This is shown in line 30 of figure 13. One dot means that the subnormal was left with someone else occasionally (about once a month), two dots regularly (about once a week or more often). The number indicates the number of people with whom the subnormal could be left. Where NA appears in line 30, this means that the subnormal could be left without anyone looking after him. In three cases the subnormal did not need to be left with anyone and in fifteen cases the subnormal was never left with anyone at all. The remaining thirty-five cases were divided fairly evenly between those who were left about weekly with some-body (nineteen cases) and those who were left less often (sixteen cases).

Thirteen of the regulars could be left with one or two other people. In only six cases were there more than two people with whom the subnormal could be left. Fourteen of those left less frequently could be left with one or two other people, and in only two cases were there more than two people with whom the subnormal could be left.

Leaving the subnormal was sometimes difficult, and often the mothers were reluctant to do so, but this does suggest that, at this level at least, the help that the mothers received tended to be rather limited.

It is possible to take a more comprehensive look at the total support the families, especially the mothers, received. The extent of the help that the mothers received from husbands, other children, whether living in the same house or elsewhere, relations and neighbours has been considered separately. Table 17.5 shows the extent of help from all of these sources. The same information is shown diagrammatically in figure 13, lines 31–5. One cross represents average help and two crosses much help. Where very little or no help was given, the space is left blank.

Table 17.5   Help and support from various sources

	Father	Others in household	Siblings not in same house	Relatives	Neighbours
Much	14	1	10	16	14
Average	17	10	11	19	25
Very little	3	8	6	7	11
None	2	4	1	8	3
Not applicable	17*	30	25	3	0
Total	53	53	53	53	53

* This includes one widower

The importance of the father's help is obvious. Others in the household were generally the subnormal's siblings, but in one case it was a lodger and in four cases some other relative.

There were five families which were extremely isolated. In one case the mother received no help from any quarter, in another only average help from another child in the same household, in another only average help from neighbours and in two more only average help from the father.

On the other hand there were five families which received much help from both relatives and neighbours, and a further two who received much help from relatives and brothers or sisters of the subnormal who had left home.

There were only seven cases where an adult sibling who had left home (line 33 of figure 13) did not give a fair amount of help. In two of these cases the siblings lived a long way from Sheffield. In one case relationships with the other children were rather unhappy and the mother said she would ask her neighbours for help in preference to her other children.

The most important point was not where the help came from but whether the help and support the mother needed was forthcoming, whatever its source. Any attempt to quantify this support is bound to be hazardous, but the method adopted in table 17.6 does agree broadly with the assessment made of the family situation. The method is to count one point for each cross in lines 31 to 35 of figure 13, that is, from each possible source of support. The maximum score possible is ten. It does not include line 30 (which shows whether the subnormal is left with anyone).

Table 17.6 Extent of support

Score	Number	
0	1	
1	4	poor
2	8	
3	11	shaky
4	12	
5	11	good
6	6	
Total	53	

Where the score was two or less, which it was for thirteen families, the position of the family, and especially the mother, was generally pretty miserable. 'Well what life have I got. . . . It's not a good life. . . . No, there's nothing to look forward to.' Seven of the fifteen mothers who felt lonely were in this group and eight of the fifteen subnormals who were never left with other people. In one or two instances, however, the parents were quite content with their lot.

The eleven families who scored 3 appeared to be in a considerably sounder position than those who scored less, but the position seemed somewhat precarious because it rested on rather a narrow base, the help of the husband, the health of a grandmother, the support of one neighbour, the solicitude of one daughter or the devotion of one sister. In almost every case the removal of one person who helped could push these families into the rather miserable, isolated position of the previous group.

The position of the families with good support was more widely based. There was almost always support from both family and neighbours. There were only three out of twenty-nine where help was from members of the family exclusively.

Examples of each group have been given incidentally in the course of describing the extent of help from the different sources. The examples which follow give an idea of the typical position of the people in each of these groups.

The aunt who looked after the very severely disabled Sybil never went out and received no help from other members of the family, except for a little help from one of her sisters. The only substantial help or support she received was from neighbours.

'You see neighbours is good and offer, if I go out I leave the key with them and they pop in and see to her.' Interviewer: How often does this happen? 'Only occasionally, you see I don't like putting on people.'

Apart from this she bore the burden of looking after Sybil unaided. She came into the group who received poor support.

The rather precarious nature of the support for the middle group is shown by the widowed mother of the severely disabled Nancy. She had had no contact for many years with one sister who lived in Sheffield. Her brother lived some distance away, though his family did give help, for instance, by having them both for their annual holidays. One neighbour who had been a great comfort and support had died a few years previously and the mother depended almost entirely on the help of just one neighbour, who was also elderly.

Bridget was severely disabled and her mother a widow, too, whose son also lived some distance away and was only able to give occasional help, mainly with holidays. However, she had a sister and brother who lived in Sheffield, who gave much support. She had lived in the area all her married life and felt accepted by those around. She gave help to them and accepted it from them. This family came in the group of those who received much support. Not all those in this group had quite such a wide range of help but, on the other hand, there were some who received more extensive support. On this reckoning, twenty-nine of the fifty-three families received much support.

The various levels of help and support

The help and support described in the previous pages has covered a wide range, from the next-door neighbour who would nod to the subnormal and say 'hello', to the friend who would look after a totally disabled subnormal for a fortnight while the mother went on holiday. It is important to distinguish these different levels because they represent the complex of contacts which go to make up the patchwork of living, and a recognition of the different levels makes it possible to indicate more sensitively ways in which help can be given.

Negative tolerance　This has been mentioned already but needs to be mentioned again here. It is concerned with not doing or saying things which upset the family, such as staring:

> 'Well there were these children next door, they used to stare at her; they used to stand on the outhouse wall. Even the mother didn't accept Judith. She used to spend all her time just sitting, watching her. Well I used to get upset.'

The behaviour of children could be upsetting as well.

> 'When we're out, boys, they can be very cruel. I try and avoid meeting with them when they come out of school. I suppose it upsets *me* more than anything.'

Two other families reported problems with children in the neighbourhood.

A related aspect is where the neighbours fail to understand the way in which the mother's social activities are circumscribed by caring for the subnormal. In this case the mother was unable to fit in with the local rules for gossiping.

> 'I don't have time . . . but I do gossip in the yard, but to gossip down the road, people can't understand this you know, because they said, "She's a funny woman her", but they can't understand, you just can't stand, I'd love to, but I just can't.'

More seriously, one mother mentioned as her main problem:

> 'The fact that bothers me about neighbours is that I was once told that if she was a nuisance to neighbours they could send her away.'

The generally favourable comments about neighbours indicated that the parents expected this sort of reaction but did not have to tolerate it very often.

Positive tolerance　Positive tolerance was more common, and was mentioned at the beginning of the chapter. It was a step further than simply not saying things which upset the family. Such positive tolerance produced such comments as: 'I've got a nice neighbour.' 'We have very good neighbours, all of them.' Some mothers were more specific.

'On the whole it's a friendly district. I did know somebody who moved out of their district to a better class district, and I was talking to the mother on one of the spastic trips, she said, "I wish I had never gone." She said, "I've been there three months, and nobody's said hello yet." When I take Henry out and I go through this estate, there's always half a dozen at least who say, "Hello luv, is he all right luv." I think I'd sooner be where people are friendly.'

Whenever the very severely disabled Terence had to be rushed to hospital,

'They'll ask "How is Terence, have you got him home yet?" I don't know whether they are interested or whether they are just curious, but at any rate they ask.'

Support and friendship of the parents together or individually The level that is being considered here is friendship with the parents not with the subnormal. Such friendship was often available to the husbands through their work. In those cases where the mother was able to do a part-time job it made a great difference, as has been mentioned already.

Membership of organizations, societies and churches was important at this level. Old-time dancing, the Philharmonic chorus, bingo and (the mother) being a member of the darts team at the local pub all had their adherents. The important thing about these contacts was their normality and the friendships to which they gave rise. One mother said that she never asked her friends for help, partly for practical reasons, but also because she valued friends simply as friends.

One mother who coped with more than most people would have thought possible found one neighbour gave her a valuable break.

'I've started popping into a neighbour's once a week for an hour, that's all. She is an old lady of seventy-odd, I find her very pleasant. We don't gossip or anything like that, we do discuss astrology and things like that, which we both enjoy. She is a very charming old lady, but I don't find anybody else has time.'

This friend could not and did not help with the subnormal, but it was clear that her contribution was a valuable one.

The restrictions that the care of the subnormal imposed on the life of the family meant that friends who did maintain relationships with the parents needed determination to do so. John's mother mentioned the effort that was needed to keep up contacts.

'You find out who your friends are. You've not much social life. We have some good friends, we haven't many but what few we have we treasure them because they have stuck by us.'

Elizabeth's mother felt they had become rather isolated.

'I think you do get a bit that way, socially you don't mix of course, you see we've got that we don't make the effort to go to a film. We used to visit different friends, we've dropped them all. In time I suppose people get tired of asking. No, it's difficult. But socially you do get outcast. I don't mean that people are nasty or cut you off, it's yourself, you build up a kind of barrier, I think we all do it, with any handicap.'

Because of this difficulty those parents who had evolved some form of routine or were members of some society were in a better position to retain social contacts of this sort. The way Henry's parents had things organized has been mentioned already on page 251. Church membership gave a few parents this kind of support.

'Many of the ministers have been very close to us, my husband to the husbands, myself to the wives.' Father: 'I should say thinking back that it's been one of the good things in our lives. Not so much being members of the church as knowing these people who came to minister. We became friendly, and it's lasted.'

Two of the families in the pilot survey had strong connections with the local Methodist church. In one case the subnormal herself was able to attend, but in the other there was no question of this. In this instance the parents appeared to have organized their lives in two circles: one centred round the subnormal, which he dominated; the other quite separate from the subnormal and centred largely on a fairly full involvement in the activities of the church.

Retaining the subnormal's family within the wider family's life   This runs parallel with the last section. The importance of the parents being kept in the mainstream of the life of the wider family was often recognized implicitly or explicitly. The mother of the severely disabled Ken met all her many brothers-in-law at the market on Saturday morning. The parents of the very severely disabled Tom met about six other members of the family every Saturday at a pub. This trip was made possible by another sister who looked after Tom. The aunts and uncles of the very severely disabled Richard did not help with him at all but they did 'visit regular'. Joyce's family 'lived in a circle' and made the annual holiday an opportunity for a family get-together.

A few families used the telephone as a means of keeping in touch. Trevor's married brother used to ring up his parents every day. This was an important part of the way Patricia's parents, who were both in their seventies, kept in touch with their brothers and sisters, who were also getting old and finding it difficult to get about.

General help but not help with the subnormal directly Much of the help referred to in the section on neighbours was help of this nature. Shopping, phoning for the doctor, getting a prescription or help with things in the house were often mentioned. 'She'd do me a phone call or a bit of shopping. She'd do things like that for me.' 'I'm never stuck fast for anyone fetching me an errand you know.' In two instances, taking one of the other children for an outing or holiday was much appreciated. One son came and did household jobs for his widowed mother. One mother mentioned how helpful the local shops were. All these things were not only valuable in themselves but also because they kept the mother in contact with the outside world.

Indirect help with the subnormal This half-way house was mentioned quite often. A typical example of such help was the neighbour who said, 'I'll keep an eye on the door' or the neighbour would keep an eye on the subnormal through the window. In two cases where neighbours had said this, both in the pilot survey, the behaviour of the subnormal was rather difficult. In another family, where there were two subnormals, the mother said:

'I've left them for half an hour, but I've never left them without popping into the neighbour to keep an eye on them. They'll look through the windows and not let the children see.'

This was only helpful with the less severely handicapped, and the big difference between this and coming into the house was made clear by Nancy's mother when talking about a former neighbour:

> 'She was good to Nancy, she would do anything for her. She would come in and see to her, say I wanted to go out, she'd come and stop with her. She wouldn't say, "I'll watch your door", she would come in.'

Direct help with the subnormal   This marks one of the major boundaries in giving support and help to the families of the mentally handicapped. In accepting the subnormal in this way the friend or relative also accepted the parents more fully than was possible otherwise.

There were two major factors concerning the subnormal which affected any direct help with him that could be given. The first was the subnormal's behaviour and physical disabilities. The second was whether he could only be looked after in his own home or whether he could go to other people's homes.

James's father gave an idea of the limitations his behaviour imposed on any help that could be given, which illustrates the first point very clearly.

> Interviewer: What about neighbours and friends? 'Well a lot have volunteered but we have never taken it up because we know what a handful he is, they wouldn't understand him.' Interviewer: Has there been anybody outside the family who has helped with James? 'Odd neighbours at our other house. At the moment the people next door are out working all the time; there is a widow next door the other way but she is not a very big person. James is quite powerful and not in any bad sense of the term, he could push you around without meaning any harm, but he is extremely powerful.' Interviewer: Were there people at the other house who could do things with James? 'Yes, there was a G.P. that lived next door that was extremely friendly with us, and she would occasionally pop in.' Interviewer: Would you think that this was because they knew James when he was younger? 'Yes, I would. This is what I wonder, what the reaction is of somebody coming in and meeting an adult of this type. I think it's different when they're grown up. In the infant stage they are all the same, like pups and kids and one thing and another. One thing that I think we are fortunate in, is that he looks normal.'

Interviewer: So here, in looking after James the neighbours play no part? 'No, we are extremely friendly with all the neighbours, but we've never called upon them at all. Next door she's a nurse and she has said, "Any time you can call upon us", but when they're in I am usually.' Interviewer: Has there ever been an occasion here when you've had to call upon people? 'Not that I can think of.' Interviewer: Would you feel you could ask them for help? 'Yes, there is no doubt that they would help, in fact the widow next door, she belongs to the church just up the road, they've got a Good Samaritan service and these people would come in and stop with James, but he is too much of a handful.' Interviewer: Would you think that any help of this nature was quite impracticable? 'If it was spasmodic and you just asked somebody to come in and they had never been before, I would say it was.' Interviewer: But suppose some people said, we do know the situation and we're prepared to get stuck into it. Would you have thought this might have been a starter? 'Yes, I wouldn't like to pitch anybody straight into it.' Interviewer: But given time and determination? 'Yes, it might have worked in a scheme over a period, once somebody had got used to the idea, if they had come once a fortnight or something, on a regular basis.' Interviewer: So James would know them? 'Yes.'

In the case of James, the limiting factor was his rather tiresome behaviour. As a result he was only left with other members of the family. Another important limiting factor was incontinence. Joyce's mother could leave her with Mrs Castle, a neighbour, 'but she doesn't know how to lift her up', which meant that she could not change Joyce and therefore could not be left with her for very long.

Lifting the subnormal was mentioned by Joyce's mother. This was important and so, naturally, was the subnormal's weight. Whether he was difficult to feed was also relevant and, possibly most important of all, whether he would accept other people. This was particularly important with non-talkers. Several mothers, especially those whose subnormal could not talk, mentioned the way the subnormal had pined while she, the mother, had been away. Another point that has to be considered is whether the mother *thought* the subnormal would accept other people.

The subnormal's disabilities also affected the second factor mentioned, whether the subnormal could be looked after only in his own home, or whether he could go to somebody else's house. The mildly handicapped Douglas, whose main trouble was epilepsy, would sometimes walk down to his aunt and uncle's house near by. The severely epileptic Jean would go and sit for hours in her grandmother's flat next door, and liked it. But James's parents found that it was far easier if his grandparents came to look after him in his own house. There was no question of the totally disabled Terence being moved. Anyone looking after him had to come to him.

The place in which the subnormal could be looked after also depended on the subnormal's relationship to the person helping. The totally disabled Joyce, whom one might think could not possibly be looked after in anybody else's home, went to stay with a friend of her mother's for a fortnight. This was acceptable to Joyce because of the strong relationship with this friend. Without such a relationship it is most unlikely that this would have been possible.

So far two factors have been considered which affect the extent to which direct help could be given to the subnormal. Both these factors were concerned primarily with the subnormal himself. There are three further factors which need to be considered which concern the person giving the help. These are: first, the willingness with which the help is given; second, the physical fitness of the person giving it; and, third, the competence with which the help is given.

The most important of these is the first, the willingness with which the help is given. In one case, where the subnormal's brothers and sisters visited as a matter of painful duty, they tended to speak sharply to the subnormal and their attitude was deeply and bitterly resented. As a result they were not in a position to give any help which was acceptable either to the subnormal or his mother. By contrast Leonard's brothers and sisters were 'very kindly disposed to him' and they 'will always see to Leonard'. Consequently this help was very acceptable. Leonard's father was a widower and, 'If I didn't feel up to the mark and I needed a little washing done they would do it. They'd keep coming in to tidy the house, which my daughter very often does, changing the bed and so on.' Then came the key phrase: 'I've never had to appeal to them to come and do it, they've always come to ask me if they could do it.' Henry's mother said appreciatively of her neighbours: 'Well they've offered.' Christine's mother was moved by the quite unsolicited and genuine help given by the wife of her late husband's employer, which has been mentioned already on page 238.

Judith's mother spoke warmly of the help two students had given.

'Up to a year ago we had two students, and one Saturday afternoon these two students came knocking at my door and they came to see me and Judith and they were grand girls. They're both outside Sheffield at college now. She looked forward to their visit on a Saturday, and they used to just sit and talk to her, and they helped me a few times to bath her, and they made her two nightgowns and a dress. They knew how difficult it was for me to get her arms in and that, it was a special dress and that, and she knew them. They used to talk and shout to her and make her register. They used to shout upstairs, "We're here Judith", she loved them to come because she was in the limelight, they like limelight you know.'

The willingness with which help was offered was generally reflected in the sort of comments made by the mother about the people concerned. 'Oh yes, they're very good', 'He's a grand lad', but however willing relatives or friends might be, the task of looking after the subnormal was physically too great in some cases. Freda's grandmother was getting old and, 'it's going to be a problem soon. She has been coming since Freda was born.' Patricia's parents, who were both over seventy themselves, had a similar problem. Her parents' generation were all getting quite old. This was making things increasingly difficult for them. This problem affected several families. In the case of Patricia's parents it was a question of the age of the parents' brothers and sisters. In other cases where the parents relied on their parents, the same problem hit them a generation earlier. Those families who tended to rely exclusively on the family, and especially the grandparents, for direct help with the subnormal were particularly vulnerable in this way.

A critical factor was whether concern for the subnormal would 'jump' the generations. We have seen that where there were siblings they generally gave their parents and their subnormal brother or sister at least some help. Apart from this there were one or two interesting cases where some other younger relative had 'the touch' for looking after the subnormal.

This leads on to the third factor, the competence with which help was given. One mother commented that her sister tended to panic when looking after the subnormal, and another that her sister would not relax and sit and watch the television but kept fussing about the subnormal. On the other hand Joyce's mother could leave her totally disabled daughter with her friend for a fortnight quite confidently.

'This Mrs Farris that I mentioned took her. Well they've a daughter, their Andrea, she's been more or less brought up with her, Andrea is more or less her age. She [Mrs Farris] has got hold of her like I have and just cleaned her and never bothered.'

The value of having been brought up knowing the subnormal, or knowing the subnormal from when he was a child, was mentioned quite often. The question of competence takes us back to the point made by James's father on page 288. Help with the subnormal is not a job to be undertaken lightly, or for just a week or two, but requires considerable patience over a long period.

One final point should be made about this direct help with the subnormal himself. That is the different length of time that different people would look after him. It ranged from: the neighbour, who was an old-age pensioner, who would sit with the very severely disabled Christine while her mother slipped out to get a prescription; to the grandparents who would come in occasionally in an evening while the parents of the very severely disabled Henry went out to a dance; to the sister who looked after the very severely disabled Tom every Saturday while his parents met other members of the family at a pub; to the son and daughter-in-law who would look after the very severely disabled Judith overnight every fortnight while her parents went out; to the aunt who would look after the severely disabled Jennifer for a whole fortnight while her sister went on holiday.

On a rather different level there were two cases where sisters of the subnormal had taken on the major part of the subnormal's care. The most total form of help was where relatives had taken over the care of the subnormal completely after his parents had died. This had happened in five cases.

Two factors affecting the acceptability of help

Some of these families needed help all too clearly but found it desperately difficult to accept it. There were no doubt many reasons for this, but two seem especially important. The first is speculative, the second has evidence to support it.

The speculative reason is that some of these families wanted to hide away the pain of their subnormal member and not let the world know about it. In cases where the subnormal's behaviour was odd or grotesque, such an attitude is readily understandable. There is, however, no direct evidence to support this, though it did appear to be evident to some extent in a few families. To say that the *family* felt stigmatized would make the same point.

The second reason was a deeply rooted reluctance to intrude on other people. This may be related to the first point but there is no clear evidence that this is so. There was a great reluctance on the part of the parents to encumber their other children with the care of the subnormal. This may well have been a correct decision but there was a rather similar reluctance to intrude on the lives of other relatives or neighbours or ask them for any help. One mother said of her sisters:

'In an emergency they'd always be willing to come, but I have an independent nature, I don't intrude upon either of them any more than is possible.'

Wanting to be independent and not wanting to put upon people was mentioned frequently. Elizabeth's mother has already been quoted.

'I think some of them [her relatives] you know are cross that I don't. I do, really, they'll say "It's no good offering help to you." Different times, years ago, they'd offer to do things but I'd never take them up on it, and I really think they got a bit cross.'

Curiously, it did seem that this feeling of intruding on the lives of relatives and friends was much less marked when the help given was regular. In this way it appears to have become a part of the regular routine of both families, and therefore it did not intrude. (The comments of James's father are relevant once again.) This underlines the importance of such help becoming part of 'the structure of coping' and 'the structure of living'. Regularity of help is one of the major bridges which make it easier for help to be given. It was both the kind of help that was needed and appeared to be the kind of help that it was easiest to give. This may have been because it made it possible for the person helping to build up a relationship with the subnormal. The bath attendant who helped to bath the very severely handicapped Christine was one example of this.

Such regular help was in quite a number of cases only part of a reciprocal relationship where the subnormal's family did not just receive help but also gave it. There is a useful description of this reciprocal relationship in Ronald Frankenberg's book *Communities in Britain* (1966, pp. 159–60). In his chapter on small towns he discusses Margaret Stacey's study of Banbury, *Tradition and Change* (1960). In the course of this he writes:

> Households of wage-earners need each other's help apart from general sociability. They expect to give and receive it in the small emergencies of daily life. If, in a working-class Banbury street, a neighbour runs out of sugar, or salt, she will borrow. If a minor accident means a visit to hospital a neighbour will look after the other children. This sort of exchange is reciprocal but not formally so. There is an informal norm that people help one another. In a situation of weekly wages this is almost inevitable. The degree of necessity varies with the stage of the life cycle that people have reached—the very old and the young married with children will have the greatest need. This, however, is aid in the acute crisis. To deal with chronic crisis requires the bringing in of kin (or in their absence social agencies). For the chronic crisis is likely to infringe on the possibility of reciprocity. Thus the so-called 'rough' working class are in perpetual chronic crisis and are in fact forced back upon their kin by the partial ostracism of 'ordinary' and 'respectable'. The 'respectable' or 'aspirant' . . . are not willing to be under obligation to their neighbours.

This concept of reciprocity fits in with the importance of the sub-normals' families being kept within the normal commerce of living. Reciprocity is an important part of the commerce of normal living and was likely to be particularly important for the subnormals' families, because they were in a state of chronic need and so were likely to run out of credit or 'infringe on the possibility of reciprocity'. Very often they did have to rely on kin but the principle of reciprocity was also important with kin. It does seem to have made it easier for families to receive help if they were also able to give it. Townsend says in his book *The Family Life of Old People* (1963, pp. 61–2): 'What seems to be an essential principle of the daily renewal of an intimate bond between adult relatives is the reciprocation of services between them.'

There was one instance which fitted the description of normal reciprocity very well. The young subnormal woman was only mildly disabled in this case.

> 'I'd never depend on anybody. When my husband was off work if money was slow in coming through, Mrs Thomas next door,

she'd lend me some money and if she is short, you know,
give back, pay back, we always help one another. I get on quite
well with Mrs Thomas next door, she is very good, we've never
had an argument or anything round here. You see we've never
bothered with anyone. She keeps herself to herself, but if
Mrs Thomas knows that we're without she'll help and if we
know she is without we'll help, we don't sit in one another's
houses, but we always help one another, we're good
neighbours like.'

Another point that fits in with the Banbury study was that none of
the four families in the professional class received extensive or regular
help from neighbours, and only one of the six in the intermediate
social class.

The exchange was generally of services. In a few cases it was help
with grandchildren. One mother in the pilot study was very clear
about it.

'I go to fetch my little grand-daughter, I look after her you see,
and she comes home from school for her dinner.'

Then later on she said:

'Well, my son and daughter-in-law, they've got a car. They
generally take us around on a Sunday. With me looking after
Linda [her grandchild] they pay it back that way.'

In another case in the pilot study the mother looked after her
grandchildren every Monday and Tuesday morning, while her
daughter did the washing or the shopping, and her daughter often
looked after Sarah (her subnormal sister) and had her to stay when
her parents went on holiday.

One very satisfactory arrangement was where the subnormal
(Jean) and her widowed mother lived in a flat on the same floor as
her grandmother.

'I wrote to Town Hall and I explained my case to them as best I
could, and they gave us two flats together. Well I've my mother
in an old-age pensioner's flat and I'm in here, and then there's
another old lady that lives on that side. Well she's a bad heart
and my mother's a bad heart, so that old lady comes and
stops with my mother at night. She goes home in day time, but
these two old people sleep together at night so if one's took
bad they can ring my bell and I can see to them. Then if she's

took bad [Jean] I can fetch my mother to sit with her while I come back.' Interviewer: And that works all right? 'Well it has up to now, you see if one old lady is took bad I can look after her, you see the other old lady comes and fetches me, and I can go in and see and give her a drop of brandy or something like that. Well I go shopping for three, I cook for three, and make them all have their meals together. I can't go and cook in here and then in here and then cook in here, we all have our meals in my mother's together, because they watch the traffic going up and down the road. She [Jean] generally sits in grandma's. Well if you cook all together you can see old ladies are getting something to eat, they are enjoying it better than they would if they were on their own, and you are not wasting as much. But they all have their own houses, you understand what I mean. When I get fed up I can just come in my own house and say, I've got five minutes. . . . Well we are all on one landing, she [Jean] goes and sits with her granny while I go and do the shopping, else I couldn't go to town shopping, and we only have to waste one bus fare, otherwise it would be three bus fares. I go in market and do shopping, and that's all there is to it.'

Another family found that having a telephone was very useful. It meant that they had some help to offer to others.

Interviewer: Do you in fact see much of your neighbours? 'Well, most of them work during the day, but when they come home from work I do see quite a lot of them, particularly the one next door.' Interviewer: And you do more than pass the time of day with them? 'Oh yes, she comes in here almost every day for a chat.' Interviewer: And is there anybody else who calls in? 'Well there is, because they all come to use the 'phone you see, and we get quite a lot of company that way.'

Perhaps what they had experienced through looking after their subnormal made some of these mothers sympathetic listeners. One of them said when she was asked if she ever felt lonely:

'Well everybody comes to me if they want a good talk. My sister-in-law comes down and has a natter. I'm not lonely.'

There was a number of other instances where the subnormal's mother was a source of help to a relative or neighbour who had been bereaved as the sister-in-law above had been. This was mentioned quite spontaneously five times. Two mothers also found mutual comfort in the companionship of other mothers who had something wrong with a child (neither was mentally handicapped).

Whatever it was, the fact that the families were not always receiving but had something to give made a big difference to the morale of the family.

There were three important aspects of this reciprocal help. First, it enabled mothers to accept help they needed. Second, it made the mothers (and fathers) feel they were needed, that they were valued as people apart from just looking after the subnormal, and, third, it helped them to feel that they were a part of life, not people who had been condemned to social euthanasia.

Conclusion

It appeared in the main that the mothers preferred to ask their other children for help with the subnormal, wherever this was possible. Husbands, whatever their social class, generally gave a great deal of help. The extent of help from the husbands serves to underline the double handicap under which the widows laboured. They had to look after the subnormal and they had no husband to help them. This is a group that needs special attention.

An important factor in the amount of help that anyone, whether friend or relative, could give was nearness. The kind of help that the families needed could be given far more easily and effectively by someone who lived near by. The families who received the strongest support were generally those who had relatives living close at hand. The importance of nearness in the giving of effective help and support is shown by the finding that neighbours appeared to give as much help as relatives to the subnormal and his family. Thirty-five of the fifty families who had relatives (three families appeared to have no relatives) received considerable support from them (70 per cent) and thirty-nine of the fifty-three families received considerable support from neighbours (74 per cent). The reluctance of some families to move from a neighbourhood where they were known and from which they received considerable support was very marked. The removal of a neighbour who had been a great help, not from Sheffield, but from the immediate locality had been a grievous blow to two of the mothers. In one case a friend had only moved quarter of an hour's walk away, but it had reduced very sharply the amount of help and support she could give.

Unfortunately the interview schedule was not as detailed about exactly how far away siblings and relatives lived as hindsight shows would have been desirable. However, this was made good by more detailed questioning in the later interviews, and the text of earlier interviews often gave the necessary information.

In a few cases the evidence is rather circumstantial but the overall pattern is clear. If one considers just those cases where siblings of the subnormal or other relatives gave much help, the importance of nearness is apparent. Out of ten siblings who gave much help, in one case all four siblings lived in another part of Sheffield but some distance away, two lived about quarter of an hour's journey away and seven lived within five minutes' walk of where the subnormal lived.

There were sixteen families where other relatives gave much help. In three cases the relatives lived in Sheffield but some distance away, in another three they lived about quarter of an hour's journey away and in ten cases they lived within five minutes' walk of where the subnormal lived. It is clear that when considering the basic needs that these families had, geographical nearness was a most important factor in meeting those needs effectively.

This indicates what an important role housing can play in giving these families the support they require.[2] A family might need to move to a house with a garden, as in the case of Stanley's family, they might need to move so that they were near to relatives, or they might need *not* to be moved from an unsuitable house because of the links they had with the neighbourhood. Instead, what might be necessary is apparently uneconomical adaptations to the house so that they could remain in it. It could be easier for the council to build a ramp and a bathroom and lavatory downstairs than for a family with a subnormal member to rebuild an extensive, sympathetic and supportive network of local relationships. Such relationships are important for any family, but particularly so for families like these. For them, they can make the difference between a life that is worth living and a life that is one long, monotonous chore.

What the mothers thought of the general practitioners and mental welfare officers

General practitioners   Most of the families were past the stage where they needed a lot of reassurance from their family doctors about the care of the subnormal. In several cases the doctors had said that the mothers knew more than they did about what dosage of a particular drug their subnormal needed, and gave the mothers considerable discretion. Out of fifty-three mothers fourteen thought their general practitioner was a lot of help, twenty thought his help was average, nineteen thought him little help.

This reflects in part the amount that the doctor was needed, and if he was not needed he was unlikely to be much help. This accounts for many cases where help was little or average. However, even where the medical help given was adequate, sometimes the doctor's manner was criticized.

'This doctor, I can meet him in the road and I'll say good morning or good afternoon, and he'll look straight through me . . . he hasn't the patience with you, and I think I get all churned up.'

This is a criticism that any person might make of a doctor, but a very few persons were highly critical of the doctor's attitude to their subnormal. In both the following instances the doctor was considered little help. The question asked in both cases was: Do you find that your doctor has been a help to you?

'No, my doctor told me straight to get rid of that boy that's daft, and have a life of your own. He's no help at all.'

'No, I do not. One [of the doctors in the practice] used to say I was a martyr, and he didn't know how I looked after her, he couldn't and he wouldn't. I said it's ridiculous, if you came to have a baby like this you'd love it and look after it. He said: "I wouldn't." Well they say things like that, that were one particular one, I'm going back some years now, but there was another one, he's not often there now, but I once had to snub him because he used to snub me. She was once really ill with measles and he said, "This is it, this is it", and I said, "What do you mean, this is it", and he said, "Well, it's a fifty-fifty chance now, she'll have to go to hospital." I said, "She won't." She were fifteen then. He said, "You can't look after her", I said, "I can, you tell me what to do and I'll do it." He said, "You'll not get the special stuff down that I want to give her." I said, "She's fifteen years old, I've looked after her for fifteen years, I'll look after her through measles", and he said, "She'll just have to go into hospital, she'll just have to do this." He's blunt with anyone normal, but he was extra blunt with her, and I just choked him off. I said, "Look here doctor, I know she is no good to the community but she's *mine*, I bore her, I brought her into this world and I love her, choose what you say." He didn't know what to say you know. He bounced down them stairs: he came again next day and he changed his tune completely. He said, "I could do with you to teach a few more mothers what to do."'

The same mother also said:

'We only contact him when her ear needs syringing, but I do think they should come now and again to give her a check-up.'

Several other mothers mentioned that they would like the doctor to call to give the subnormal a check-up. In addition there were one or two cases where it seemed that a more detailed and thorough study of the subnormal's epilepsy might have made it possible for the fits to be better controlled. Where the doctor did call regularly it was much appreciated.

'Well this new doctor, he calls in twice a week to see him. He's told me if I'm worried during the night I am to ring him during the night.'

Another doctor called in once a month to see that the subnormal was well. This was considered much help in both cases. Sheila Hewett's observation on the feelings of the mothers of cerebral palsied children (1970, p. 158) is apt: 'Their comments on helpful and unhelpful general practitioners seem to indicate that their perception of their relationship with their medical advisors is influenced very much by the doctor's ability to convey the idea that he is an ally, working *with* the parents, not against them.'

Mental welfare officers Mental welfare officers came out rather worse than the general practitioners. Out of fifty-three families:

10 thought that the mental welfare officer was a lot of help
16 that he was average help
27 that he was little or no help.

We encountered the same problem as Sheila Hewett of the families being very uncertain who was a mental welfare officer and who came from some other department. However, these families did not receive as many visits from official agencies as the children in Mrs Hewett's survey, and so it was easier to decide who any particular visitor was.

Almost exactly half reckoned the mental welfare officer was little or no help. 'We never see anybody; we haven't had anyone for eight or nine years.' 'We never see him.' 'Well, I used to get them once a year when I was down at my mother's, but I've never had anyone up here.' (She had been 'up here' for seven years.) The families may have forgotten about more recent visits but visits can hardly have been frequent.

However, sometimes the mother saw no reason for visits. 'I couldn't say they have not been helpful, but there hasn't been any necessity to help.' 'Well visits are few and far between. We hardly ever see anybody for years. But that could be partly our fault because apart from the short stay home we don't really bother anybody.'

However not all the parents who had not been visited felt like this.

'That's what I say, they don't come. They ought to come visiting me but the last one that came, she said, "We know that Nancy is well looked after." We just seem to be the forgotten two.'

'Well they're supposed to come to your home once a month, but now they don't. They don't come once in every moon, and as you say, who do I talk to? Well, who can I talk to if they don't come? He's under them isn't he?'

Both these families needed help. Another family was managing perfectly well and could have got in touch with the mental health department if help had been needed, but the father said, 'You have mentioned this short-term care. Actually the thing has never been put to us.' One mother had stronger views.

'No, I found them more of a nuisance than anything. They, like you, said, "What's going to happen?" They pressed the point

more, "When you die, what is going to happen to her?" and then
they go into all sordid details, but I prefer to leave it in God's
hands.'

In all the cases quoted so far the mental welfare officer's help was
considered to be little or none. Where help was considered average
the parents' comments tended to be rather non-committal. 'They
come to see me. If there was anything I needed they would be the
people I got in touch with.' 'He's very nice and Mrs Percival before
him, she were very nice.'

It was sometimes difficult to decide between whether the help was
average or much because, while the mental welfare officer was giving
much help at the time of the visit, this, in some instances, had not
always been the case. This was so with Helen's family.

'Well as a matter of fact I never heard a word from them, and
[they said] now that Helen isn't going to school you'll get a
visit about every two months. I never heard a thing for three
years, then I went to a meeting up at Lodge Moor and there
was some member there who mentioned it. Next day a person
from the Town Hall came, and they said, "Do you want her
to go away?" Well, she came twice, then I never had another
visit of any description until about February, and he said,
"I am Mr X from Mental Health", and he has been goodness
itself. He calls as regular as clockwork once a month. Well you
feel somebody is taking a note of you then, don't you. He'll
call and say, "Do you want anything? How are you going on?"
He got us to see Dr Leakey and I said, "What am I going to do
when you go? I suppose I am going to be left again high and
dry." [He is going on a course.] He said, "Well I'll be back in
a year", but a year is a long time, isn't it, and I can ask him
anything and he'll tell me where to go. Well I knew nothing
before, I was just at a dead loss.'

It was the situation at the time of the visit which was taken into
account, so this was considered to be much help. So was the help
given to Judith's mother.

'I were just going through a phase with my nerves, I were crying
and crying and crying, I were going silly with me head, I were
feeling terrible, and nobody had been to see me. . . . Mr
Pinkerton I told you about, he's a real use . . . you know he's
for these children. He came to see me and he *knew* me, he knew

the difference in me and he went into action straight away and he had Dr Leakey from the hospital come to see me and she were grand. She held my hand and said, "You let me look after Judith for you, let me arrange for Judith to be looked after for three, four or five weeks", you know she were marvellous. That's how she came to be known at the hospital. The ordinary mental welfare, they weren't going into it properly until Mr Pinkerton come to see me. When Dr Leakey came I wouldn't let her [Judith] go because I was getting a bit better, but she [Dr Leakey] said she'd always arrange a bed for Judith. You know the Town Hall could never guarantee me a fortnight's holiday, whereas Dr Leakey has guaranteed me one, more or less has, you know.'

Julian's mother also found the mental welfare officer a help.

'This gentleman that comes now doesn't talk down to Julian, we're on the same level. We discuss sideboards and whose are longest now. He's very patient and very good. I kind of feel I've got a friend there now.'

There were two instances in the pilot study where the mental welfare officer was clearly a very great help to the mother, and each of these persons echoed Julian's mother when she said, 'I kind of feel I've got a friend there now.'

A glance at figure 13 shows that the help given by the mental welfare officers (line 27) was not related in any obvious way to the families' need. There were clear instances where help from a mental welfare officer was needed and it had not been given, though it is true that in no case had the family asked for a visit and not received one.

The amount of help given by the mental welfare officers is not impressive, especially when one considers the burdens under which many of these families were labouring, but there is more to it than the mental welfare department simply not doing its job. Some of these issues are considered in the next section.

Factors influencing the effectiveness of help from social workers

Relationship of social workers to the provision of services The visits underlined the importance of the point made in chapter 10, that the social workers were put in an impossible situation when they were

not in a position to offer to the family the help that they needed.
The help needed most acutely was day care for the very severely
disabled. There was no day care available for these adults apart
from the four cases where the subnormal was looked after for one
or two days a week in hospital or at the session for spastics run by
the Spastics Society one day a week.[1] As one parent who had received
very few visits said:

> 'You can cope on your own and any difficulties you come up
> against, you call on your own doctor, and that's more or less it.
> We've never felt there's been any particular need to get in touch
> with them. We've never felt there's anything they could do.
> I heard that when he finished at Norfolk Park [the special care
> unit] at sixteen, that they just stay at home and that was it.'

One of the reasons that the doctors were considered more helpful
than the mental welfare officers is probably because the families
had a better idea of what the doctor was for. If the social worker
was unable to do anything about the family's most pressing need, and
the parents seemed well adjusted and did not want to talk about
'problems' with the mental welfare officer, it is not surprising that
contact was dropped.

It is interesting that in several of the cases where the mental
welfare officer was considered helpful, he had been able to *do*
something. One mother said:

> 'A few years ago I was having all this noise and it was through
> them that I got the notice [it said "No ball games allowed"].
> It isn't a playground this grass, it wasn't supposed to be, but
> there was football until ten o'clock at night, it was dreadful.
> And through the mental health people they got the notice put
> up, and it has improved from there. Well, they've done a thing
> which has helped me most, that is to get this bit of quietness
> which I need at night to relax myself to cope.'

In the first example of much help quoted above, the mental welfare
officer 'got us to see Dr Leakey' and in the second 'he went into
action straight away'. But there appeared to be few instances where
the mental welfare officers did anything practical which related to
the immediate needs of the subnormal. The main exception to this
was arranging short-term care, but even this was sometimes arranged
directly with the administrative staff of the Mental Health Service.
True, there were a few instances where, as in the case already quoted,

'If there was anything I needed they would be the people I got in touch with', but such basic aids as incontinence pads, a cot bed, or a bath attendant seem to have been suggested most often by a neighbour or health visitor rather than by the social worker.

This is a pity because the provision of some basic help of this kind appeared in some instances to be the basis upon which other help became more acceptable—especially the sort of help a social worker is trained to give. More will be said about this shortly.

There seemed to be two factors which lay behind the rather limited contacts the mental welfare officers had with these families. The first was the powerlessness of the mental welfare officers to offer what was needed, especially day care for the very severely disabled. The second was the general training, the attitude to the relationship between casework practice and practical assistance, and the lack of knowledge of some mental welfare officers about what physical helps and aids were available for the family.

The result of this was often few visits or complete loss of contact.

Where the social worker's casework skills seemed relevant This loss of contact by the social worker was sometimes most unfortunate. Two instances of this have been given already. There were cases where the mother *did* want to talk to somebody who came from outside her immediate environment. The value placed on regular visits by Helen's mother, 'You feel somebody is taking note of you', was echoed by others, but as Helen's mother said to the mental welfare officer, when she learned that he was going on a course for a year, 'What am I going to do when you go . . . a year is a long time.'

No sooner was contact established than the social worker was off. A fundamental aspect of work with these families is its long-term nature, and a high turnover of social workers makes it far more difficult to give the families the sort of help they need.

Related to this is the point made by one of the mothers in the pilot survey. She was very eloquent about her need for a 'mother figure, a sort of mother confessor' to whom she could talk and unburden herself. 'Not these young dollies that come in their mini-skirts but more someone like myself who would know what I was going through.' She mentioned how valuable it would be to have someone, perhaps middle-aged like herself, who was not a member of the family and who could come and look after her very severely disabled son for a while every now and again. It may be hard to criticize a social worker for being young and dressing accordingly but this very articulate mother did express a need which was evidently not being met by the Mental Health Service. It is not difficult to see why an experienced married woman who has brought up a family and is extremely busy looking after her subnormal child should be irritated by a young social worker who wants to explore the mother's feelings but has no experience of bringing up children and has no practical help to offer.

There was one area in particular where it seemed that the skilled help of a social worker could be most important but was rarely given. (This leaves on one side the problems the mother of a *young* subnormal child may have in accepting her child for what he is.) This was to help the mothers deal creatively with the extremely close bond which generally grew up between the subnormal and herself. This was discussed at some length in chapter 14. One dangerous aspect of this relationship appeared to be that the mother could become the subnormal's only contact with the outside world. In these circumstances the removal of the mother from the subnormal, whether by death or illness, could have a devastating impact on the subnormal. However, judging from the comments of some of the mothers, and on the evidence of some of the files, the situation where the parents and the subnormal or a widow and the subnormal were jogging along without presenting the authorities with any problems was likely to be viewed as 'good care', and they would be left to get on with it. If the subnormal was not going to training centre, as the more disabled and many of the older ones were not, the situation tended to encourage the growth of an over-intense and exclusive relationship between the subnormal and his mother.

Such a relationship needs handling with great care because there is much in it that gives the subnormal a sense of well-being. For this situation to be dealt with creatively, skilled help over a long period, with adequate facilities for day care, and short-term care which is readily acceptable by the mother, are essential.

On the same general issue, there appeared to be a too-easy acceptance of defeat if the subnormal refused to go to training centre, or the family were for some reason unable to get him ready in time. The way the problem of getting the subnormal up in the morning was solved, in at least two cases, was by him ceasing to attend training centre. This solved the immediate problem but the long-term price was likely to be very high. In two other cases the life of the subnormal and his family had been transformed by him starting to attend training centre.

In the very few cases where the family presented more typical social work problems, the contact between the social worker and family was generally good.

The level at which social workers operate There appeared to be a general uncertainty among the mental welfare officers about the sort of service they should be trying to offer to the subnormals and their families, let alone how to offer it. This appeared to be the basic reason for the poor or indifferent opinions of the mental welfare officers' services. The problem is partly due to the very different demands made by the mentally ill and the mentally subnormal. It may be that a rather different approach is required to help the mentally subnormal from that which is required to help the mentally ill. It may be that the training is too much devoted to understanding the acute problems of the mentally ill, not the long-term living of the mentally subnormal. It may be that the psycho-dynamic bias of social workers and social work training does not make them sufficiently aware of the mundane 'slog' of caring for the subnormal.

But, fundamentally, I am convinced that the social work help which was offered was simply irrelevant. It was not related to the everyday situation of the lives of the families of the subnormal. The overwhelming fact of caring for the subnormal was the everyday 'slog', the daily grind which was sketched out in chapter 15. It was because the help offered did not take account of the fact that the subnormals had to be got up, dressed, fed, put to bed and generally cared for every day that so many had to be admitted to hospital, because for all their weaknesses the hospitals do take account of this basic fact.

There was, however, one part of the help offered by the Mental Health Service which did take account of this. It fulfilled two of the vital requirements for help that related to the families' daily routine— regularity and reliability. This was the training centres. Where the subnormal was able enough to attend, this made an enormous difference. The mother of the moderately disabled Ronald said:

'It gives you that relief during the day.' Interviewer: Does Ronald enjoy it? 'Oh yes, he comes down in the morning and says, "Here goes the bus." He is ready for it in the morning. See at the weekend he doesn't know what to do with himself, it's something to occupy his mind, and he doesn't know what to do at home.'

Mark was mildly disabled. His sister made a similar point.

'It gives him something to do, it occupies his mind, he has
something to look forward to the next day.' Interviewer: Does
he enjoy it? 'Yes, he really does.'

Arthur was moderately disabled. His mother had a very high
opinion of the training centre.

'It's a wonderful place, a wonderful atmosphere. The atmosphere
I think is terrific, they're obviously cared for, and that's the
main thing.'

This high opinion of the training centres was general, but only
seventeen out of fifty-three attended. A few had done so in the
past and had ceased to do so. In a few cases there was unfavourable
comment, but, for the most part, this is a service which works well,
is appreciated and well used, because it relates to the actual pattern
of living of the families concerned and meets the needs of both
the subnormal and his family.

The families of the very few very severely disabled who received
some day care in hospital also appreciated this service.

'Up to me starting to go for outpatient treatment it didn't
matter what I wanted, I had to depend on somebody either
to go for me, or come and sit in while I went. Well you couldn't
do your shopping like that, it were one mad dash while you
got back. You're thinking "Are they waiting to go." Well it
does give you these two days, you think, "Oh I haven't got
to dash back."'

But in one important respect the service was lacking—punctuality.

'Sometimes it could be half past eight, another time she's been
here nearly twelve o'clock, it's the same with her coming home,
that's only point I've got with it. I once went out and I got
in at four o'clock, and I'd not been in three minutes and
ambulance was back. Well it doesn't give you much time
really, because them is your only two days, you can go out,
but then you can't go out comfortable.'

There is one other point about training centres. A place must be
available there when it is needed. Ruby was in her middle thirties.
Her mother said:

'No, she's never had any training of any kind.' Interviewer: Would you like her to? 'Well I am afraid it's a bit late now, she is too set in her habits now, that's the one thing that ought to have happened years ago. Had she gone when she was younger and took it as a matter of course, yes. Now it would be an upheaval and she'd go all to pieces and nobody would get any benefit from it.'

We can see that the help provided by the training centres was much appreciated and well used. This is because it was, in the terms used about the daily grind, structural help which was directly relevant to the daily routine of the subnormals and their families. This help also fulfilled the requirements of regularity and reliability, which were essential if it was to fit into the family's routine. This was not true in general of the help given by the mental welfare officers.

The overwhelming impression given by the visits was that the sort of help which either made or would have made a difference to the lives of the subnormals and their families was help with the small details of daily or weekly routine. It was these details which affected the quality of life of the subnormal and his family far more than the occasional visit of a mental welfare officer.

This is not to imply that social workers are failing in their duty by not lifting a heavy subnormal woman in and out of bed every morning and evening, or by not playing football with an over-active young man for half an hour every day. But if the way the services are organized leads the client to assume that the social worker will, by some miraculous powers, do just this, they will be disappointed. Moreover, while much help might be given by home helps (but only one mother received such help), various domiciliary nursing services (five cases)[2] and physical aids, such as chairs, ramps and handrails, the value of such services, when they were offered, was often reduced considerably by their irregularity and lack of punctuality.

Among the families visited, the position in almost every case was that the theoretical statutory responsibility for the well-being of the families rested on the shoulders of the mental welfare officers. Because the families' well-being depended so much on aspects of daily living, this was a totally unrealistic burden to expect them to bear. It is true that the social workers could have known more about what services and aids were available, but, basically, they were in as impossible a position here as they were with the lack of day care for the very severely disabled.

The organization of the Mental Health Service, and the mental welfare officers in particular, was not geared to providing this sort of service, with the one notable exception of the training centres. The Mental Health Service was not meeting the *basic* needs of these families, that is the needs connected with the daily grind (chapter 15). The same criticism could be made in general terms about the help given with the wider aspects of living, recreation and suchlike which were considered in chapter 16. This is a criticism of the way the service was organized. Since the visits were made, the social services have been reorganized into the new unified social service department. There is little evidence to suggest that the reorganized department is better equipped to help with these *basic* needs.

The radical implications of a policy of community care find little place in the way the social services operate, or even in thinking about how they should operate. The services have grown and been modified from an originally paternalistic and authoritarian basis, which assumed that at a certain stage the client would *not* be cared for in the community. The care of the mentally defective in the past is a good example of this. There have been modifications to the way the services operate but no radical reorientation. One of the modifications was to tag on an idea called 'community care' but the lack of fundamental rethinking can be seen all too clearly.

The assumption about the way the social services should operate still appears to be that, first of all, the social services will try to help a certain group of people, and then the general public should be asked to help the social services. Such an understanding seems implicit in the 1971 White Paper *Better Services for the Mentally Handicapped*. Voluntary service is not mentioned until the seventh of eight chapters. The heading of the second section in that chapter is 'Supplementing official services'. The position of these families shows that this approach is the wrong way round. It is not a question of the community 'supplementing official services'; it is a question of the official services helping and enabling the community to do better the caring it does already, with more help and less strain on individual members of it.

The pattern of such help is already there. There were cases where the subnormal and his family were helped, sustained and kept in the mainstream of the life of the community by extensive, regular and reliable help from relatives, neighbours and friends. Two of the most remarkable instances of this were Joyce and Terence, both of whom were almost totally disabled. In both cases the care of the family was assisted by official help. Both received various forms of nursing aids. In addition Joyce received twice-weekly day care in hospital and Terence was admitted to hospital very quickly and informally whenever he was ill.

These and the many other instances of the help and support that were given indicate the way in which the official services can help the family and community to care for their subnormal. The help needs to be regular, reliable, relatively permanent, accessible, acceptable and, whenever possible, reciprocal. Wherever families received help which measured up to this formidable specification, it was nearly always also *local* (see page 297).

Administratively this is the key to giving these families help that relates to the business of everyday living. It does not mean that all services must be locally based. Some, for instance training centres and assessment centres, would have to be organized centrally. It does mean that the fundamental thinking and organization of the services needs to start from the locality where the subnormal lives. It would be impossible to organize centrally help of the kind and scale which is required. To accept that the service which these families need should be based locally has wide implications. The pattern of the needs of these families suggests very strongly that if more than minor administrative tidying up is to be done, some way of providing a service which is locally based must be found.

This is considered further in the final chapter of conclusions and recommendations.

19   Conclusions

An outline of the pattern of service proposed in the White Paper
Better Services for the Mentally Handicapped **and the Sheffield Development Project**

The White Paper published in 1971 proposes far-reaching and radical changes in the whole pattern of services for the mentally handicapped. Any recommendations need to be related to these extensive changes proposed by the Government.

One of the most impressive parts of the White Paper is the list in chapter 3 of general principles on which the proposals are based. These principles establish firmly the rights of mentally handicapped people and their families to the same social contacts and the same health and welfare provision as other members of society, the only provisos being according to their capacity and according to their needs. In the light of the latter it is good to see a clear statement of the handicapped person's needs for initial assessment, reassessment and 'stimulation, social training and education and purposeful occupation or employment in order to develop to his maximum capacity'. The needs of the family are also recognized. 'Each handicapped person should live with his family as long as this does not impose an undue burden on them or him, and he and his family should receive full advice and support.'

When the handicapped person has to leave his home, there is frequent emphasis on the need for the substitute home to be homelike and the importance of 'constant human relationships', including links with his own family. The importance of hospital services being 'accessible to the population they serve' is also stressed.

There is a refreshing statement that the administrative machine must serve the individual not vice versa. 'There should be proper co-ordination in the application of relevant professional skills for the benefit of individual handicapped people and their families, and in the planning and administration of relevant services, *whether or not these cross administrative frontiers*' (my italics). In view of this 'hospital and local authority services should be planned and operated in partnership'.

312

The importance of voluntary service and 'understanding and help from friends and neighbours and from the community at large' is also recognized. In practice I feel that it is inadequately recognized but its importance does not pass unnoticed.

These principles are made more impressive by the fact that they are backed up with specific figures, albeit tentative, which show a clear change in policy (see table 5 of the White Paper). The number of hospital places for adults is to be nearly halved (from 52,100 in 1969 to 27,000) and the number of residential places provided by local authorities is to go up almost sevenfold (from 4,300 in 1969 to 29,400). For children, hospital places will be cut by a thousand (from 7,400 in 1969 to 6,400) and the number of local authority residential places increased from 1,800 in 1969 to 4,900. In addition, fostering, lodgings and other forms of residential care are to be increased for children from 100 places to 1,000, for adults from 550 to 7,400. As well as this, day care and training centre provision is to be increased. For instance, the number of training centre places for adults living in the community is to go up from 24,500 to 63,700.

This extensive programme is expected to be spread over as many as fifteen to twenty years, though the White Paper expects some authorities to complete it in ten years.

Possibly the biggest question mark to be put against the White Paper is money. This will depend very largely on the local authorities. 'The Government will play its part, but the main responsibility lies with the local authorities themselves' (para. 198).

It is the implementation of the policy, rather than the policy itself, which raises the questions. For this reason the Sheffield Development Project is important. It is, as its sub-title tells us, a 'feasibility study report proposing a new pattern of service for mentally handicapped people in Sheffield County Borough'. It was published in its final version in February 1971, four months before the White Paper. A summary of the proposals in the Development Project sent out in October 1971 after the White Paper was published says: 'The study was undertaken during the period when the policies described in Command 4683 (the White Paper) were being developed and this influenced the team's thinking to an important degree.'

The summary of the Sheffield Project also carries a careful disclaimer. 'It must be emphasised that the proposals contained in the study report are recommendations for services in Sheffield

County Borough and are not intended necessarily as a blueprint which the Department would like to see universally adopted in other areas.' It may be that this is directed in particular to the fact that the proposed Sheffield pattern has no separate hospitals at all for the mentally handicapped, whereas the White Paper perches carefully on the fence on the question of whether or not there should be any 'larger specialized hospitals as in the present hospital service' (para. 191). However, the Sheffield Project is clearly going to have important implications for the way the services will develop over the country and most of the discussion that follows is directed to considering the way in which the pattern proposed for Sheffield, based on small units rather than larger specialized hospitals, might function most effectively.

It will be clear from the discussion which follows that the writer favours the small unit rather than the larger specialized hospital. The reasons for this preference derive in large part from the visits that were made during the research to the families where the mentally handicapped member was living at home. It should be made clear, however, that no special visits for the purpose of the research were made either to handicapped people in hospital or to their families, and so this preference does not arise from a direct comparative study.

The proposals for Sheffield in the Sheffield Development Project are summarized in more detail in appendix E. They provide for comprehensive assessment of all mentally handicapped children by a multidisciplinary team, increased provision of day care, in particular for very severely disabled adults, and a fourfold increase in training centre places.

Residential care will include four twenty-four bed hospital units for children, two on general hospital sites and two in a community setting. There will be two additional local authority homes of fifteen to twenty places with the possibility of a third.

There will be twelve hospital units for adults with twenty-four beds in each. Four units will be on an existing district general site, four on the site of a proposed district general hospital and four in a community setting. In addition there will be a twenty-four bedded unit on a mental hospital site for emotionally disturbed adolescents and adults. The local authority will provide about 350 residential places in the community in a variety of ways, including residential homes, group homes and boarding-out arrangements.

The study also recommends a joint local authority and hospital social work service and a jointly appointed organizer of voluntary services.

One of the most important features of the Sheffield Development Project from the planning point of view is that it attempts to draw the line between those who are the responsibility of the local authority and those who are the responsibility of the hospital authorities, when residential care is needed. The basis of this division is 'the degree of functional handicap suffered by the potential residents' (para. 3.3). They suggest three groups:

A. Those who, because of heavy physical handicaps or severe behaviour problems, require the support of a full hospital service fairly close at hand;

B. Those who, because of less obvious physical handicaps, possibly some degree of incontinence and behaviour problems, require limited medical supervision;

C. Those who could be cared for within a normal home if such a home were available to them.

The division of responsibility is based on the hospital authorities providing beds for groups A and B and the local authorities for group C. It is admitted that 'the lines between the groups may be found to have been drawn in the wrong places'. This uncertainty about where the line should be drawn also appears in the White Paper. The White Paper envisages that 'in future, when only those really needing hospital care are admitted to hospital, local authority homes will receive residents in need of more personal care and help than most present residents' (para. 167).

The figures in the Sheffield Development Project differ in a small way from those in the White Paper, having a slightly heavier bias towards hospital provision. The main difference is that the White Paper proposes only thirteen places for children in hospital per 100,000 population, whereas the Sheffield Project plans twenty places, half on a hospital site (group A), half in a community setting (group B).

Despite this difference (and the Sheffield plans may be modified in the light of experience), the Sheffield proposals are an indication of the way in which the division of responsibility proposed in the White Paper may work out in practice. The three groups of 'functional handicap' which the Sheffield Project adopts as the basis for its recommendations for residential care have wide implications. These are considered below (pp. 317–20).

A summary of the main findings from the visits

(a)   *The attitude of the parents*

The attitude of the parents, and especially the mother, to the mentally handicapped person affects everything else. The attitude of the family to the wider family, friends, neighbours, doctors or social workers is bound to be influenced profoundly by the sort of person the mother is, her attitude to the handicapped person and to life in general. A range of attitudes was traced from a negative refusal to accept the reality of the subnormal's handicap and withdrawal into fantasy, to a positive, warm, loving acceptance of the subnormal for what he or she was. For those who could not talk, a close relationship with the person or people caring for him was often very important. This was especially significant because of the pattern of non-verbal communication which frequently developed between the handicapped person and those caring for him.

(b)   *The concept of the structure for coping*

In chapter 15 the impact of the daily grind of looking after the subnormal was outlined. It was seen that the way the families managed was by creating a 'structure for coping'. This led to the use of the phrase 'structural help' for help which related to the 'structure for coping'.

(c)   *The concept of the structure of living*

A consideration of the families' social activities, holidays and suchlike gave rise to the concept of 'the structure of living'. This is closely related to, but separable from, the 'structure for coping'. The importance of the attitude of the parents was noticed once again. The factor of central importance in this 'structure of living' appeared to be the extent to which this structure incorporated the subnormal and his family into the general commerce of living and the life of the wider community. The outline of different levels of help given by family, friends or neighbours shows how various levels of help related to the 'structure for coping' and the 'structure of living'.

(d) *The need for effective help to fit in with the structure for coping or the structure of living*

Such help needed to be regular, reliable and punctual. The training centres were a good example of official provision which met these requirements.

(e) *The importance of nearness in giving effective help*

Where effective help was given which related to the structure for coping or the structure of living, it was given most often by people who lived close at hand.

(f) *The general ineffectiveness of social work help*

This may have been in part due to ineffectiveness in providing practical assistance, but of far greater importance was the fact that the social work help offered was *not* related to the everyday needs of the families, i.e. to the structure for coping or the structure of living.

(g) *The potential help available from the community*

Some of the families were very isolated, but most received a fair amount of informal help, and some a great deal, from family, friends and neighbours. Given the will, the right approach and some assistance, the visits made it clear that the actual help already given by the community was considerable and the potential even greater.

A commentary on the Sheffield Development Project and the White Paper

This commentary concentrates on issues about which this study has something relevant to say. It does not deal with every aspect.

(a) *The profoundly handicapped*

Both the White Paper and the Sheffield Development Plan assume that the profoundly handicapped, especially those with additional physical handicaps, will need care in hospital. For instance, the Sheffield Development Plan says that for such people 'the need for hospital in-patient services seems unequivocal' (para. 3.2). The White Paper is less dogmatic: 'There are different opinions, even among the experts, on the extent to which local authority services can meet the needs of people with substantial but not profound mental handicap.' However, the White Paper appears to assume that the profoundly handicapped will need full hospital care.

This study questions any such assumption. It has shown that care at home can be of positive value for the profoundly retarded, and from this it can be argued that residential care in a locally based unit may be particularly important for this group of people. In all fairness it should be noted that the Sheffield Development Plan did recognize that the families of some severely handicapped people might want to look after them at home (para. 3.3). This does, however, give the impression of being an afterthought.

What are the advantages of care at home for the profoundly retarded? It will not always be a good thing for either the subnormal or his family. Among the fifty-four families visited, over half of whose mentally handicapped members could be described as severely or very severely disabled, there was one case whose immediate admission to hospital would have helped both him and his family, and the family wanted him admitted. In addition, in some of the few families (seven at the most) where the relationship with the subnormal appeared to be near the negative end of the positive/negative axis described in chapter 14, the subnormal might have been better off in residential care. With these possible exceptions the visits showed that, while the families might pay a high price for keeping him at home, the subnormal was generally cared for and loved as a valued person. This was of special importance where the subnormal was unable to speak. The relationship of the subnormal with his mother and other members of the family enabled him to have a measure of non-verbal communication which would be difficult to equal in most institutional settings.

The difficulties and dangers of this relationship becoming over-close and too exclusive were mentioned in chapter 14, but it is not the difficulties of nursing or the possible emotional problems which are most important. The most important factor is the positive value of the human relationship which enables the subnormal to lead as fully a personal and satisfying life as possible. This is not to say that even the very severely retarded must be looked after at home; nor is it to say that a life which is as fully personal and satisfying as possible cannot be achieved in a residential setting; but it does mean that the care these families gave to their subnormal member showed, especially in the case of the very severely disabled, how vital a factor this relationship is. Any pattern of care for the very severely disabled needs to build on this relationship, not deny it. This may not be easy because an important part of the relationship often appeared to be the physical care given to the subnormal. The fact remains that if human values are to be the determining ones in the care of the mentally handicapped, the positive value of intimate personal relationships cannot be denied.

The positive advantages of care at home should not be taken to deny that the very severely disabled will often need residential care and will often need it from childhood. This was evident from the analysis of the files in Part I. But such residential care needs to be planned on a basis which acknowledges the prime importance of the relationships that the severely disabled can have with their family or friends. The White Paper recognizes this in its list of general principles.

It is recognition of this that lends force to the argument that serious consideration should be given to the possibility of looking after the profoundly handicapped in locally based residental units. Residential care in such units would make it possible for existing contacts with family and friends to be maintained far more easily. The importance of nearness in enabling friends or family to give effective help to subnormals and their families at home has been pointed out already (page 297). The same can be expected to be true when the mentally handicapped person is in residential care. In view of the particular value to the profoundly handicapped of existing close personal relationships, special consideration should be given to how these relationships can be maintained in good working order. Residential care in a locally based hostel may be one way in which this can be done.

(b) *The relative importance of medical, social and geographical factors*

The discussion about the profoundly handicapped, above, may have indicated one weakness in the approach adopted both in the Sheffield Development Project and in the White Paper. This is an excessive medical bias in their categories. In both documents overmuch administrative weight is given to factors which can be described broadly as medical (e.g. 'functional handicap' in the Sheffield Development Project), and too little weight is given to social factors. This is a question of balance. The importance of physical and medical factors is not disputed. It is a question of the relative weight given to each in the planning.

The insufficient weight given to social factors can be illustrated most clearly in the Sheffield plans for residential accommodation. This is planned on the basis of 'the degree of functional handicap suffered by the potential residents', which was explained on page 315. On these grounds it was recommended that two hospital hostels with twenty beds for children in the moderately disabled group B 'will be most conveniently situated outside the hospital boundaries and close to the children's own homes' (para. 7.19). These hostels would serve a population of over a quarter of a million, and so would be unlikely to be close to many of the children's homes, and certainly not as close as this study indicated was desirable. The same point applies to a slightly lesser degree to adults (para. 7.34).

The choice can be put very simply. A hostel based on the prior importance of social factors (in particular the importance of nearness and contacts with family and friends) would serve a *smaller* population, and therefore would have to cater for a *wider* range of handicaps. A hostel based on the prior importance of 'functional handicap' would have to serve a *wider* population but would cater for a *narrower* range of handicaps.

(c) *Lack of a clear proposed pattern of care for those at home*

(i) *Importance of the structure for coping and the structure of living* Both the Sheffield Development Project and the White Paper fail to do justice to the unremitting nature of the attention that the subnormal needs and the indefinite period for which he needs it. It was pointed out at the end of chapter 15 that if the subnormal was in hospital, society would provide twenty-four-hour care for a lifetime. The needs of people at home should be considered in the same way. However, the White Paper does not attempt the same specific targets for support within the home as it does for residential care and training centre and day care places. It says: 'It is not possible to set similar targets for increasing the numbers of social workers, home helps, play group organizers and similar staff. The need for more such staff is great, but the mentally handicapped and their families are only one group among many for whom their services are required: any estimate of numbers related to the mentally handicapped alone would not be meaningful' (para. 199).

The Sheffield Development Project gives even less thought to this, and the section on 'Local Authority Supporting Services' (paras 7.51 to 7.64) deals only with the services of health visitors and social workers.

This in no way measures up to the overall support these families need for their task, that is a pattern of regular, reliable and punctual help which fits in with the structure for coping or the structure of living.

In some respects, however, the services do make, or plan to make, a substantial contribution to the structure within which the subnormal is cared for. Part of that contribution is the provision of training centres and day care. Both the White Paper and the Sheffield Development Project envisage a considerable expansion of the number of training centre places (see appendix E). This increased provision is to be welcomed warmly. In some ways even more important is the provision to be made for the severely handicapped adults at home who cannot attend a training centre. At the moment there is no provision in Sheffield for such people, apart from admission to hospital, except for a very few who are taken into hospital one or two days a week. The Sheffield plans (see appendix E) will go a long way to meet possibly the most serious single gap in present provision.

In conjunction with this increased provision, more transport will be needed. In two of the families that were visited, the irregularity of the time at which the ambulance arrived seriously reduced the value of the day care given in hospital. It is most important that *punctual* transport should be provided, along with the increased day care provision. This is not mentioned in the Sheffield Development Project report.

Provision for the education of children, formerly excluded from the educational system and catered for in junior training centres or a special care unit, has, since 1 April 1971, been the responsibility of the Education Department. This will call for close co-ordination between the hospitals, the local authority health department and the Education Department.

(ii) *Short- and long-term care*   Short-term care made a big difference to the lives of some of the families, but only nine out of fifty-three had made regular use of it, and a further nine had used it less often. To provide families with the break they need, the care must be acceptable or parents will not be prepared to use it. It was noticeable how many families mentioned the one local authority hostel. In one case this was the *only* place to which the mother would let her son go for short-term care. The comparative smallness and homeliness of the hostel were obviously appreciated, and it appeared to offer the kind of care that parents hoped for. Short-term care in hospital had been satisfactory in some cases but not in others. If one is concerned about the acceptability of short-term care, there is no doubt that the parents as a whole would choose the hostel rather than a hospital. The existing hostel cannot deal with the very severely disabled, but even so, this type of care would appear to be far more acceptable for them as well. The large-scale increase in the provision of hostels planned for Sheffield makes it likely that short-term care in hostels will become more readily available.

Similar considerations apply to long-term residential care. Many parents were anxious about the future. The importance of the parents and the subnormal being happy and confident that the subnormal will be well looked after when the parents die can hardly be exaggerated. If the parents' reaction to the one local authority hostel which is already (1972) in operation is any indication, then the plans of the Sheffield Development Project will make a lot of parents, and one hopes a lot of the mentally handicapped as well, much happier.

All this can be considered in structural terms. The training centres contributed to and fitted in with the family's structure for coping with their daily and weekly routine. Short-term care did in a few cases contribute to and fit in with the family's annual routine. The knowledge that there will be good and acceptable residential care when it is needed fits in with the pattern of an acceptable life-cycle for the mentally handicapped person and his family. Furthermore, it would appear that, by removing a source of considerable anxiety, the provision of such residential care would make the present position of the family much happier.

(iii) *Practical aids*   The importance of practical assistance is mentioned in the White Paper (para. 143), though not in the Sheffield Development Project. Some families had found various aids and devices were particularly helpful, and there were other cases where help of this nature could have been very useful. The importance of such aids in helping to care for a mentally handicapped person at home should not be underestimated.

A cot bed had made a great difference to the life of Judith's parents.

Several mothers were very grateful for incontinence pads, though it does seem unreasonable to ration them, a point one mother made. Large disposable nappies were helpful in one instance.

An extra handrail had enabled one young man to get up and down stairs without help. Gates at the top and bottom of stairs were frequently mentioned as one of the devices which made care of the subnormal easier.

Some parents, generally where the subnormal was epileptic, were anxious about them going to the lavatory. Removable door panels or a door which opened outwards could prevent an emergency if the subnormal collapsed behind the door.

Advice and help about apparently trivial details could be helpful. For instance, one or two wirelesses had lasted longer than their predecessors by being put on a high shelf. There were instances where the care of the subnormal had been made much easier by fitting a bolt to his bedroom door. Some parents could have done with advice about when a bolt could be fitted safely and when not. If the mother were a widow, she was likely to need help with fitting such things as shelves and bolts.

A neat device which saved Jennifer's sister, who looked after her, a lot of anxiety was a buzzer. Jennifer used to get out of bed to go to the lavatory and often failed to cover herself up afterwards. This had led to her getting a number of very heavy colds. Her sister had a buzzer fitted in her bedroom which buzzed when Jennifer opened the bathroom door. This meant she could slip out of bed and see that Jennifer was covered after she had returned to bed.

Expert help with bathing helped a great deal in two cases and could have been used in others. Joyce's mother wanted the sort of chair that ambulance men use, to help her take Joyce into the bathroom. A bathroom and lavatory in the right place, generally on the ground floor, did sometimes, and could often, help enormously. The need for a wheelchair that would fit over the lavatory, and a lavatory that it could fit over, was mentioned by Christine's mother.

Steps, stairs and kerbstones sometimes became obstacles of huge proportions. Patricia's father mentioned the obstacle course of five-inch-high kerbstones over which he had to take her every time he took her shopping. He and other parents mentioned the need for a properly sloped kerb edge at all crossing places. This does not affect only mentally handicapped people but many others, especially the elderly, and could usefully become standard practice. In some cases it was a great help if the subnormal could go straight out into the garden without going up or down any steps. Once he was outside it was a great help if the garden was secure. It was sometimes possible to do this by erecting a gate in a strategic position.

Home helps were notable by their absence. Only one widowed mother received the services of a home help and the doctor had spoken about trying to get a home help for Christine's widowed mother. This potentially most important form of help is mentioned again in the section on 'A co-ordinated, integrated, locally based service' later on in this chapter (see p. 333).

The possibility of assistance of a more generous nature should also be considered. The suggestions made so far relate to the basic routine of living, the daily grind. Help which would improve the quality of life can also be given.

Telephones were a great help to those fourteen families that had them, and the installation of a telephone under the provisions of the Chronically Sick and Disabled Persons Act would be appropriate in several cases.

The behaviour or condition of some of the subnormals made the use of public transport impossible. In such cases the provision of a car, in the same way that a car is provided for physically disabled people, should be considered. This could make an immense difference to the life of some families. Help of this sort would only help those families where there was a member who could drive a car. In a fair number of the families visited, especially when the mother was a widow, there was no member of the family who could drive. We have seen already that widows tended to get out very little in the evenings or at weekends. There is a strong case for providing enough money for such families to be able to hire a taxi to go out into the country on a fine day in the summer. It is permissible to give help of this nature under the Chronically Sick and Disabled Persons Act.

Money was often short and the care of the subnormal was often expensive. Every means to help financially should be sought. The White Paper says:

> Some families may also qualify for the new tax-free attendance allowance of £4·80 per week, where a severely disabled person at home requires care or attention day and night, or continual supervision for his own safety or that of others.

Some of these families would certainly qualify.

Practical aids and help are important, and the families should be made aware of what is available. One father suggested that a booklet about services available would be valuable. Practical assistance of this nature is an important part of any adequate pattern of service for those at home.

(iv) *Connection between domiciliary and residential services* An element which appears to be lacking in both the White Paper and the Sheffield Project is adequate integration between residential and domiciliary services. It is true that the White Paper urges that 'admission to hospital should have no air of a final break with the patient's family, as it often does at the present' (para. 185). It also says about local authority residential accommodation: 'Contacts with their own family or with social workers they already know should be maintained' (para. 164). However, apart from short-term care, no attempt seems to have been made to see if there are ways in which the resources available in residential units could contribute to the care of those at home. However, it may be that the residential units, which of necessity offer twenty-four-hour care, may be able to play a greater part in the care of those at home than the occasional offer of short-term care. The pattern of service suggested later in this chapter (see p 328) puts forward a way in which this might be done.

(v) *The role of the social worker* Both the White Paper and the Sheffield Development Project give the key role in providing an effective pattern of service to those at home to the social worker, and they assume that he or she can do this effectively.

The White Paper says that 'the person best placed to act as co-ordinator is likely to be the social worker, who should take her part in the multi-disciplinary team as soon as handicap is suspected and thereafter maintain a continuing relationship with the handicapped child and his family' (para. 141). A little further on it says: 'The essence of good community care is the availability of someone, usually the social worker, from whom they can confidently expect understanding and help to meet any situation' (para. 145).

The Sheffield Development Project takes a similar line. 'The main responsibility for social support of the individual and his family falls on the social worker giving help with problems of adjustment, emotional relationship difficulties and practical support through childhood and adult life. . . . The social worker should be responsible for making available to the family the whole range of social services, both statutory and voluntary' (paras 7.55 and 56).

It has been shown in chapter 18 that this assumption is unjustified. The social work help was not related to the everyday situation of the lives of the families. This was undoubtedly made more difficult by a shortage of social workers, but this was basically a function of the way in which the social services were organized. The Mental Health Service was not geared to meeting the basic needs of the families, that is the needs connected with the daily grind.

Here, above all, we can see the inadequacy of the pattern of service proposed for those at home. It is no use expecting social workers, even if their numbers are increased, to fulfil a role the service is not designed to meet. The expectations in the White Paper and the Sheffield Development Project of what the social worker will be able to do to support these families at home are unrealistic. In view of the key role given to social workers, it is unlikely that the mentally handicapped living at home and their families will receive a service which measures up to their needs.

(d) *The contribution of the subnormal's family and the wider community*

The White Paper and the Sheffield Development Project have both gone to considerable trouble to consider ways in which voluntary service could help in the care of the mentally handicapped. The White Paper devotes a whole chapter to it (chapter seven) and has many imaginative suggestions to make. The Sheffield Project also stresses the importance of the participation of volunteers, and recommends the appointment of a whole-time organizer of voluntary services (para. 7.50).

However, the criticism which was made near the end of chapter 18 still holds good. 'The assumption about the way the social services should operate appears to be that, first of all, the social services will try to help a certain group of people, and then the general public should be asked to help the social services. . . . The position of these families [who were visited] shows that this approach is the wrong way round. It is not a question of the community supplementing official services; it is a question of the official services helping and enabling the community to do better the caring it does already, with more help and less strain on individual members of it' (page 310).

To ask the social worker to work in this way is to ask that he should abdicate a position he does not generally hold anyhow, namely that of providing first-line care for the family. He does not and cannot, and it is more realistic for him to assist those who do, or encourage those who are in a position to do so. Furthermore, it is important that he should be working in an administrative and organizational framework in which he is able to be in good contact with those who are providing the front-line care.

Many social workers already do work in this sort of way, but this is a very different position from that envisaged by the White Paper or the Sheffield Project. It involves a different approach, which takes as one of its basic assumptions that the social services work with, encourage, enable and support the caring that the community already does. Such an approach might go a long way to meet the criticism made about the general ineffectiveness of the social workers' service to these families, and could provide the basic plan for a realistic pattern of service for those at home.

A similar criticism can be made about residential care. It is not that the importance of voluntary help is ignored but the possibility of, for instance, involvement of the family in the actual running of the residential units does not appear to have been considered,[1] neither does the way in which it is necessary to build the home or hostel into the life of the locality in which it is set. This needs to be done from the earliest planning stage, not added on as an afterthought when all the critical decisions have been taken. Many planning and administrative decisions will affect the extent to which a hostel is integrated into its local area. The one local authority hostel in Sheffield and both the hospital hostels, one for men, one for women, are all somewhat isolated in this way. Research on hostels in Lancashire showed a similar isolation. While the hostels enabled the residents to maintain relationships with kin, friendships in the locality of the hostels did not *grow* (Campbell, 1968).

Integration of residential units into the area in which they are set will not be easy. A pattern of service which might go some way to doing this is suggested in the next section.

(e) *Summary of commentary on the White Paper and the Sheffield Development Project*

A number of criticisms have been made of the White Paper and Sheffield Development Project. They can be summarized as follows:

(i) The need for the profoundly retarded to be looked after in hospital units was questioned and the value of them being looked after in a locally based hostel was suggested.

(ii) The wisdom of using 'functional handicap' as a basis for planning residential provision was questioned and an alternative of having a hostel catering for a much *wider* range of handicap from a more *limited* area was put forward.

(iii) The proposed pattern of service for those at home was criticized as being inadequate in that it did not measure up to the daily grind of looking after the subnormal.

(iv) The main reason for this weakness was held to be the key role given to the social worker—a role which it was organizationally impossible for him to carry out.

(v) It was suggested that there was inadequate integration between residential and domiciliary services.

(vi) It was felt that inadequate account was taken of the possible contribution of members of the subnormal's family, friends, neighbours and other members of the community in the proposals for both the services for those at home and the running of the residential units.

A co-ordinated, integrated, locally based service

(a) *An outline*

Earlier in this chapter (see pp. 316–17) the main conclusions from the visits were listed. The main criticisms made about the White Paper and the Sheffield Development Project have been summarized above. These criticisms were made in the light of the conclusions drawn from the visits. On this basis it is possible to draw up a list of features that should be included or tested in a service for mentally handicapped people. No claim is made that this is the only model possible, but this particular model incorporates the insights of this particular study in relation to current official policy.

(i) The official services should complement, assist and work in with the care and help which is given or which could be given by members of the mentally handicapped person's family, friends and other members of the community.

(ii) The total pattern of service offered, by whatever combination of sources of help, must meet the basic needs of the whole family and, in particular, must take account of and fit in with the structure for coping and the structure of living, and provide a satisfactory life cycle for the subnormal and his family.

In order to meet these requirements:

(iii) Care of those at home and those in residential care should be integrated as closely as possible.

(iv) With this in view the practicality of a hostel which would cater for a wide range of disabilities, including the most profoundly handicapped, should be tested.

(v) In this way the hostel could cater for a limited local area.

(vi) Social workers should be based on or near the hostel to work in the same area as that covered by the hostel.

(vii) The close contact of hostel, hostel staff and social workers with the locality should make it possible to link a service on this pattern with informal, local resources through the families of the mentally handicapped and other local contacts.

(viii) The resources of the hostel should be available for those at home and the hostel should be used as a source or agency for a wide range of practical assistance.

In short, the basis for the planning of both domiciliary and residential services should be the local area. This does not mean that all services would be provided locally but the locality would be seen as the basic unit for planning.

(b) *The context within which an integrated locally based hostel would operate*

Many other services and facilities would obviously be necessary which could not be provided on a local basis. The pattern of what would be needed is substantially what is proposed in the White Paper and the Sheffield Development Project. Wherever possible, for instance with the special schools and adult training centres, a close tie-up with the locality would be important.

It is assumed that the mentally handicapped, including those in the hostels, would have the usual recourse to general medical facilities. This would generally be the local general practitioner, but normal use would be made of specialist help and facilities.

There may be some handicapped people who, because of particularly difficult behaviour or, for instance, sexual offences, may not be able to be catered for in a local setting. Provision for such people would be essential. The number is likely to be small and the unit planned for Sheffield for twenty-four emotionally disturbed adults or adolescents seems likely to be adequate.

No mention has been made of those less severely handicapped who need a less supervised form of residential care. The Sheffield Project plans a number of group homes, of about six people, and extensive use of lodgings. These would fit well into the locally based pattern which is suggested.

A locally based hostel dealing with a wide range of handicaps would pose a number of administrative problems and would need close co-operation between the hospital and local authorities. Questions would arise about staffing and who would take ultimate responsibility. In practice it might prove extremely difficult to limit desperately needed beds to people from a local area, and this might be made worse by the difficulty of finding sites in the right places. Further problems would arise over fitting the area served by a hostel into the existing areas of the social services department and the health department. Co-ordination with other residential accommodation, for instance for children and old people, would be needed. It would also have to be decided whether the case-load of a social worker based on a hostel would be mixed or whether he would deal entirely with the mentally handicapped.

Doubtless other problems would arise, but the fact that there would be an obvious need to co-operate and a clear focus for it, namely the integrated hostel, should make this difficult task somewhat easier. Once the local authority areas and the hospital areas become co-terminous in 1974, one serious obstacle to joint planning will have been removed.

The pattern of service which is recommended in connection with an integrated hostel is consistent with the lines laid down in both the Seebohm Report and the White Paper. Both these advocated greater involvement with the community, better co-ordination between the helping services, and planning in smaller units. For instance, the White Paper bases its figures on areas of 100,000 and the Seebohm Report envisaged an area office for a population of 50,000–100,000 (para. 590). It also considered that some provision might be necessary at a more local level than this (para. 593). A development on the lines proposed would be a useful exploration of the implications of this general policy. There remain three questions of fundamental importance which must be looked at in more detail. It is hoped that in doing so the positive advantages of an integrated locally based service will be apparent. The three questions are: Why should social workers be locally based? What contribution could a local hostel make? What is meant by local? They are considered in the next three sub-sections.

(c) *Why should social workers be based locally?*

The argument here turns on a point made in the Introduction. There, it was said that the prime understanding of community implicit in this study was the small-scale one of the intimate, face-to-face relationships of the social network of kin, friends and neighbours who helped to care for the subnormal and gave support to him and his family. When this support was examined in chapter 17, it was seen that when effective support was given it was given most often by people who lived near at hand. Effective support was support which related to the basic essentials of everyday living, or the structure for coping, and incorporated the subnormal and his family into the life of the wider community, or the structure of living. In practice what had happened was that those who did give regular help and support had become part of the structure.

It was the general inability of the social workers to give this kind of support themselves *or to be instrumental in helping the family to build up such a structure* that lay at the root of their ineffectiveness, but if the social worker was locally based, this would enable him to acquire a good working knowledge of a wide variety of local sources of help. In the first place he could be aware of the families' existing network of care and support, and be able to get to know some of the people who made it up and become known by them. In this way he could become a part of the existing team of friends and kin who were supporting the family, and be able to give other members of it help and encouragement.

However, the support that some families received was sparse, and he would need to be aware of other sources of help and support. This would include knowing what help was available from tenants' associations, churches and other organizations, and the personalities of the people concerned. Sometimes such organizations might be able to offer just the sort of help that was needed.

But it is important that the social worker should be aware of smaller, more local, more informal groups than these organized ones. By their very nature, such informal groups are difficult to describe. In some cases they are so lacking in cohesion and awareness of a corporate identity that they cannot really be described as groups at all. Jane Jacobs draws a sketch of this level of local life in her book *The Death and Life of Great American Cities* (1961). In her chapter on 'The uses of sidewalks', she describes what goes on outside her own house (pp. 50–2):

> The stretch of Hudson Street where I live is each day the
> scene of an intricate sidewalk ballet. I make my own first
> entrance into it a little after eight when I put out the garbage
> can, surely a prosaic occupation, but I enjoy my part, my little
> clang, as the droves of high school students walk by the center
> of the stage dropping candy wrappers . . . [Shortly] numbers of
> women in housedresses have emerged and as they criss cross
> with one another they pause for quick conversations that sound
> either laughter or joint indignation, never, it seems, anything
> between. . . . The heart-of-the-day ballet . . . becomes more and
> more intricate. Longshoremen who are not working that day
> gather at the White Horse or the Ideal or the International for
> beer and conversation. . . . Mr. Lacey, the locksmith, shuts up
> his shop for a while and goes to exchange the time of day with
> Mr. Slube at the cigar store. Mr. Koochagian, the tailor, waters
> the luxuriant jungle of plants in his window . . . and crosses the
> street for a bite at the Ideal where he can keep an eye on
> customers and wigwag across the message that he is coming.
> The baby carriages come out, and clusters of everyone from
> toddlers with dolls to teen-agers with homework gather at
> the stoops. When I get home after work the ballet is reaching
> its crescendo. This is the time of roller-skates and stilts and
> tricycles, and games in the lee of the stoop with bottletops and
> plastic cowboys. . . . As darkness thickens . . . the ballet goes
> on under lights eddying back and forth but intensifying at the
> bright spotlight pools of Joe's sidewalk pizza dispensary, the
> bars, the delicatessen, the restaurant and the drugstore.

The street that Mrs Jacobs describes is obviously very different from the Sheffield streets in which the mentally handicapped people and their families live. But she does catch the essence of the delicate fabric that makes up the life of a locality in a town. The details are different, but the main point is the same—the need to be aware of the threads which make up the fabric of the life of the neighbourhood.

Awareness of such elements in the neighbourhood is only conceivable if the social worker is locally based. A vital part of the service such a social worker could offer would be a real knowledge of what went on locally. Which hairdresser would be prepared to call and cut the subnormal's hair at his home. Which local publican might be in a position to give the subnormal's mother a part-time job. Which launderette might dry sheets during the winter for a reduced price. Which grocer might be persuaded to deliver an order.

If the services of a home help were needed, the social worker might know, or be in a position to find, a sympathetic and competent person locally who could be employed to help and get to know one particular family. The important point is that it would be local and, one hopes, relatively permanent. Because it was local the relationship with the family might grow. When the help went away on holiday, her sister from the next street but one might take over. By doing as much as possible at the local level there is a greater chance of the family being involved in the web of relationships which make up the life of a locality. If the home help was arranged locally by a locally based social worker with a local person, it could become another thread strengthening the fabric of local life.

So far everything suggested has dealt with people who make a living by offering a service (the shops) or paying someone to offer a service. This is different from offering a service simply out of goodwill, but the use of money in this way should not be despised. Apart from the obvious encouragement that even a small payment offers, it may have the effect of breaking the barrier of reserve which prevents people offering help from shyness or fear of what the neighbours might think. In Hertfordshire[2] a scheme was started a few years ago of making a small payment to neighbours for going in to old people first thing in the morning and last thing at night, lighting their fires, getting the coal in and generally seeing that they were all right.[3] One might wish that such neighbourly help could be given spontaneously without payment, but it is far better that it should be given for payment than that the old people should not receive help which they need; furthermore, it creates a contact from which a relationship may grow. Help on these lines might be tried for some families with a mentally handicapped member.

It has been suggested so far that a locally based social worker would be in a good position to organize effective local paid help and also to bring about some contact between the subnormal or his family and local organizations.

It may be necessary to take a more positive initiative than this, and encourage the formation of a small group of people who would be prepared to help specifically and directly with the subnormal.

What such help would involve was made very clear by James's father (see p. 288). Such help would need to be given regularly over a long period if it was to be effective. The demands likely to be made on people helping in this way suggest that such help could be given best by a small group of people rather than by an isolated individual. This would also help to ensure continuity in the event of a member of the group moving away or having to drop out. Several parents stressed the time and patience needed to establish a relationship with the subnormal. The two students who visited Judith (p. 291) seemed to establish an excellent relationship quite quickly, but inevitably, because they were students, the contact lasted for only a year or so. If the more difficult task was attempted of bringing such help into existence locally, then there would be a chance of the sort of spontaneous growth which, it was suggested, could happen with a local home help. This is not to say that there is no value in outside help of the sort the two students gave to Judith, but if such help could be integrated with help locally, it would stand a far greater chance of becoming relatively permanent. It would be ideal if such outside help could act as a catalyst for more local support and contacts.

There remains one vital person who so far has been left out of the discussion completely—the mentally handicapped man or woman. It would be foolish to pretend that all the subnormals who were visited were obviously lovable, but it would be equally misleading to imagine that they could not inspire affection. The subnormals themselves may be a creative element in the community.

One final point should be made about the advantage of the social worker being based locally. The importance of help being reciprocal was emphasized in chapter 17. A locally based social worker might well know not only who might help the subnormal's family, but also to whom the subnormal and his family might themselves give help. In some cases it was the giving of service to others that forged the strongest links that the family had with the people among whom it lived.

It could be that help of this nature might enable some of those parents who were very isolated to overcome their deep reluctance to accept help or friendship from informal contacts outside the family. The attitude of the mother to such informal contacts could be the rock on which all attempts to foster local community support might founder. The possibility of help being reciprocal might enable some mothers to accept help which they needed desperately, without feeling that their independence was being threatened. Many of the families not only needed help but also needed help with accepting help. If genuine and effective care by the community is going to grow, such apparently trivial points are important.

(d) *What would the contribution of a local hostel be?*

Such a locally based service fits in well with the pattern of residential hostels being evaluated in Wessex by Dr Kushlick and his team. At the moment they are concentrating on provision for children. These hostels are based on an area of approximately 100,000 population. Kushlick (1967a) estimated that a unit of about twenty would cater for all subnormal children, whatever their disability, in need of residential care in an area of that size. He points out the advantages of hostels over traditional institutions for the subnormal (pp. 39ff):

> These hostels would be sited in towns having their own
> specialist medical, social and educational facilities. . . .
> Education and training [could] be provided in the same training
> centres as are attended by those children who live in their own
> homes.

In addition:

> Because of the size of the catchment area they would be
> comparatively short distances from the family they serve. . . .
> The proximity of the children's families to the units might
> allow the parents to maintain contact with their children where
> such contact is otherwise rendered difficult by the formidable
> problems of visiting a child in a distant institution.

The first locally based unit was opened in Southampton in 1970. Dr Kushlick writes about this unit (1970, p. 260):

> The children in the new unit all come from a defined local area,
> and local authority social workers, child care officers, educational
> psychologists and teachers from this area have easy, direct
> access to all of their clients and to the head of the living unit
> at a single visit. A local general practitioner, a member of the
> clinical team, is responsible for their primary medical care;
> when investigation or treatment is required for physical
> conditions, this is undertaken by the paediatrician at the
> children's hospital. Half of the children attend the junior training

centre together with local children who live with their families. Similarly, parental and volunteer participation from the neighbourhood is rendered easy and encouraged by an open-visiting policy.

Dr Kushlick's Wessex experiment is the complement, in terms of residential care, to locally based support for the care of those still at home. In fact it could become very much more. Such a locally based residential unit could become *part* of the locally based support for those at home. The boundary between the two would no longer be hard and fast. The local residential home could play a key role in the care of *all* mentally handicapped people in the locality. It might be a suitable place for the local social workers to be based, though possibly such a use might make it less of a home. Whatever solution was reached in terms of buildings and offices, close contact between hostel staff and the local social workers would be essential. Equally close contacts with health visitors would also be necessary. It is important that they should regard one another as fellow members of the team which is providing subnormals and their families with the service they need, whether it is at home or in residential care.

It would be important for there to be places for short-term care in these local homes. Their nearness would mean that in the case of both short- and longer-term care, the subnormal would not be cut off from all the people he knew. Indeed it would be possible for some relative or neighbour who had helped with caring for him at home to help care for him in the residential home. This might be one way in which the residential home could build up its contacts with the locality it served. Where locally based support for the subnormal and his family had led to a real incorporation of the subnormal in the life of the area while he was living at home, a pattern of care like this would mean that when the subnormal had to go into residential care, he would not be cut off from this support, but it could provide an important element of continuity.

In practice continuity would, one hopes, be provided in other ways as well. The subnormal might go into the residential home not only for short-term care but possibly over a weekend while his parents went out by themselves. The files recorded one case of the subnormal being looked after in the one existing local authority hostel while his parents went out together on a Sunday afternoon. In fact the residential home might be able to provide just that sort of practical first line assistance that the social worker by himself cannot. Looking after the subnormal for shorter or longer periods might well figure large in the help that could be offered to those at home.

A close connection between the residential home and locally based social work help could be helpful in another way. Dr Kushlick, speaking about the administrative advantages of hostels, stressed the value of easier access for those in the hostel to 'existing facilities for children living in their own homes'. He continued: 'In this way an ad hoc team might be set up of hostel matron, teacher, educational psychologist, specialist in subnormality and paediatrician.' By the same token the residential home might be a source or agency for specialist skills for those living at home.

The specialist skills needed are not just those mentioned by Dr Kushlick. Some more practical skills are required, such as advice about foods and methods of feeding, advice about types of clothing which make it easier for the subnormal to dress himself, clothing suitable for the incontinent or aids for dealing with the periods of an over-active subnormal woman, detailed and expert advice about the use of bathing aids, walking aids, and lavatory chairs, techniques for lifting the subnormal correctly and bathing him. The teacher or educational psychologist might be able to give advice to the parents about how they can train their subnormal to be as independent as possible, or how to keep him occupied, and suggestions on what toys and games he could manage.[4] It may be that people who have worked in hospitals for the subnormal may have valuable experience of this sort which could be of great use in a community setting.

If the residential home were to make available and easily accessible to those at home assistance and support that related directly to the daily grind of looking after the subnormal, the burden on the families could be greatly eased. It would make it possible for the social worker to offer a service that could meet the needs of the subnormal and his family, and would provide a context within which his specific skills could be used more creatively.

However, the fundamental argument in favour of this integrated approach is that it seems to offer the best chance of providing the 'sympathetic and constant human relationships' that the White Paper emphasizes so rightly. For the mentally handicapped person himself it should mean that he need never be moved far from his family and friends, whether he remains in his own home or has to go into residential care. He would get to know the social worker or social workers and, even if individual members of it changed, the *team* of social workers responsible for him would remain the same, whether he were at home or in the residential unit. In the residential unit he would get to know the staff through going there for a variety of shorter periods of care.

His family too would have the opportunity of getting to know the staff of the residential home, through taking the subnormal there to be looked after for shorter or longer periods, through meeting them in the district simply because it was in the same area, and possibly through having sought specific advice from them about some aspect of caring for their subnormal. It was evident that some of the mothers had a good relationship in this way with some members of the staff of the training centres. The family would also continue to deal with the same team of social workers. A further possibility is that once the subnormal did have to go into residential care, his family, especially his mother or the woman who had been caring for him, would be able to continue to take a part in caring for him. His mother might, for instance, come and give him one of his meals every day. This could make it far easier for the mother to allow the subnormal to go into residential care, and would also be of real assistance to the staff.

A simple activity like this, helping to feed the handicapped person, could assist in providing him with a continuing relationship with his family, and make it easier for his family to maintain their relationship with him. It would help the staff of the residential unit, offer them the chance of a good working relationship with the family of one of the residents and be one more valuable tie with the locality which the hostel served. It could in fact be instrumental in helping to provide a complex of 'sympathetic and constant human relationships'. It could do this, not only for the subnormal and his family, which is of prime importance, but also for the professionals concerned with them, which, apart from making their job more worth while, would make their help more effective because it would be given in a full social context. It is with an attitude which sees the value of making it possible for a mother to come and give her severely disabled son his evening meal every day that a service could be built that provides 'sympathetic and constant human relationships', and it would be by a series of such apparently trivial minutiae, underpinned by this basic concern, that the value of an integrated locally based service would be shown.

What can be done by a full involvement of families and other members of the community in a residential setting has been shown in Sheffield by St Luke's Nursing Home, which gives terminal care to the dying. Members of the patient's family are given every opportunity to be of service to him, for instance, feeding him, and over 200 volunteers help with a wide variety of specific, well-defined tasks, from helping with the accounts or with the meals to the actual nursing of the patients. The volunteers are an integral and highly valued part of the Home. The situation is not quite the same as in a hostel for the mentally handicapped, but it does illustrate the basic point that a residential unit which recognizes the fundamental importance of the role of the families of the residents and other volunteers has much to offer to both the residents and those who help.

Such an integrated locally based service would be in a position to provide the basic services needed for the large majority of the mentally handicapped in that area over their whole life-span. The harsh division between home and institution would have a chance of becoming care within, by, and as part of, the community, whether the mentally handicapped were living with their family or in a residential home.[5]

(e) *What is meant by local?*

Much use has been made of the word 'local', but what is meant by this? It was said in the Introduction that the study was concerned to look, in the first instance, at the network of family, friends and neighbours who give help and support to the subnormal and his family, and then to consider the geographical implications of those networks. We have seen that where effective help was given which linked in with the structure for coping or the structure of living it was generally close at hand, and when, for instance, a particularly helpful neighbour moved a quarter of an hour's walk away, this reduced very substantially the amount of help and support that she was able to give. There were cases where people from further afield gave considerable help. These people were generally members of the subnormal's family. However, the general rule was the closer the better, and frequently this meant not more than a street or two away.

This shows a very similar pattern to what the authors of *Helping the Aged* found about the experience of old people (Goldberg *et al.*, 1970, p. 193).[6]

It is now gradually realized that the very old, who have lived for the most part of their lives in one small neighbourhood, are most successfully rehoused within the familiar streets to which they have grown attached and which constitute their world imbued with many memories. . . . A move, even ten minutes away, can mean the end of his accustomed way of life; for example, the life-line services of a neighbour may be disrupted which can be more vital than the occasional visits from children.

The smallness of the area in which people feel 'at home' is given further support by Dr W. A. Hampton's study of politics in Sheffield, *Democracy and Community* (1970). The respondents were asked if there was an area around their home address in which they felt 'at home'. Nearly three-quarters of the Sheffield respondents described their 'home' area as the few streets surrounding their address, and a total of 85 per cent described an area no larger than a local authority ward. What the respondents expected of a 'home' area in practical terms is not considered, but a community development project in one part of Sheffield also found that neighbourly interaction and mutual help tended to be concentrated in a limited area of a few streets (Skipper: Sheffield Council of Social Service).

If one is considering areas as small as this, the number of people involved is unlikely to exceed about 1,000, and this is clearly far too small as an administrative unit for planning services. It does, however, indicate the size of area with which the administrative unit must be capable of establishing effective contact.

Dr Kushlick (1970) has shown that a hostel catering for a population of 100,000 makes some involvement of members of the community possible. The Seebohm Report has been quoted already as advocating an area office for a population of 50,000–100,000, but the report also suggests that some provision at a more local level than this might be needed. The Association for Neighbourhood Councils thinks in terms of a neighbourhood council for a population of 5,000–15,000 (Baker and Young, 1971). This figure is very similar to the population of the areas for the Home Office Community Development Projects. A figure in the range of 5,000–20,000 is mentioned. The Coventry Community Development Project in Hillfields, for instance, has a population of about 10,000 (Benington, 1970). As one of the aims of these projects in areas of high social need is the active involvement of the local people themselves, the size of population envisaged would seem to be an important guide. A sub-committee of the Standing Medical Advisory Committee on the Organization of Group Practice (1971) suggested that a group of five or six doctors was the optimum and that such a group would be responsible for a population of approximately 15,000 people (paras 38 and 39).[7] The upper limit suggested for a Community Development Project area (20,000) is about the same size as a local authority ward. The Sheffield figures indicate that there might be twenty-four adults from a population of that size in need of residential care, a figure very similar to those in the White Paper (table 5). For children, the position is not so simple. The White Paper figures suggest that about five residential places for children might be needed for a population of 20,000. This means that for children it would be more difficult to look after them in a residential unit near their family; and at the same time one might argue that it is even more important for them to be near their families than it is for adults. This needs careful study. One possibility is that mentally handicapped children might be looked after in the same unit as other children. This is being carried out already with a few less severely handicapped children. The figures are discussed in more detail in appendix F. On balance, for adults at least, a hostel serving a population of 20,000 appears a reasonable proposition.

However, 20,000 could only be taken as a guide. A wide range of factors would have to be taken into account in deciding on the specific areas. It is clear from this study that the type of area, especially in terms of social class, would be important because of the greater concentration of the mentally handicapped at the lower end of the social scale. Social class would also affect the proportion of families having cars and telephones, both of which would be of direct relevance in deciding what size the area should be. The availability of public transport and the bus routes, the position of shopping centres and existing social welfare facilities and many other physical factors would have to be considered. In addition less obvious factors, such as local patterns of neighbouring and social activity, would have to be looked at. It is more difficult to make reliable generalizations about an area of 20,000 than it is for an area of 100,000, because it is more likely to be dominated by one particular section of the population rather than be representative of the whole. This means that careful study of such factors would need to be made when deciding on the areas.

Further consideration of this is beyond the scope of this study and could usefully be the subject of further research. However, it would be quite possible to test the value of an integrated locally based service by choosing a very few areas where circumstances appear to favour such an approach.[8] Appropriate areas will tend to suggest themselves more by centres than by boundaries, and it may be possible to build up a service based on local areas by gradually introducing more local centres until the right degree of 'local-ness' for that district has been reached.

The question of what is meant by 'local' and what areas could best be served by local centres is important and complex, but this research can only point to the need for experiment and continued study along the lines that have been suggested.

Conclusion: community care—the relevant preposition?

The social service departments which will be involved in the implementation of the policies of both the White Paper, *Better Services for the Mentally Handicapped*, and the Sheffield Development Project are the reorganized social service departments outlined by the Seebohm Report. The report was rightly emphatic about the importance of the relationship between the social service department and the community (paras 475 and 478):

> Our interest in the community is not nostalgic in origin, but based on the practical grounds that the community is both the provider as well as the recipient of social services and that orientation to the community is vital if the services are to be directed to individuals, families and groups within the context of their social relations with others. . . . The staff of the social service department will need to see themselves not as a self contained unit but as part of a network of services within the community.

The report made it clear that it expected the social service department to take an active role in community development. 'A clear responsibility then should be placed upon the social service department for developing conditions favourable to community identity and activity.' The report goes on to say in the same paragraph (para. 483): 'We are not suggesting that "welfare through community" is an alternative to the social services but that it is complementary and inextricably interwoven. . . .'

This study has tried to spell out some of the ways in which the social services might interweave themselves with the community so as to provide a more effective service. It has in fact gone a little further than the Seebohm Report suggested, in that it has sought to involve the hospital service in the process, which fell outside the terms of reference of the Seebohm Committee.[9]

The simile of the interweaving of the informal helping and caring process active throughout society, and the contribution of the social services, is a sound one. It takes one beyond the stage of care *in* the community at home but living in isolation from those round about. It takes one beyond care *in* the community *in* institutions, even small ones, which have little involvement or share in the community. It takes one beyond care *by* the community, if by that one is suggesting that members of the community, untrained and unaided, should be left to get on with it. It takes one to the point where a partnership of the community at large and the social services is seen as essential by both. The caring done by families, friends, neighbours or larger, more organized groups of people is seen, recognized and acknowledged. An attempt is made to see both particular needs, and the strengths and limitations of the informal resources available. The social services seek to interweave their help so as to use and strengthen the help already given, make good the limitations and meet the needs. It is not a question of the social services plugging the gaps but rather of their working with society to enable society to close the gaps.[10]

The understanding by the White Paper, *Better Services for the Mentally Handicapped*, of the role of voluntary service (chapter seven), for all its imaginative ideas, is epitomized in the sub-heading 'Supplementing official services'. It does not appear to appreciate adequately that the basic caring is the care already being given by families throughout the country, the basic helping is the help already being given by countless relations and friends. It is on this that all other help is based and should be seen to be based. This requires a reorientation in the approach of the helping professions and helping services on the lines suggested by the Seebohm Report, which saw that the caring already done and the caring of the official services needed to be seen as 'complementary and inextricably interwoven'.

This study has shown something of the network of unofficial care and support with which fifty-four severely mentally handicapped adults were surrounded. We saw that effective official help was help which was interwoven with these networks. A model integrated, locally based service was put forward as a pattern designed to make it possible for unofficial and official caring to work together and support one another more effectively. Possibly the strongest argument for development along these lines is that it offers the chance for the service to grow according to local strengths and local needs.

Whatever the original slogan 'community care' was supposed to mean, we have now reached the stage where care in, by, as part of, and in co-operation with the community can develop most fruitfully if it is linked with the insights of community development. This study has suggested an administrative framework which might enable this to happen.

It might be argued that however desirable this may be, it is unrealistic. On the contrary, the lack of realism lies in expecting the social services, as generally organized at present, to offer an adequate service, not just to the mentally handicapped but to other groups in need, especially the elderly. The community can care. It is up to the professional helpers and the helping services to help it to do so.

Appendix A
Additional tables

Table A1   Agency reporting mildly subnormal

Age reported	Home Male No.	%	Female No.	%	Institution Male No.	%	Female No.	%
Education	322	82·6	243	69·0	37	59·6	27	47·4
Family	4	1·0	11	3·1	4	6·5	4	7·0
Other local authority service	17	4·4	17	4·8	4	6·5	6	10·5
Police or prison	20	5·1	8	2·3	7	11·3	2	3·5
Hospital or G.P.	0	—	8	2·3	5	8·1	5	8·8
MSS	14	3·6	48	13·6	3	4·8	13	22·8
Other	13	3·3	17	4·8	2	3·2	0	0
Sub-total	390	100·0	352	99·9	62	100·0	57	100·0
Not known	1		3		0		1	
Total	391		355		62		58	

χ^2 on Education, MSS and the rest = 65·301   p = 0·001

Table A2 Socio-economic group by type of housing, showing redistribution of cases where SEG not known

	MSN								SSN							
	Home				Institution				Home				Institution			
	Council	Urban	Suburban	Total	Council	Urban	Suburban	Total	Council	Urban	Suburban	Total	Council	Urban	Suburban	Total
Non-manual	9	3	8	20	0	1	3	4	16	7	60	83	7	4	16	27
Manual	190	188	18	396	18	30	8	56	223	141	31	395	47	67	17	131
SEG not known but type of housing known	77	62	6	145	9	19	5	33	42	28	8	78	6	22	4	32
H.M. Forces	2	0	0	2	2	1	0	3	0	1	1	2	0	0	0	0
Type of housing not known				183				24				116				33
Total	278	253	32	746	29	51	16	120	281	177	100	674	60	93	37	223

Redistribution of cases where SEG not known but type of housing known (line 3 above)—the numbers which have been added are in bold

	MSN								SSN							
	Home				Institution				Home				Institution			
	Council	Urban	Suburban	Total	Council	Urban	Suburban	Total	Council	Urban	Suburban	Total	Council	Urban	Suburban	Total
Non-manual	3	1	2	6	0	1	1	2	3	1	4	8	1	1	2	4
Manual	74	61	4	139	9	18	4	31	39	27	4	70	5	21	2	28
Total	77	62	6	145	9	19	5	33	42	28	8	78	6	22	4	32

Table A3 Socio-economic grouping including those classified by type of housing

	MSN Home	Institution	Total	SSN Home	Institution	Total
Non-manual	26 + 6 = 32 (4·7%)	6 + 2 = 8 (7·7%)	40 (5·1%)	98 + 8 = 106 (16·6%)	30 + 4 = 34 (16·3%)	140 (16·5%)
Manual	515 + 139 = 654 (95·3%)	65 + 31 = 96 (92·3%)	750 (94·9%)	463 + 70 = 533 (83·4%)	147 + 28 = 175 (83·7%)	708 (83·5%)
Sub-total	686	104	790	639	209	848
SEG and type of housing not known*	60	16	76	35	14	49
Not known as % of total	8·0	13·3	8·8	5·2	6·3	5·5
Total	746	120	866	674	223	897

* Includes ten in H.M. Forces

Table A4 *How many subnormals who could be living with a sib were doing so? Adults only*

	MSN Home			Institution			SSN Home			Institution		
	Male	Female	Total	Male	Female	Total	Male	Female	Total	Male	Female	Total
Living with sib and no parent	22	35	57	6	13	19	20	22	42	3	8	11
Living with a parent and not taken on by a sib on parent's death	0	0	0	3	4	7	0	0	0	11	6	17
Living with other relative or friend	17	40	57	8	5	13	6	1	7	4	1	5
Total	39	75	114	17	22	39	26	23	49	18	15	33

Note: The figures for living with a sib and no parent are in all cases, except for the mildly subnormal in an institution, lower than the equivalent figures in tables 8.2 and 8.3. This is due to the fact that the death of the subnormal's parents might not have taken place before the subnormal lived with one of his sibs.

Table A5 Subnormality of mother: adults

| | MSN | | | | | | SSN | | | | | |
| | Home | | YIG | | OIG | | Home | | YIG | | OIG | |
	No.	%	No.	%	No.	%	No.	%	No.	%	No.	%
Nothing adverse known	508	81·4	38	73·1	29	96·7	375	87·8	53	84·1	50	96·1
'Dim'	107	17·2	12	23·1	1	3·3	44	10·3	7	11·1	2	3·9
Known to be subnormal	9	1·4	2	3·8	0	0	8	1·9	3	4·8	0	0
Sub-total	624	100·0	52	100·0	30	100·0	427	100·0	63	100·0	52	100·0
Not known	106		18		7		23		4		9	
Not known as % of total	14·5		25·7		18·9		5·1		6·0		14·8	
Total	730		70		37		450		67		61	

Table A6 Age of mother at birth of subnormal: children

	MSN Home No.	Institution No.	SSN Home No.	%	Institution No.	%
Under 30	5	9	76	45·5	54	65·0
30–34	3	1	31	18·6	13	15·7
35+	4	1	60	35·9	16	19·3
Sub-total	12	11	167	100·0	83	100·0
Not known	4	2	57		12	
Not known as % of total			25·4		12·6	
Total	16	13	224		95	

χ^2 (SSN) = 9·397 p = 0·01

Table A7 *Age of mother at birth of subnormal: adults*

| | MSN | | | | | | SSN | | | | | |
	Home No.	%	YIG No.	%	OIG No.	%	Home No.	%	YIG No.	%	OIG No.	%
Under 30	282	51·0	22	59·5	13	43·3	197	50·1	26	46·4	15	28·8
30–34	141	25·5	5	13·5	9	30·0	74	18·8	13	23·2	7	13·5
35 +	130	23·5	10	27·0	8	26·7	122	31·0	17	30·4	30	57·7
Sub-total	553	100·0	37	100·0	30	100·0	393	99·9	56	100·0	52	100·0
Not known	177		33		7		57		11		9	
Not known as % of total	24·2		47·1		18·9		12·7		16·4		14·8	
Total	730		70		37		450		67		61	

χ^2 on Home v. YIG (MSN) = 2·674 NS χ^2 on Home v. YIG (SSN) = 0·627 NS
χ^2 on Home v. OIG (MSN) = 0·671 NS χ^2 on Home v. OIG (SSN) = 14·639   p = 0·001

Table A8 *Live births by age of mother—England and Wales 1963*

Age of mother	No.	%
Under 30 years	602,440	70·5
30–34	153,696	18·0
35+	97,917	11·5
Total	854,053	100·0

* Derived from Table C143 'Live Births by age and parity of mother and place of confinement 1963, England and Wales' in the Registrar General's Statistical Review for 1963, Part III Commentary.

Table A9 *Type of offence: adults*

	MSN Home		Institution		SSN Home		Institution	
	No.	%	No.	%	No.	%	No.	%
Trivial or petty stealing	102	47·4	14	35·0	21	34·4	9	31·0
Threatening behaviour	13	6·0	3	7·5	3	4·9	2	6·9
Sexually assaulted	10		1		7		0	
Exhibitionism	22 } 77	35·8	8 } 17	42·5	15 } 29	47·5	3 } 9	31·0
Sexual assault	10		4		5		1	
Prostitution	35		4		2		5	
Running away	15	7·0	5	12·5	8	13·1	9	31·0
Other	8	3·7	1	2·5	0		0	
Sub-total	215	99·9	40	100·0	61	99·9	29	99·9
Not known	8		2		2		3	
Not applicable	507		65		387		96	
Total	730		107		450		128	

Note: Those in the 'Not applicable' row are those whose file did not record any offence. The numbers in this row are slightly lower than for those who had no criminal record. This is because in a few cases committing some minor offence did not involve any contact with the authorities.

Table A10 *The relative strength of association with admission to hospital of physical characteristics and behaviour: severely subnormal children and adults*

SSN children					SSN adults Younger institution group					Older institution group				
Strength of association with admission	Factor	Level at which associated with admission to hospital	Number Home	Inst.	Strength of association with admission	Factor	Level at which associated with admission to Hospital	Number Home	Inst.	Strength of association with admission	Factor	Level at which associated with admission to hospital	Number Home	Inst.
0·5319	Behaviour problem at home	Moderate or severe	15	49	0·6035	Behaviour problem at home	Moderate or severe	14	36	0·2580	Incontinence	Any incontinence	53	24
0·4986	Behaviour problem in locality	Moderate or severe	3	25	0·3872	Supervision needed	Few minutes or constant supervision	80	44	0·2107	Feeding	Can with help or not at all	41	16
0·4460	Supervision needed	Constant supervision	71	75	0·3795	Behaviour problem in locality	Moderate or severe	8	15	0·1838	Dressing	Can with help or not at all	82	24
0·3618	Incontinence	Total	35	47	0·2695	Mentally ill	Clear evidence	8	11	0·1477	Supervision	Few minutes or constant supervision	80	22
0·3284	Feeding	Not at all	39	46	0·2156	Epilepsy	Weekly or more often	16	12	0·1425	Speech	Any defect	208	41
0·3104	Behaviour problem at training centre	Moderate or severe	6	9	0·2076	Incontinence	Any incontinence	53	22	*0·0835	Walking	Severe defect or not at all	29	8 }
0·2576	Epilepsy	Monthly or worse	20	27	0·1775	Feeding	Can with help or not at all	41	17					
0·2461	Dressing	Not at all	74	56	0·1623	Dressing	Not at all	22	11					
0·2420	Speech	Total disability	55	45	*0·0858 }	Speech	Total disability	21	7 }					
0·1729	Walking	Severe defect or total disability	39	31		Blind								
0·1445	Blind	Severe handicap	12	13										
Total in group			224	95	Total in group			450	67	Total in group			450	61

*0·0858

* The difference was not significant

Note: The numbers do not add up to the total in the group because some cases do not appear in the table at all and others appear

Appendix B   Figures 1-13

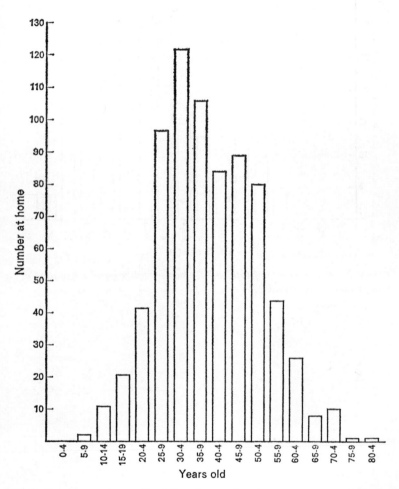

Figure 1   Age structure of mildly subnormal at home on 1 September 1968 (total 746)

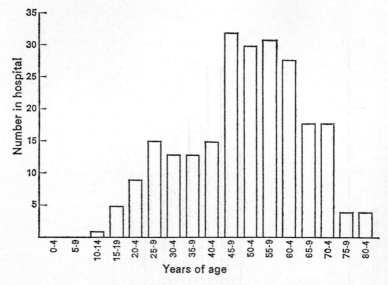

Figure 2   Age structure of total mildly subnormal hospital population at 1 September 1968 (total 236)

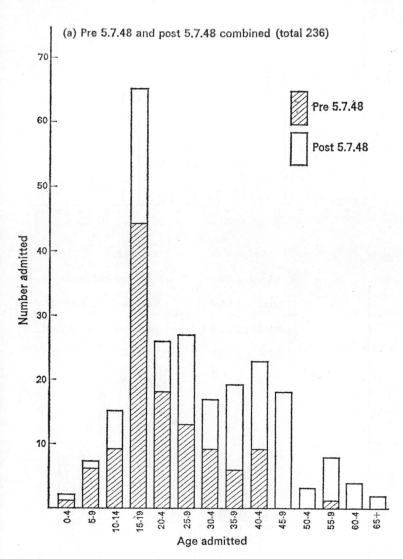

Figure 3a   Age mildly subnormal admitted to hospital

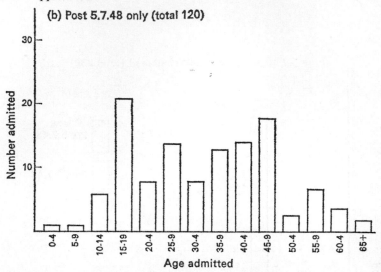

Figure 3b   Age mildly subnormal admitted to hospital

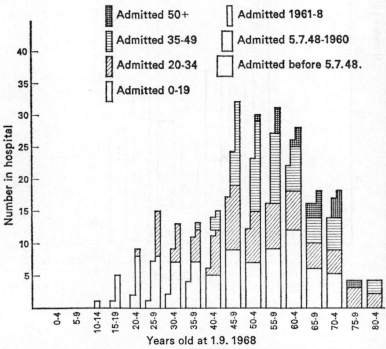

Figure 4   Age structure of total mildly subnormal hospital population at 1 September 1968 by age admitted and period admitted

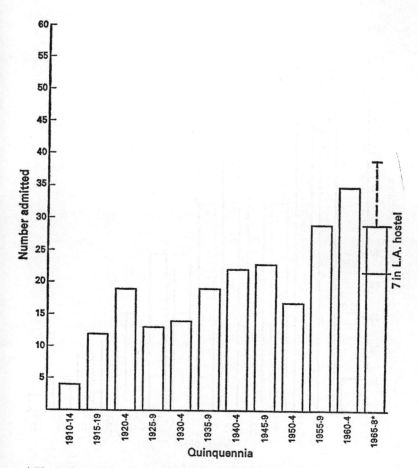

* The 'quinquennium' was only $3\frac{2}{3}$ years long, i.e. 1 January 1965 to
1 September 1968

*Figure 5   Quinquennia in which mildly subnormal admitted to hospital
(including pre 5.7.48) (total 236)*

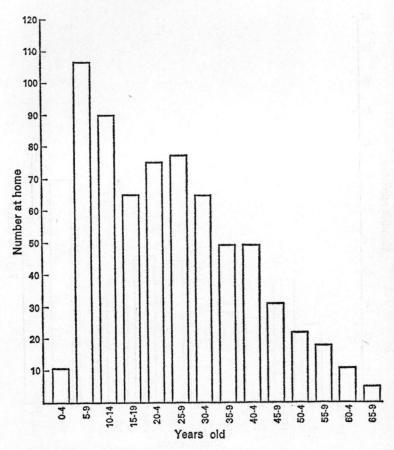

Figure 6   Age of severely subnormal at home at 1 September 1968
(*total 674*)

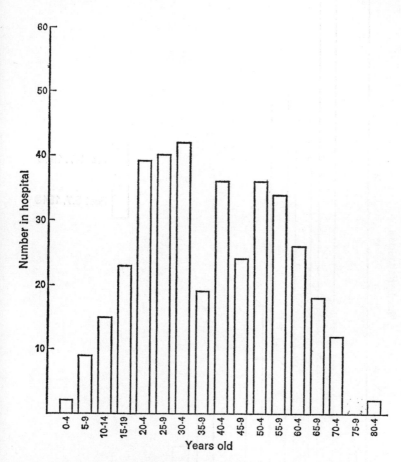

Figure 7   Age structure of total severely subnormal hospital population on⌉ 1 September 1968 (total 377)

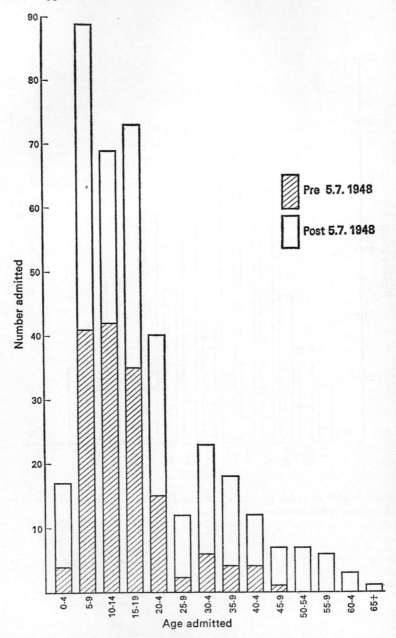

Figure 8a   Age severely subnormal admitted to hospital: pre 5.7.48 and post 5.7.48 combined (total 377)

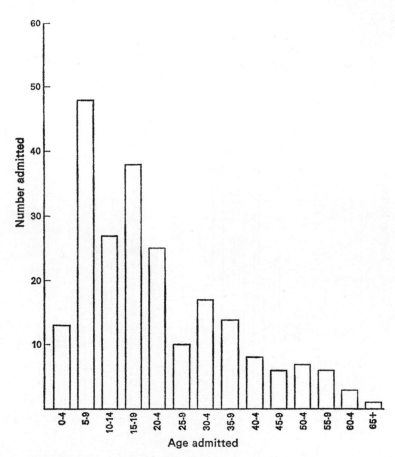

Figure 8b Age severely subnormal admitted to hospital: post 5.7.48 only (total 223)

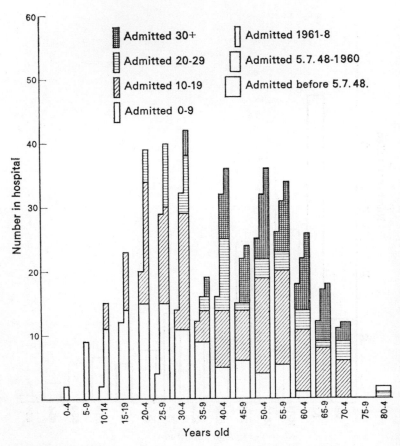

Figure 9   Age structure of severely subnormal hospital population at 1 September 1968 by age admitted and period admitted

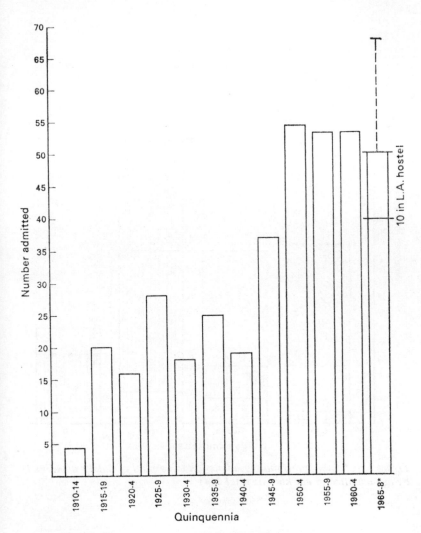

* The 'quinquennium' was only 3⅔ years long, i.e. 1 January 1965 to
1 September 1968

Figure 10 Quinquennia in which severely subnormal admitted to hospital (including pre 5.7.48) (total 377)

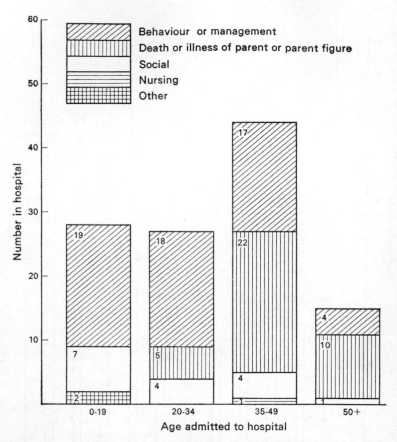

Figure 11   Factors precipitating admission to hospital of mildly subnormal by age admitted (6 not known: total 114)

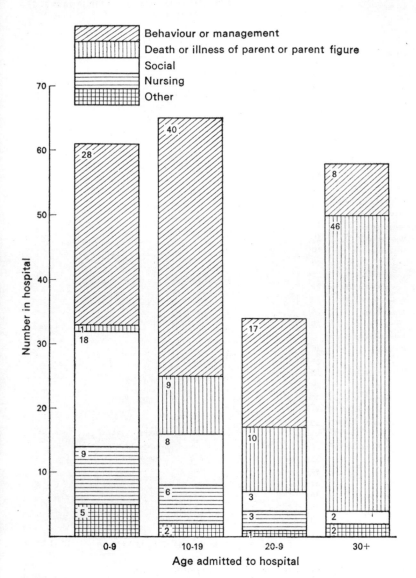

Figure 12   Factors precipitating admission to hospital of severely subnormal by age admitted (5 not known: total 218)

Ref No		1	2	3	4	5	6	7	8	9	10	11	12	13	14	15	16	17	18	19	20	21	22	23
Sex	1	F	F	M	F	F	F	M	M	F	M	M	F	M	F	F	F	F	F	F	M	M	M	F
Disabilities																								
Epilepsy	3	x		xx	x		x		x		x			x	xx	x				x	x			xx
Blind/deaf	4	x							x				x		x									
Mobility	5	xx	x	x	x			x	xx	x	x	x		x		x	x	x	xx	x			xx	xx
Continence	6	xx	x	x	x	x	x	xx	xx	x	x	xx	xx	x	x			x	xx	x	x		xx	xx
Talking	7	xx	x	xx	xx	x	xx	xx	xx	x	xx	xx	xx	xx	xx	xx	x	x			x	x	xx	
Dressing	8	xx	xx	xx	xx	xx	xx	xx	xx	xx	xx	xx	xx	xx	xx	xx	xx	xx	x				xx	xx
Washing	9	xx	xx	xx	xx	xx	xx	xx	xx	xx	xx	xx	xx	xx	xx	xx	xx	xx	x				xx	xx
Feeding	10	xx	xx	xx	xx	xx	xx	xx	xx		x	xx	xx	xx			x				x	x	xx	
Temperament	11		xx		x																	x		
Daily grind																								
Sleep of family	12	x	x	x	xx	x	x	xx			x		x		x	xx	x	x	x	x	xx	x		
Getting N. up	13	x/	x		x	x/	x/		x/		xx			x/	x/	x		x		x/	x			x/
Putting N. to bed	14	x/	x		x/		x	x/	x/	x/	x/		x		x/			x				x/		
Mother cooking meals	15	x/		x		x			x		xx	x/									x	x		
Behaviour at meals	16		x	x	x	x	x/	x/			x/	x	x/	x/			x				x	x		
Destructiveness	17		x		x			x/			x		x								x	x		
N. out by self	18																					x		
Transport Problem	19	xx	x		x/	x	x	x/	x/		x		x	x		x	x			x	x	x/	x/	xx
Shopping	20	x/	x/	x/	x/	x/	x/	x/	x	x	x	x		x		x/	x		x/			x/		x/
Leaving N. in a room	21	x	x	x		x		x	x	x	x	x	x	xx	xx	x		x	xx	xx	x	x		
Leaving N. in the house alone	22	xx	xx	x	x	x	x	x	xx	x	x	x	x	xx	xx	xx	x	xx	xx	xx	x	xx	x	xx
Mother's health	23	x	x		x		x		xx	x					xx	xx	x				xx	x	x	
Father's health	24	x	x		x	x																		
Mother lonely	25	x				x				x											x	x		
Positive factors of help																								
G.P. help	26	++						++	++	++	+	+			++	++	++		+		++		++	++
M.W.O. help	27	++		+				++	+	++	+						+			++	+			+
Short-term-care	28			++	++	+				++							+			++	++	++		+
Training centre	29	+						+	+											++	+			+
Leaving N. with other people	30	+4	+5	+1		+2	+1	+2	+3	+1	+1	+2		+2		+2		+5	+1					+2
Neighbours' help	31	+				+	+	++	+	+	+	+	++	++	+		+		+		+	+		
Relatives' help	32	++	++					++	+	+	+	+	++	NA	+	+	+	+	+			++	+	
Sibs' help	33	NA	A	NA	+	A	NA	NA	NA	++	+	NA	+	NA	NA	++	NA	++	++	NA	NA	NA		+
Others of household help	34	NA			NA			+	++	NA	NA	NA	NA	NA	NA	NA	NA	+	NA	NA			++	NA
Father help	35		NA	++	++	+		++	++	NA	++	++	++	NA	NA	NA	++	NA	NA	NA	++	+	++	NA
Parents out	36			++	++			++	+		++	++				+								
Mother out	37	+	++	++		+		++	++	+					++		++							
Out at weekends	38		++	+				+		+	+	+				+				+	+			
Holidays	39	++	++	++	+			++	+	++	+				++	++	++		+	++	++	+		++
Own car	40		++	++	+			+		+	++					+						++	++	
Father/figure alive	41	+		+	+	+	+	+	+	+	+				+					+		++	++	
Ref No		1	2	3	4	5	6	7	8	9	10	11	12	13	14	15	16	17	18	19	20	21	22	23

Figure 13   The combination of factors (families visited)

Notes on Figure 13

The figure in line 30 refers to the number of people with whom the subnormal could be left.

In lines 3–11 one cross (x) represents a mild disability, two crosses ($\substack{x\\x}$) a severe or total disability.

In lines 12–25 one cross represents a lesser problem, two crosses a marked problem. In either case a diagonal line indicates that the problem has been resolved.

	24	25	26	27	28	29	30	31	32	33	34	35	36	37	38	39	40	41	42	43	44	45	46	47	48	49	50	51	52	53
1	M	F	M	F	F	F	F	M	M	M	F	F	M	M	M	M	M	M	F	F	M	M	M	M	F	M	F	F	M	M
3	xx		xx		xx	xx	x			xx				x				x		xx			xx	xx					x	
4	x										x									x	x			x						
5				x		x	x		x	x		x	x							x										
6	x	x				xx	x		xx				x		x		x		x											
7		x			x		x	xx	x		x	x	x	x		x	xx	xx	x		xx	x			x		x			
8	xx	xx	x	xx	x		xx	x	xx	x		x	xx	x		x	x	x	x	x			x				x			
9	x	xx	xx	xx	x	x	xx	xx	xx	x	x	x	xx	x		xx	x	x	x				x				x			
10		x	x	x		x	x	x	xx	x	x							x	x											
11		x	x								x		x	x	x							x								
12	x/			x	xx	x/	x/				x/	xx			x					x	x/	x/								
13	x		x	x/x	x/	x/		x/	x/			x/								x/	x/	xx			x/					
14	x/			x/x					x/					x/	x			x/			x/									
15	x/					x/															x/									
16		x/								x				x/					x/x											
17		x	x												x		x/													
18	x/		x											x	xx									x/		x				
19		x/x	xx	xx	x	x/	x/x	x/x	x	xx	xx	xx	x/			xx	x/		x/x	x	x			x/		x/				
20		x/			x/		x/x	x/x			x/x				x/	x/x	x/									x/				
21	x	x	x	x	xx	x		x		x		x		x		x		x				x	x		x			x		
22	xx	x	xx	xx	xx	x		x		xx	xx	x	x	x	xx	x	x	x				xx	xx		x			xx		
23	x		x	x	x	x					x		xx	x	x	x				x				x				xx		x
24	x				xx								x	x						x	x	x			x					
25	x				x							x		x	x	x			x	x			x							x
26	+	+	++	++			+	++		+	+	++	++	+	+	++	+	+	+		+	+		++	+			+		
27	+	++	++					+		+	++	+	++	+		+	++				+	++		+		++	+			
28			+	+				+		++		+		++				++				++			+					+
29	++	+		+	++			++		++			++	++				++			++	++	++		++	++	++		++	++
30	++2	++1	+2	++2			++3	+3	++2	+2		+1	+1	+2		+1	.	++5	+1		NA		++1	NA	++2	NA	+1	++1	++3	+1
31		+	+	++	+	+	+		+	+	+	++	+	+			++	+	++	+	++		+	++	++			+	+	+
32	++	++	+		NA		NA	++	+		+	++	++	+		+	+	++	+		+		+	++	++		+	++	+	
33	NA	NA	NA	++	NA		+		+	NA	+	+		++		++	NA	++	NA	+	NA	+	NA	NA	+	++	NA	NA	++	NA
34	+	NA		NA	NA	NA	NA	NA	+			NA	+	NA	+	NA	NA	NA	NA	NA	+	NA		NA	NA	+	NA		+	
35	++	+	+	NA	+	+	NA	+	+	++	++	NA	++	++		NA	+	NA	NA	++	+	+		+	+	+	+		W NA	NA
36	++	+	++					+		+										+	++		++	+			++	++		
37		++	+	+			+	+	++		++						+	+			++			+	++	NA			NA	++
38		+			+		+	+					+	+			+	+		+		+	+	+			+			
39		++	++	++	++	+	++	++		++		++		++			++	++	++	++	+		++	++	+		+		++	+
40		+			+		+							+			+		+	+		+	++							
41	+	+	+		+	+		+	+	+	+		+	+	+		+			+	+	+	+	+	+	+	+	+	+	
	24	25	26	27	28	29	30	31	32	33	34	35	36	37	38	39	40	41	42	43	44	45	46	47	48	49	50	51	52	53

In lines 26–41 one plus (+) represents some help, two plusses (++) represents much help (NA = not applicable).

Line 18 concerns only those able enough to go out by themselves and refers to any problems which arose in connection with this.

A in line 33 indicates any sibs living a long way away from their parents.

W in line 35 case no. 52 is where the father was a widower.

Minor alterations have been made to preserve the anonymity of the families.

Appendix C Discussion of strength of association using the phi test and coefficient of contingency

In tables 9.9 and A10, a rating was given to a variety of different factors. This rating used either the phi test or the coefficient of contingency. Strictly speaking, these measures are not comparable.

Both tests assume knowledge of the value of χ^2 but unlike the χ^2 test they measure the *strength* of the relationship. The phi test is only applicable to 2×2 tables. The formula is very simple ($\phi = \sqrt{\chi^2/N}$ where $N =$ the total of observations). However, for more complex tables (for instance 2×3) the contingency coefficient has to be used ($C = \sqrt{\chi^2/N + \chi^2}$).

The difficulty arises in comparing the results from tables of different sizes (for instance 2×2 and 2×3). '[They] can only be compared directly under certain circumstances . . . [the] maximum value [of C] will vary with the number of categories of observation studied: for a 2×2 table the maximum value of 1 is 0·707, for a 3×3 table it is 0·816 and so on. . . . The maximum values associated with rectangular tables such as 2×7 or 3×4 are as yet unknown. The general conclusion must be that only C values resulting from similar contingency tables may be compared.' (Yeomans, 1968, p. 292f.)

In practice this did not prove to be a problem. Almost all the factors appearing in these tables were 2×2 or 2×3 tables. In many cases it was possible to treat the tables either as 2×2 or 2×3. For instance in table A10 in the section for children it was possible to treat feeding as a 2×3 table which meant taking 'Feeding by self', 'With help' and 'Not at all' separately or as a 2×2 table which meant taking 'Not at all' against 'With help' and 'Feeding by self' together. Because of this it was possible to draw up a table comparing the strength of association between the 2×2 and the 3×2 tables. This gave the following results for the middle section of the table for SSN children in table A10:

2 × 2 tables		3 × 2 tables
0·3284	Feeding	0·3120
0·3104	Behaviour problem at training centre	
0·2576	Epilepsy	0·2578
0·2461	Dressing ←	
	Speech	0·2420
		0·2391

It can be seen that the difference between the results for the 2×2 and 3×2 tables is small and generally of no importance. The case of dressing coming above speech on the 2×2 score and below speech on the 3×2 score is the only case where the difference between the two affected the order. In every case the 2×2 score was used where there was a choice, and thus dressing appears above speech.

It is the order which is important rather than the score itself. The figures in the two right-hand columns of those at home or in an institution with that characteristic fit in with the order suggested by the ratings.

Appendix D Guided Interview Schedule

1–2 Ref. No.   Date . . . .
      Name: Time begun . . . .

3–4 Date of Birth:
      Home Address:
      Person Interviewed:

Section I

5 Can you tell me if N has any special physical condition?
   For instance is he a Mongol   or Spastic   or Autistic

6 Does he ever suffer from epileptic fits?   None/Mild/Severe

7 Is he Blind ⎫
         or ⎬ None/Mild/Severe
       Deaf ⎭

8 Is he normally fairly healthy or do you find he is frequently
   under the weather?   YES/NO
   Does he suffer from:
     Weak heart
     Weak chest
     Overweight
     Other

9 Does he have any difficulty with walking?
     No handicap
     Can with help
     Crawling and wheelchair
     Crawling only or wheelchair only
     Not at all

10 Does he need help with getting dressed?
     No handicap
     Can with help
     Not at all

11 Does he need help with washing?
     No handicap
     Can with help
     Not at all

12 And what about feeding. Is N able to feed himself?
  No handicap
  Can with help
  Not at all

13 Does N need any help when he goes to the toilet?
  Fully continent
  Fully continent but needs help
  Nocturnal enuresis only
  No bladder control
  Totally incontinent

14 And does he have any difficulty with talking?
  Can join in general conversation
  Simple conversation
  Simple sentences
  A few words
  Gestures/grunts/noises
  Not at all

15 Do you find that he has any habits or mannerisms that are difficult to live with?
  PROMPT: For instance does N like everything to be tidy or bite his nails, or is there something he always likes to be doing?

16 And (if a girl) how does she manage with her periods?

17 Does N attend Training Centre? YES/NO
  If yes: Do you find this a help? YES/NO
     Does N seem to enjoy it? YES/NO
  If no: Has he ever? YES/NO
    (Why did he stop going?)
    Would you like him to now? YES/NO

Section II

I wonder if you would mind if I asked you for some details about members of the family such as age, employment, the places where you have lived and about this house?

18 First of all is your husband living?
  YES   NO

19 In what year was he born and How long ago did he die?
  where was this?

20 Can you tell me what his job is? Can you tell me what his job was?
               (Go to 25)

21 And what sort of hours does he work?

22   Does he ever have to work nights? How often?

23   What about weekends. Does he ever have to spend them away?
       How often?

24   Is he disabled or handicapped in any way?

25   And yourself—could you tell me your year of birth? Where
       were you born?

26   Now can you tell me—whether you have the whole of this house?
                                —is this flat self-contained?

27   Are you the owners?   YES/NO
                                             L.A./Privately rented

28   Perhaps I could just run through a list of items and you could
       then tell me whether you have them or not:
          Separate kitchen
          Fixed bath
          W.C. outside/inside
          Refrigerator
          Washing machine
          Vacuum cleaner
          Car
          Telephone
          Television

29   Can you tell me which if any of these are a particular help to you?

30   If interviewing parents:
       (a) Were you living in this house when N was born?
           NO   YES
           Were you living in Sheffield when N was born?
              NO   YES
           How many moves have you   Have you had any moves
           had in the last 10 yrs?   in the last 10 yrs?
                                         NO   YES
                                                     How many?
           How long have you been living in Sheffield?←
           OR
           And I suppose you've been living in Sheffield all
           your life?

30   If N is living with sib or others:
       (b) How long had N been living with you?
           Have you moved since he came?   YES/NO
           If yes: How many times?
           How long have you been living in Sheffield?

31   Are you satisfied with your present housing from
       the point of view of looking after N?   YES/NO

Section III

Can I now go through a list of possible problems you may have in looking after N?

32 First of all does he disturb the sleep of the family?
    In what way?
    How do you cope with this?
    Does he have his own bedroom?   YES/NO

33 Does he have any difficulty in getting up in the morning?
    PROMPT: Is he perhaps rather slow?
    How do you cope with this?

34 And what about N going to bed at night—do you have any trouble here?
    How do you deal with this?

35 When you're cooking a meal do you find that having N around makes it difficult?
    If NO—is this because you do most of the cooking while he is at Training Centre?
    But is there a problem when he is around?
    If YES—how do you overcome this?

36 Does N's behaviour at mealtimes present difficulties?
    PROMPT: For instance does he behave so badly that he makes it difficult for other members of the family to eat?

37 Do you find you have a lot of washing because of N?
    Is there any problem with doing the washing?
    If NO—is this because you do all the washing while N is at Training Centre?
    If he were there would it be difficult?

38 And with cleaning—is there any difficulty here?
    Does N ever help you?

39 Do you find that N will help himself to food when he shouldn't?
    What do you do about this?

40 Is N destructive? Do you have to keep knives and breakables out of his way?
    How do you deal with this?

41 I wonder if you have any difficulties with transport—for instance can N travel on public transport himself?   YES/NO
    Can he be taken on a bus?   YES/NO
    If attends Training Centre how does he get to the Training Centre?   Ord. Bus/Special Bus

42 Do you have the use of a car during the day or only at weekends?

43 Do you feel that transport is a problem?

44 Can N go out by himself at all?   YES/NO
    If so does he ever get into trouble?

45 Do you find it difficult to get the shopping done?
    How do you manage?

46 Do you feel able to leave him with other people?

    YES   NO
    How many people are there   Does this make things
    with whom you can leave   difficult for you?
    him?
    How often do you do this?   How do you get round
                                           this?

47 Can you leave N in a room by himself?
    About how long for?

48 Do you normally leave N alone in the house?

    YES   NO
    How long do you feel you   Why not? what might
    can leave him?   happen?
                                           Has it ever happened?
                                           Even though you may be
                                           worried do you ever go
                                           out and leave him?
    Are there any precautions you can take?

49 Are you ever able to get out together?
        How often?—regularly/occasionally/never
        Where do you usually go?
        or
        Would you like to?

50 Do you or your husband ever go out on your own?
        OR (if widow) Do you ever go out on your own?
        PROMPT: Bingo, football, pub   Husband: Reg./Occ./Never
                                               Wife: Reg./Occ./Never

        If not: Would you like to?

51 What about the weekends—do you ever get out as a family? YES/NO
    Would you like to?

52 Do you find there are any problems specially connected with
    weekends?
        PROMPT: For example no Training Centre

53 Do you ever go away for a holiday?

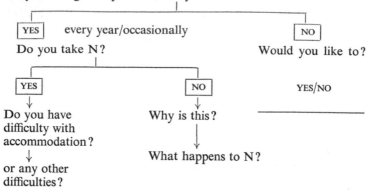

Do you have
difficulty with
accommodation?
↓
or any other
difficulties?

54 Do the problems of looking after N affect your husband's work?
In what way?

55 If applicable:
Would you like to go out to work if it were not for N?
or
Would you work full time if it were not for N?

56 Now how about yourself—are you keeping fairly well at the
moment?
Have you been under the doctor for any length of time?
What's been the trouble?
Do you think looking after N has affected your health
at all?

57 If husband living:
And your husband—does he keep fairly fit?
Has he been under the doctor for any length of time in
the last 10 years?

58 If applicable:
Do . . . . (the other members of the family) keep well?

59 If husband living:
You must have had to make a lot of decisions about N. Do you and
your husband ever find it difficult to agree on what to do for the
best?

60 Now when N's at home do you find it difficult to keep him occupied?
Do you find that N insists on a lot of attention from you or your
husband?
What does he do?

61 Do you find you have suffered financially from keeping N at home?

62 Well Mrs. X we've been through many possible difficulties. What
do you see as the main problem in your case?

Section IV

We've talked about the problems you have—could we now see what help you have in coping with them?

63   If applicable: What help is your husband able to give?

64   If applicable: And what about the others? Do they help?

65   Would you now mind if I run through a list of things which N might need help with and ask you who it is who gives the help?

	MOTHER	FATHER	SN	OTHER
a. Getting up in the morning				
b. Washing him				
c. Shaving him				
d. Dressing him				
e. Feeding him				
f. Getting him ready for Training Centre				
g. Taking him to Training Centre				
h. Collecting him from Training Centre				
i. Keeping him occupied				
j. Taking him out for a walk or drive				
k. Bathing him				
l. Washing his hair				
m. Cutting his hair				
n. Cutting his nails				
o. Putting him to bed				
p. Getting up to see to him at night				

66 Has N any brothers or sisters?

Brother or Sister	Married	Children	Living In			Support
			Same Home	Sheffield	Else-where	

What sort of attitude do they have towards N?
PROMPT: Are they good with him or are they not much help?

67 And your relations? Do you have any brothers and sisters?

How many?

Do they live in Sheffield?

(Much: Adequate: Little: None)

Does your *husband* have any brothers and sisters?

How *many* does he have?

Do they live in Sheffield?

(Much: Adequate: Little: None)

What sort of attitude do *they* have towards N?
Are any of them, or any other relations, particularly
good with N or helpful to the family?
PROMPT: How do they help?
Do you feel you can ask for help if you need it?
Have you ever done so?
What has been the response?

68   Do you have any problems with your neighbours or are they quite friendly?

>   I wonder if you could tell me whether any of them are particularly good with N or helpful to you and the family?
>   Do you feel you can ask them for help?
>   Have you ever asked them?
>   If so what has the response been?

69   Do you ever think that having N has made you feel lonely and cut off from other people?

70   Is there anyone you can go to if things get on top of you?

>   PROMPT: Is there anyone with whom you are particularly friendly?

71   If they have moved recently—
Were things very different where you used to live?

72   Does N have any particular friends of his own?   YES/NO

73   Do you or your husband belong to a parents group or society for handicapped children?

	Mother	YES/NO
	Father	YES/NO
Do you find this a help?		YES/NO

74   What about any other society, group, club or church?
Are they helpful in any way?   YES/NO

Section V

75   Do you have any definite plans for N for the future?

76   Have you made any use of short-term care?

>   If so where and when and for how long?
>   Has this helped in any particular way?

77   Do you find your doctor (G.P.) has been a help to you?

78   And the MWO is he any help?

79   Is there anything else you would like to tell me that I haven't asked?

Time recorded interview completed................................

Interviewer's Notes

Difficulty in doing the interview.

Reliability of informants.

Co-operativeness of informants.

Ability to accept help.

Central factor in being able to help N at home.

Assessment of mother's mental health.

Assessment of N's temperament—almost completely apathetic
underactive
as lively as most
livelier and more energetic
uncontrollably excitable

Main problems as seen by the interviewer.

Appendix E Summary of the Sheffield Development Project

The Sheffield Development Project plans a radical reshaping of the services for the subnormal in Sheffield County Borough. The capital cost of the project for the first five years at 1970 prices totals £3,524,000 and the additional running cost of the hospital services is estimated at £175,000 per annum and the local authority more than £500,000 per annum when it has been implemented.

The plans can be split into three sections, one dealing with assessment and training, one with various forms of residential care, and a third with other administrative matters.

Assessment and training

Children

(a) The existing centre for handicapped children called the Ryegate Centre and associated with the Children's hospital should become the Comprehensive Assessment Centre where all children found to have a mental defect should be assessed by a multidisciplinary team of professional people (para. 7.5).

(b) Day care places for children under five should be provided by the local authority in nursery classes in junior training centres or in day nurseries or in nursery schools or in a combination of these (para. 7.14).

(c) Existing local authority education or training places for children may be adequate but their adequacy will need to be assessed as the case register is built up (para. 7.29).

(d) There will be two twenty-five place day care centres at Ryegate and the Northern General Hospital associated with the twenty-four bed units on those sites (see next section) (para. 7.26).

Adults

(a) Local authority will expand provision from the present 255 places to about 1,000 places with a far greater variety of regimes than at present, e.g. advanced industrial units and an adolescent work assessment unit (para. 7.46).

(b) Two 115-place day care units (for the very severely disabled) to be built alongside the ninety-six hospital beds at the Northern General Hospital and the ninety-six on the Norton site (para. 7.42) (see below).

382

Residential care

The following provision is proposed:

	Local authority	Hospitals	
Children (paras 7.21 & 7.22)	8 present hostel places for short-term care only	24 places Northern General Hospital	} Group A
		24 places. ? at Ryegate	
	Hostel with 15 beds providing five-day-week care	2 hostels with 24 beds (outside hospital boundaries)	} Group B
	20-place hostel for full-time care ? possibly one further hostel		
Adults (paras 7.36, 7.38 & 7.39)	One existing hostel (34 places)	96 beds Northern General Hospital	} Group A
	One hostel already planned (36 places)	96 beds Norton District General Hospital site	
	Two residential homes for working men and women (25 places each)	4 hostels (25 beds)	Group B
	7–8 hostels (25 places each)	24 beds for emotionally disturbed adults and adolescents at Middlewood Mental Hospital	
	Group homes (max. 6 people) and lodgings	230 places	

In addition

(a) Voluntary help should be encouraged and a whole-time organizer of voluntary services should be shared between hospital and local authorities (para. 7.50).

(b) More health visitors should be recruited and a joint mental health social work service should be established between the local authority and hospitals (paras 7.52 and 7.60).

(c) A local co-ordinating committee with members representing voluntary bodies, general practitioners, hospital and local authorities and, initially, the Department of Health and Social Security should be established (para. 7.65). This committee is seen as being of the first importance, though not having any executive powers.

Appendix F   Potential residents for hostels based on a population of 20,000

In relating residential units to local areas it is the children who pose the greatest problems. If one were to have a hostel for mentally handicapped children drawn from a population of 20,000, there would be about 1·2 children in it on average. This figure is based on the number of severely subnormal children from Sheffield in hospital on 1 September 1968. There is a marked difference between Sheffield and Wessex in the rates per 100,000 of severely subnormal children in institutional care. The rate for Sheffield is ±6/100,000 but for Wessex is ±20/100,000 (Kushlick, 1969). (The number of places planned in the White Paper is 25/100,000.) However, when the total rates are compared, that is for both those at home and those in an institution, they are quite close. The rate for Wessex was ±48/100,000 and for Sheffield ±53/100,000.

The Sheffield Development Project plans two, possibly three, local authority hostels, two hospital hostels and two hospital units for children. Even if all children whatever their handicap were taken together, this would still give only about six children per 20,000 population, if one takes the Sheffield Development Plan figures of thirty residential places for children per 100,000. It might be possible to reduce this problem by careful siting of a hostel but sites are difficult to find and the children needing residential care tend to be widely distributed. The possibility of mixing them with other children was mentioned in chapter 19 but there are other possibilities, such as more extensive fostering or even trying out a residential home for only five or six children.

The picture is rather different when the adults are considered. The total number of severely subnormal adults from Sheffield in hospital on 1 September 1968 was 347. This includes those admitted before 5 July 1948. This works out at a rate of seventy-two per 100,000. There was a total of 233 mildly subnormal adults in hospital, and this gives a rate of forty-eight per 100,000. This would give a total rate per 100,000 for all subnormals in an institution of 120. This in turn gives a rate of twenty-four per 20,000.

But a number of those at present in institutions could not be moved either because of their behaviour or because they had been in an institution for so long. McKeown and Leck (1967) in an investigation of the medical, nursing and social needs of all Birmingham patients (1,652) in hospitals for the subnormal showed that only about half needed the kind of care which made it necessary for them to be in hospital. Included in those needing hospital care were those who needed only basic nursing. Hostels could probably provide this in most cases. If those needing only basic nursing were added, 60 per cent of those in hospital, according to McKeown and Leck's figures, did not need hospital care. In a subsequent investigation

384

(McKeown and Teruel, 1970), in which patients were assessed on a different basis, namely the consultant's classification, this proportion was rather lower. If those needing only home nursing are included, 46 per cent of the children and 47 per cent of the adults, according to the later survey, did not need hospital care. According to the consultants, approximately one-third of the patients did not need hospital care and about one-fifth were considered suitable for discharge to their own homes or, more commonly, to hostel accommodation. However, the proportions given make certain assumptions about the kind of person who can be looked after in a hostel, which is one of the points at issue.

This study of subnormals in Sheffield considered only people in hospital at the time they were admitted. It can therefore offer no evidence about the *present* condition of those in institutions. However, the analysis of the files did show that there was one group most of whom had no need of hospital care when they were admitted. This was the old institution group, admitted because of the death or illness of a parent. They accounted for roughly one-third of those in hospital. Moreover, it seems likely that the behaviour of a considerable number of those admitted because of a behaviour problem (45 per cent of the total) will have calmed down as they have grown older, and they too could be cared for outside hospital. It seems reasonable to assume that the same would be true of many of those admitted for social reasons. In addition the case was argued in chapter 19 for looking after the very seriously physically disabled within the local hostel wherever possible.

There would certainly remain a number who did need specialist hospital care, generally for reasons of behaviour. Any realistic policy of community care has to recognize this. Also, it might be necessary to leave in an institution some of those who had been there for a very long time and for whom it had become home. On the other hand, residential care in small local hostels would very likely provoke increased demand from families whose subnormal was at home. It is impossible to be precise about the numbers of subnormal who could be cared for in hostel-type accommodation, but this consideration of the numbers involved shows that a hostel serving a population of 20,000 is far from unreasonable.

Notes

Chapter 1 Introduction

1 A study carried out about the same time in Sheffield by Dr K. S. Holt showed the considerable effect that subnormal children could have on their siblings (Holt, 1957). The PEP follow-up study indicated that the effect might not be as serious as Holt's study suggested.

2 Two large-scale projects carried out in New York by Saenger (1957; 1960) dealt in some detail with factors, including social factors, which led to admission to an institution and with the integration of the subnormal into the community. These studies covered both the mildly and the severely handicapped, but the two are not always considered separately, and at times this confuses the issue. They do go some way in considering care by the community, as shown by, for instance, the subnormal's friendships, or the number of subnormals who had tried to get a job, or the characteristics of the different communities, e.g. Jewish compared with Puerto-Rican.

   Another interesting American study was carried out by Jane Mercer (1966) in which she looked at the patterns of family crisis which led originally to the subnormal being admitted to an institution, in relation to whether the family took him back home later or not.

3 This is even more marked in the studies by F. M. Martin and G. F. Rehin. They concentrate almost entirely on services in the community, especially social work services (Martin, 1960; Martin, 1961; Rehin and Martin, 1968). They do, however, acknowledge the need for planning to 'be firmly related to clinical and social realities'.

   A study by Sheila Hewett (1970) of 180 cerebral-palsied children, of whom the larger part was mentally handicapped, gave a most valuable account of the practical problems of caring for such children in their own homes and a critical account of the various services intended to help the mothers and their children, and made also some useful comparisons with bringing up ordinary children. This drew on the work of John and Elizabeth Newson, with whom the book was written. The whole book is based on the mother's experience, in a very similar way to the second half of this book, and in view of the fact that this study concentrates on adult subnormals and Mrs Hewett's on children, the two are in many ways complementary.

A recently published study of physically handicapped children and their families by Joan McMichael (1971) shows the very considerable stress to which the families were subjected. When families were subjected to the degree of stress indicated by some of the cases in Dr McMichael's study, it is unlikely that the handicapped would remain at home until adulthood, even if they survived as long as that. As the mentally handicapped members of the families visited in this Sheffield study were all adults, the greater stress sometimes present in families with younger handicapped members, who would most likely be admitted to hospital before reaching adulthood, needs to be borne in mind.

Chapter 3   A profile of the survey population

1 This is worked out as follows—Modal age of reporting = sixteen. The youngest person likely to be excluded is therefore someone who was sixteen in 1948, someone therefore who was thirty-six in 1968.
2 These figures are taken from A. Kushlick's chapter on 'Social Problems of Mental Subnormality' in *Foundations of Child Psychiatry* (ed. Emanuel Miller), Pergamon, 1968, p. 376, table 3.

Chapter 4   How the subnormal were reported

1 This was the case until the passing of the Determination of Needs Act (1941), which made parents responsible for dependent children only (i.e. those under sixteen) and children were no longer responsible financially for parents and grandparents.

Chapter 6   Social class

1 The classification of socio-economic groups follows that of the Registrar General as laid down in the Classification of Occupations (1966, pp. x–xii). The actual titles used are those for the five broad categories of social class. However, the social class was determined by the socio-economic group into which the father or father figure fell. This is why the term socio-economic group has been retained. The table below shows how socio-economic groups and the five broader categories are related.

Definition of socio-economic group

  I 'Professional' includes socio-economic groups 1, 2, 3, and 4.
 II 'Intermediate' includes socio-economic groups 5, 6 and 8.
III 'Skilled' includes socio-economic groups 9 and 12.
IV 'Semi-skilled' includes socio-economic groups 7 and 10.
 V 'Unskilled' includes socio-economic group 11.
    H.M. Forces includes socio-economic group 16.

No one fell into the agricultural categories 13, 14 and 15 and if the occupation was inadequately described (S.E.G. 17) they were coded 'not known'.

2 I am indebted for these figures and for much help in the whole of this chapter to my colleague Mr Trevor Noble.

Chapter 8 The family background

1 This relates to the original home sample of 150 visited by Tizard and Grad between 1954 and 1957. Thirty-seven of these had been admitted to hospital at the time of the further study about eight years later. These were compared with the 113 who had remained at home.
2 This study supports this suggestion. Among the children, only nine out of eighty-nine mongols presented a serious behaviour problem (10 per cent), but among the non-mongols seventy-one out of 259 did so (27 per cent). The contrast was not so marked among the adults. Seven mongol adults out of a total of 108 presented a serious behaviour problem (7 per cent). Among the non-mongol adults 119 out of 1,307 did so (9 per cent.)

Chapter 9 The subnormals themselves

1 These figures are the chronological figures for those under sixteen or over fifteen on 1 October 1968. They have been taken in order to work out the rate per 1,000. For this reason no percentage has been given. If the usual definition of children is adopted for those in an institution, i.e. someone who was under sixteen when he was admitted, the number of SSN mongol children in hospital goes up to twelve and the number of SSN mongol adults in hospital goes down to twenty. On these latter figures there was a significantly higher proportion of mongol children at home ($\chi^2 = 14 \cdot 262$ $p = 0 \cdot 001$) but no significant difference in the case of adults.

Chapter 10 The help and services the subnormals and their families received

1 The total numbers shown in the training centres or at the special care unit in tables 10.1, 10.3(a) and 10.3(b), and 10.5(a) and 10.5(b) are less than the total number actually attending training centres in Sheffield. The position is rather complex. The number shown attending a junior training centre is greater than the centres' registers showed, because all children were coded as attending a junior training centre if they were under sixteen, even though in some cases they were attending a senior training centre. It is easier, therefore, to consider the total numbers attending all training centres. The number on the books of all the training centres and the special care unit on 31 August 1968 was 477. The total number shown as attending in the tables is 375. The difference is due to those who were excluded from the survey or those for whom only limited information was coded. These exclusions were explained in

chapter 2. Most of the difference was accounted for by those who lived in the 'new' areas of Sheffield and those who had moved into Sheffield from other local authority areas.

Chapter 12   Introduction to the visits

1 Seventeen visits were carried out by Mrs J. P. Lee and thirty-seven by M. J. Bayley.

Chapter 13   The subnormal people who were visited

1 The results of one interview were not coded, as explained on p. 178.

Chapter 16   The quality of life

1 In the exceptional case the text of the interview suggests that there was in fact one daughter who would look after the subnormal on the very rare occasions that the parents went out.
2 This is shown diagrammatically in figure 13, lines 36, 37, 38 and 41.
3 In the two cases in figure 13 where there was no father or father figure and a single dot appears in line 40, this refers to the fact that a relative or friend had a car which was generally available for them.

Chapter 17   Family, friends and neighbours

1 Young and Willmott (1957) showed that when the mother died: 'The first and most obvious effect is that, since her children no longer visit her home, they see less of each other. Of the 162 married, widowed and divorced women in the general sample with their mothers alive, 35 per cent had seen a sister in the previous day, against 16 per cent of the 242 where mothers were dead.'
2 Townsend has shown how important this was for old people and their families (Townsend, 1963, pp. 216–19).

Chapter 18   The professional helpers

1 Two other people attended a centre for the physically handicapped once a week.
2 According to health visitors' records eight of these families were visited during the period the visits were being carried out.
In one case weekly visits were made, in four other cases visits were paid quarterly, in one case only one visit had been made and in the remaining two cases the frequency of the visits was uncertain.

Chapter 19   Conclusions

1 An account of the work of a residential unit for disturbed or maladjusted children in the United States in Wisconsin, where

the parents are involved very closely, is given by Kemp (1971).
In this unit the parents are expected to play an active part in the
centre for at least six hours a week. Parents are concerned not only
in the care of their own child but also take some interest in teaching,
playing with, or caring for a group of children. The staff use
concrete situations and daily routine to help parents to find better
ways of handling their child, for instance a constructive way of
coping with a temper tantrum.

The author concludes by saying: 'It is helpful when the family
can be involved in concrete programs designed to change a child's
behavior. We start with a behavior that really "bugs" the
parents and have them take part in forging and carrying out new
approaches.'

The work of Dr Peter Mittler in Manchester with the parents of
mentally handicapped children also involves the parents in the
educational process (Hester Adrian Research Centre & National
Society for Mentally Handicapped Children, 1971).

2 I am indebted to Mrs Beverley Freeston for this information.

3 The Sheffield Home Warden scheme provides a similar service, but
its basis is rather different. It evolved from the home helps who only
work on weekdays. The home warden is paid more and works at
weekends and in the evenings. She is trained in simple first-aid and
home care.

4 The Disabled Living Foundation (346 Kensington High Street,
London W.14) publish a series of pamphlets about practical details
of this nature.

5 One of the gravest difficulties such an approach would face would
be the increasing mobility of an increasing proportion of the
population. However, this is hardly an argument against forging local
contacts, but rather an argument for making local contacts easier
to establish, and this such a pattern of service might be able to do.

6 Another important study of old people was published in 1972, too
late to be considered in the text. This is the study of geriatric
patients in Glasgow by Isaacs, Livingstone and Neville (1972).
Many of the points they raise about the aged and their families
in Glasgow are as relevant for the mentally handicapped and their
families in Sheffield; for example, the importance of the home help
service, the role of the nurse in training relatives and the value of a
daughter going out to part-time employment. They do not advocate
a service quite on the lines suggested here, but it would meet a
number of the points they raise.

7 This raises further possibilities for fruitful co-operation at a local
level, for instance such a group practice might well look after a local
hostel. The committee themselves say in the same paragraph
(para. 39): 'It would also be large enough to justify the
attachment, as advocated by the Seebohm Committee, of one or
more social workers whose work would be related to the population
of the group practice and who would be able to communicate
effectively with the doctors, nurses and health visitors.'

8 It is interesting that Tizard and Grad (1961) mentioned in the conclusion of their study of 250 mentally handicapped people and their families that: 'There is at present a growing support for the view that a general, family case worker should deal with most of the problems of families who need social assistance of any kind. Such family caseworkers would work in a clearly defined locality in which they would be known to and would know all the families.'

9 The Association of General Practitioner Hospitals makes a plea for locally based hospitals in their pamphlet, 'Your local hospital— Near? or Far?' (Obtainable from Dr R. M. Emrys-Roberts, 1 Red House Lane, Walton-on-Thames, Surrey.)

10 This approach is quite different from that of the Aves Report (1969) to which the Seebohm Report looked forward. Near the beginning, the Aves Report referred to the work 'carried out by numberless friends and neighbours, who became aware of individual needs and met them in a completely informal and unorganized way', only to go on to say: 'But this brief reference to the importance of the good neighbour may perhaps explain why it seemed desirable to focus our attention mainly on the role of the volunteer within the framework of some form of organization' (para. 10). It is true that a little later the report says (para. 32):

> We can imagine that eventually much of the work done by organizations which draw on the help of volunteers from outside their own areas may be undertaken by local groupings which involve residents in whatever action is needed.

But they imagine that this is in 'the shadowy future'. The report does not, however, indicate how this can be encouraged, and the serious limitations of the approach they have adopted is shown in the all-too-familiar comment about the middle-class predominance in the organized voluntary services. In response to this they point to the need to widen the field of recruitment, rather than to question the adequacy of their interpretation of voluntary help (paras 165–7).

Bibliography

Public general statutes

49 and 50 Vict., c.25	Idiots Act, 1886
53 Vict., c.5	Lunacy (Consolidation) Act, 1890
3 and 4 Geo. V, c.28	Mental Deficiency Act, 1913
17 and 18 Geo. V, c.33	Mental Deficiency Act, 1927
19 Geo. V, c.17	Local Government Act, 1929
20 and 21 Geo. V, c.23	Mental Treatment Act, 1930
9 and 10 Geo. VI, c.81	National Health Service Act, 1946
7 and 8 Eliz. II, c.72	Mental Health Act, 1959
18 and 19 Eliz. II, c.44	Chronically Sick and Disabled Persons Act, 1970

Books, articles, reports, etc.

Aves, G. M. (1969), *The Voluntary Worker in the Social Services* (The Aves Report), London: Allen & Unwin.

Baird, Sir Dugald (1962), 'Environmental and obstetrical factors in prematurity, with special reference to experience in Aberdeen', *Bulletin of the World Health Organisation*, 26, 291–5.

Baker, J. and Young, M. (1971), *The Hornsey Plan: A role for neighbourhood councils in the new local government*, 3rd edn, published by the Association for Neighbourhood Councils, 18 Victoria Park Square, London E.2.

Benington, J. (1970), 'Community Development Project', *Social Work Today*, 1 (5).

Birch, H. G., Richardson, S. A., Baird, Sir D., Horobin, G., Illsley, R. (1970), *Mental Subnormality in the Community*, Baltimore: Williams & Wilkins.

Bott, E. (1971), *Family and Social Network*, 2nd edn, London: Tavistock. (1st edn 1957.)

Bowlby, E. J. M. (1951), *Child Care and the Growth of Love*, Geneva: WHO.

Campbell, A. C. (1968), 'Comparison of family and community contacts of mentally subnormal adults in hospital and local authority hostels', *British Journal of Preventive and Social Medicine*, 22 (3), July 1968.

Dennis, N. (1958), 'The popularity of the neighbourhood community idea', *Sociological Review*, n.s.6, 191–206.

Dennis, N. (1962), 'Secondary group relationships and the pre-eminence of the family', *International Journal of Comparative Sociology*, 3, 1962.

Dennis, N. (1963), 'Who needs neighbours?', *New Society*, 43, 25 July 1963.

Department of Health and Social Security (1971), *Better Services for the Mentally Handicapped*, Cmnd 4683, London: HMSO.

Department of Health and Social Security (1971), *Sheffield Development Project: Feasibility Study Report proposing a new pattern of service for mentally handicapped people in Sheffield County Borough*, MO (MS) 46 (cyclostyled).

Department of Health and Social Security (1971), *The Organization of Group Practice: A report of a sub-committee of the Standing Medical Advisory Committee*, London: HMSO.

Edgerton, R. B. (1967), *The Cloak of Competence*, Berkeley: University of California Press.

Feversham Report (1939), *Departmental Committee on the Voluntary Mental Health Services*, London: HMSO.

Frankenberg, R. (1966), *Communities in Britain*, Harmondsworth: Penguin.

General Register Office (1966), *Classification of Occupations 1966*, London: HMSO.

Goldberg, E. M. with Mortimer, A. and Williams, B. T. (1970), *Helping the Aged*, London: Allen & Unwin.

Gould, J. and Kolb, W. L. (1964), *A Dictionary of the Social Sciences*, (UNESCO), London: Tavistock.

Hampton, W. A. (1970), *Democracy and Community: a study of politics in Sheffield*, Oxford University Press.

Hester Adrian Research Centre and National Society for Mentally Handicapped Children (North West Region) (1971), *Working with Parents: Developing a workshop course for parents of young mentally handicapped children*, published by the National Society for Mentally Handicapped Children (North West Region), 1 Brazennose Street, Manchester, 2.

Hewett, S. with Newson, J. and E. (1970), *The Family and the Handicapped Child*, London: Allen & Unwin.

Holt, K. S. (1957), *The impact of severely retarded children upon their families*, unpublished M.D. thesis, University of Manchester.

Home Office Department of Education and Science, Ministry of Housing and Local Government, Ministry of Health (1968), *Report of the Committee on Local Authority and Allied Personal Social Services* (The Seebohm Report), Cmnd 3703, London: HMSO.

Howe Report (1969), *Report of the Committee of Inquiry into Allegations of Ill-Treatment and other Irregularities at Ely Hospital, Cardiff*, Cmnd 3975, London: HMSO.

Isaacs, B., Livingstone, M., Neville, Y. (1972), *Survival of the Unfittest*, London: Routledge & Kegan Paul.

Jacobs, J. (1961), *The Death and Life of Great American Cities*, London: Cape.

Jones, K. (1960). *Mental Health and Social Policy 1845–1959*, London: Routledge & Kegan Paul.

Kemp, C. J. (1971), 'Family Treatment within the Milieu of a

Residential Treatment Centre', *Journal of the Child Welfare League of America*, 50 (4), April 1971.

Kushlick, A. (1964), 'The prevalence of recognized mental subnormality of I.Q. under 50 among children in the South of England with reference to the demand for places for residential care', paper to the *International Copenhagen Congress on the Scientific Study of Mental Retardation*, August 1964.

Kushlick, A. (1966), 'A community service for the mentally subnormal', *Social Psychiatry*, 1 (2), 73–82.

Kushlick, A. (1967a), 'A method of evaluating the effectiveness of a community health service', *Social and Economic Administration*, 1 (4).

Kushlick, A. (1967b), 'The Wessex Experiment—comprehensive care for the mentally subnormal', *British Hospital Journal and Social Service Review*, 6 October 1967.

Kushlick, A. (1968), 'Social problems of mental subnormality', in *Foundations of Child Psychiatry* (ed. E. Miller), Oxford: Pergamon.

Kushlick, A. (1969), Letter to *Lancet*, 29 November 1969, 1196f.

Kushlick, A. (1970), 'Residential care for the mentally subnormal', *Royal Society of Health Journal*, 90 (5), September/October 1970.

McKeown, T. and Leck, I. (1967), 'Institutional care of the mentally subnormal', *British Medical Journal*, 3, 2 September 1967, 573–6.

McKeown, T. and Teruel, J. R. (1970), 'An assessment of the feasibility of discharge of patients in hospitals for the subnormal', *British Journal of Preventive and Social Medicine*, 24 (2), May 1970.

McMichael, Joan K. (1971), *Handicap: A Study of Physically Handicapped Children and Their Families*, London: Staples.

Mann, P. H. (1965), *An Approach to Urban Sociology*, London: Routledge & Kegan Paul.

Martin, F. M. (1960), 'Community mental health services', *Planning* (PEP), 26 (447).

Martin, F. M. (1961), 'Mental subnormality and community care', *Planning* (PEP), 27 (457).

Mercer, J. R. (1966), 'Patterns of family crisis related to reacceptance of the retardate', *American Journal of Mental Deficiency*, 71 (1), July 1966.

Minar, D. W. and Greer, S. (1969), *The Concept of Community*, London: Butterworth.

Ministry of Health (1962), *A Hospital Plan for England and Wales*, Cmnd 1604, London: HMSO.

Ministry of Health (1963), *Health and Welfare: The Development of Community Care*, Cmnd 1973, London: HMSO. Revised 1964 and 1966 (Cmnd 3022).

Ministry of Health (1966), *The Hospital Building Programme: A revision of the hospital plan for England and Wales*, Cmnd 3000, London: HMSO.

Mitchell, G. D., Lupton, T., Hodges, M. W., Smith, C. S. (1954), *Neighbourhood and Community*, Liverpool University Press.

Moncrieff, J. (1966), *Mental Subnormality in London: A survey of community care*, London: PEP.

Morris, P. (1969), *Put Away*, London: Routledge & Kegan Paul.
National Association for Mental Health (1961), *Annual Report for 1960–61*, London: NAMH.
National Council for Civil Liberties (1950), *50,000 outside the Law*, London.
Olshansky, S. (1965), 'Chronic sorrow: A response to having a mentally defective child', in *Social Work with Families* (ed. E. Younghusband), National Institute for Social Work Training Series, no. 4, London: Allen & Unwin.
Pahl, R. E. (1970), *Patterns of Urban Life*, London: Longmans.
Payne Report (1972), *Report of the Committee of Inquiry into Whittingham Hospital*, Cmnd 4861, London: HMSO.
Rehin, G. F. and Martin, F. M. (1968), *Patterns of Performance in Community Care: A report of a mental health services study*, London: Oxford University Press for Nuffield Provincial Hospitals Trust.
Robb, B. (1967), *Sans Everything*, London: Nelson.
Saenger, G. S. (1957), *The adjustment of retarded individuals in the community*, New York Inter-Departmental Health Resources Board.
Saenger, G. S. (1960), *Factors influencing the institutionalization of mentally retarded individuals in New York City*, New York Inter-Departmental Health Resources Board.
Scottish Council for Research in Education (1949), *The Trend of Scottish Intelligence*, University of London Press.
Stein, Z. and Susser, M. (1963), 'The social distribution of mental retardation', *American Journal of Mental Deficiency*, 67, 811.
Shaw, C. H. and Wright, C. H. (1960), 'The married mental defective: a follow-up study', *Lancet*, 30 January 1960, 273–4.
Skipper, J. *Out into the community*, first and second reports, Sheffield: Sheffield Council of Social Service. (Duplicated, no date.)
Stacey, M. (1960), *Tradition and Change: a study of Banbury*, Oxford University Press.
Tizard, J. (1964), *Community Services for the Mentally Handicapped*, Oxford University Press.
Tizard, J. and Grad, J. (1961), *The Mentally Handicapped and Their Families*, Oxford University Press.
Tönnies, F. (1955), *Community and Association*, London: Routledge & Kegan Paul.
Townsend, P. (1963), *The Family Life of Old People*, Harmondsworth: Penguin.
Vernon, P. E. (1960), *Intelligence and Attainment Tests*, University of London Press.
Watkins Report (1971), *Report of the Farleigh Hospital Committee of Inquiry*, Cmnd 4557, London: HMSO.
Willmott, P. (1963), *The Evolution of a Community: a study of Dagenham after forty years*, London: Routledge & Kegan Paul.
Wood Report (1929), *Report of the Mental Deficiency Committee, being a Joint Committee of the Board of Education and the Board of Control*, London: HMSO.

Yeomans, K. A. (1968), *Applied Statistics. Statistics for the Social Scientist: Vol. 2*, London: Allen Lane, The Penguin Press.
Young, M. and Willmott, P. (1957), *Family and Kinship in East London*, London: Routledge & Kegan Paul.

Index

Acceptance
positive/negative axis, 190–1
realistic, 191
of the subnormal's handicap, 186–191
see also Attitude
Admission to hospital
age at and precipitating factors, 67–9
factors associated with, 21, 57–69, 167–8
strength of various factors associated with, 138–43
Age of mother at birth of subnormal, 110–12
Association for Neighbourhood Councils, 340
Attendance allowance, 324
Attitude
'closed', 205–6
of families to subnormal, 186–207, 240
'open', 205–6
of parents to subnormal, 316
of realistic expectation, 192–3
resigned, 190–2
of society, 34, 262–3
see also Acceptance
Aves, G. M. (The Aves Report), 392

Baker, J. *et al.*, 340
Bath attendant, 217, 305
Bathing the subnormal, 213, 215–17, 229, 323
Bed
cot, 210–11, 305, 322
getting subnormal out of, 211–14
putting subnormal to, 214–15
Beds, shortage in subnormality hospitals, 46, 160–1
Behaviour, 329
aggressive, 58–60, 62
and bad home conditions, 64
destructive, 58–60

and other children, 61–2, 66
factor in hospital admission, 58–62, 67–9, 123–30, 139–43, 167–8
problem, definition
moderate, 124–5
severe, 125–6
slight, 124
problems
at home, 126–7, 175
in the locality, 127–9, 175
men and women compared, 129
possible exaggeration of, 129–130
at training centre, 127–9
at work, 127–9
promiscuous, 61
sexual, 61, 130–2
threatening, 132
Benington, J., 340
Better Services for the Mentally Handicapped, (White Paper, 1971), 6, 9, 43, 312–15, 317–30, 342–3
Birch, H. G. *et al.*, 80
Blindness, 119
Board of Control, 3, 162
Bott, Dr Elizabeth, 12, 17–19, 206
Bowlby, E. J. M., 4

Campbell, A. C., 327
Car, 146, 222–3, 230, 231, 246–8, 324, 341
Career
of mildly subnormal, 150–4
of severely subnormal, 154–9
Central Association for the Care of the Mentally Defective, 3
Central Association for Mental Welfare, 3
Central Government, 11
Children
chronological definition, 70
definition, 70
other, anxiety about, 61–2, 66
see also Sib/Sibling

Children's homes, 36, 65
Chronically Sick and Disabled
    Persons Act 1970, 232, 324
Churches, 285–6, 289, 331
Clothes
    expense, 230–1
    washing, 219–20, 231
Communication
    non-verbal, 196–200, 316
    by subnormal, 195–200
Community
    ambiguous meaning of, 10–12
    face-to-face level of, 11–20, 331
    general discussion, 10–19
Community care
    comprehensive basis for, 19–20
    in, by, and *out of* the community,
        1–20 *passim*, 343–4
    lack of rethinking about, 310
    as positive principle, 5–6
Community development, 344
Community Development Projects,
    10, 340–1
Contact with research families, 177–
    178
Continence (and incontinence), 119–
    120, 140, 142–3, 168, 171, 175–
    176, 231, 289
    see also Incontinence pads
Co-ordination of services, 330
Coventry Community Development
    Project, 340
Crime, 130–2
    see also Sexual offences

Day care for severely handicapped,
    159, 184, 204, 219, 221, 227,
    229, 304–5, 313, 321
Deafness, 119
Death
    of father, 62–3
    of mother, 62–3
    of parent as precipitating factor
        in hospital admission, 62–4,
        67–9
Dennis, N., 13–16
Department of Education and
    Science, 146
Department of Health and Social
    Security, 146
Depression (economic), 34, 52–3,
    71
Destructiveness, 227
Disabled, definition
    mildly, 182–3

moderately, 182
severely, 181–2
very severely, 180–1
Doctor, *see* General practitioner
Domiciliary services, 309
    relation to residential care, 325,
        328–9
Dressing, 122–3, 140, 142, 144, 175,
    213, 337

Edgerton, R. B., 33–4
Education, 146–50
    authorities, 43
    department, 47, 51–2, 55–6, 321
Ely Hospital, Cardiff, 7
Employment
    of father, 112, 285
    of mother, 112–13, 249–51, 285
    of subnormal, 150–8
Epilepsy, 58, 61, 120, 140–1, 175
Evenings, parents going out in,
    242–6

Family
    large, 98, 100
    problem, 98, 173
    relationships, 107–10, 113–14,
        167, 179, 200–7
    size of, 99–101, 112
    support, 165–6, 167, 201, 213,
        223, 229, 249, 252, 286–92
    see also Relatives of subnormal
Farleigh Hospital, 7
Father
    going out, 244–5
    health, 104, 114, 233–4
    help, 63, 214–15, 216–17, 222–3,
        229, 265–7
    retirement, 234
    subnormal, living with, 93–6, 194
Feeding
    mother helping with in residential
        care, 338–9
    of subnormal, 123, 168, 175, 220–
        221, 237–8
Female
    agency reporting to Mental Health
        Service, 50–4
    more at home, 53–4
Feversham Report, 3
Files, use of, 21–3
Financial cost of care, 6, 230–2
Frankenberg, R., 18, 293–4
Friends, support from, 165–6, 215,
    229, 251–2, 278–80, 285–6

Functional handicap, 315, 319–20, 327

Future, fear of and parents' death, 257–61

Garden, 224, 323–4
General practitioner, 12–13, 299–300, 304, 335, 340–1, 391
Goldberg E. M. *et al.*, 339–40
Gould, J. *et al.*, 11
Grad, Dr Jacqueline, 22, 143

Hampton, W. A., 19, 340
Handrail, 215, 323
Health
    of father, 104, 114, 233–4
    of mother, 101–5, 113, 232–4
    of subnormal, 120, 143
Health and Welfare: The Development of Community Care, 1963, 5–6
Health visitors, 56, 305, 390, 391
Help
    direct with subnormal, 288–92
    indirect with subnormal, 287–8
    reciprocal, 293–7, 334–5
    by subnormal in home, 152–3, 157–9, 218, 221
    from various sources, 281–3
    see also Father, Neighbours, Family, Sib/Sibling
Hewett, S. *et al.*, 176, 203–4, 252, 300, 387
Holidays, 160, 231, 252–5
Holt, K. S., 145, 176, 387
Home
    definition, 35–6
    unsatisfactory conditions, 64–5
Home help, 6, 216, 324, 333, 391
Home Warden, 391
Hospital(s)
    long stay, 7–8
    patients discharged from, 28, 170–171
    subnormality, 256, 260, 314
    Hospital Plan, 1962 (revised 1966), 5–6
Hostels, 8, 11, 43, 46, 160, 260–1, 319–22, 327–31, 335–41, 384–5
Household tasks
    cleaning, 218–19
    cooking, 217–18
    washing clothes, 219–20, 231
    see also Housekeeping, standard

Households
    size of, 97–9
    subnormal in charge, 135, 138
    of two, vulnerability, 98–9
Housekeeping, standard, 84–7, 90, 167
Housewives, subnormals who were 150–2, 154
Housing
    importance of, 298
    and social class, 73–4
    types, 82–4, 90
Howe Report, 7

Idiots Act, 1886, 2
Illegitimacy of subnormal, 110
Immigrants, from other local authority areas, 74, 78–9
Incontinence pads, 211, 229, 231, 305, 322
    see also Continence
Institution
    care in, 5
    definition of, 35–6
Intelligence
    distribution, 115
    I.Q. below 40, 76, 79
    testing, 32
Interview schedule, 177–8
Intolerance by neighbours, 263–4
Isaacs, B. *et al.*, 391

Jacobs, J., 332
Job(s), *see* Employment
Jones, Professor Kathleen, 3, 4

Kemp, C. J., 391
Kerbstones, 323
Kushlick, Dr A., 7, 8, 9, 31–2, 74, 79, 111–12, 115–16, 177, 335–7 384

Labelling, 32–4
Lavatory, 323
Law, contact of subnormal with, 61, 130–2
Leaving the subnormal
    with other people, 280
    reluctance of parents, 253–7
Life cycle, 16, 322
Local
    meaning of, 339–42
    support, 311, 336
Local education authority, 146
Local Government Act, 1929, 3

Local health authority, 30, 146
Locality, 16–19, 20, 392
Lunacy Act, 1890, 2

Male, agency reporting to Mental
    Health Service, 51
Management problem, 6, 58
Mann, P. H., 16
Married subnormals, 92–6, 169–
    171
Martin, F. M., 387
McKeown, T. *et al.*, 384–5
McMichael, Joan K., 388
Meals,
    behaviour at, 237–8
    need for help with, 220–1
Medical officers, 3
Menopause, 234
Mental Deficiency Acts, 40
    1913 and 1927, 2–4
Mental Deficiency Committee, 3, 4
Mental Health Act, 1959, 4–5, 33,
    34, 39, 40, 161
Mental Health Bill, 1959, 4
Mental health of parents, 64–5,
    104–5, 233–4
Mental health service(s)
    growth, 3–5
    Sheffield, 21, 177–8
Mental illness of subnormal, 120–2,
    139–40, 171, 175
Mental Treatment Act, 1930, 3
Mental welfare officers, discussion
    of role, 301–11
Mildly subnormal, age,
    those at home notified, 37–40,
    50–3
    those in hospital admitted, 41–2
    those in hospital notified, 50–3
    structure, those at home, 37–40
    structure, those in hospital, 40–2
Mercer, J. R., 387
Middlesex, prevalence rates in, 48
Minar, D. W. *et al.*, 13
Ministry of Health, 4
Ministry of Social Security, 51–2,
    55–6, 87–90
Mitchell, G. D. *et al.*, 19
Mobility, geographical, 78, 391
Moncrieff, Jean, 6–7, 99, 111–12,
    143
Money, shortage, 87–90, 253
Mongol, 115–16
    age of mother at birth, 111
    social class distribution, 76–7

Moral defective, 33
Moral imbecile, 33
Morris, P., 7, 32
Moss Side Hospital, 130
Mother
    age of at birth of subnormal,
        110–12
    going out, 244–6, 248
    health of, 62–3, 101–5, 113, 167–
        168, 232–4
    and household of more than two,
        93–5
    and household of two, 93–4
    subnormal living with 92–6, 194
    subnormality of, 105–6, 167

National Assistance Board, 51, 89
National Association for Mental
    Health, 5
National Council for Civil
    Liberties, 4
National Health Service, 12–13
National Health Service Act, 1946,
    4
National Society for Mentally
    Handicapped Children, 8
Nearness, importance of in giving
    effective help, 297–8, 317, 319,
    320, 335, 336
Neighbourhood, 14–16, 263–4, 279,
    332
Neighbours
    relations with, 251–2, 263–4, 284–
        285
    support from, 12–13, 229, 274–
        298, 333, 339–40
    see also Friends
Network(s), social, 16, 17–22, 82
Nursery, day, 146–7
Nursing, problems leading to
    hospital admission, 66, 69, 142

Occupation centres, 3, 42, 145
Old people, 13, 339–40, 344, 391
Old people's home, 6, 36, 53, 330
Older institution group, definition,
    103
Olshansky, S., 189
Organisation of Group Practice,
    Standing Medical Advisory
    Committee on, 340–1, 391

Paediatrician, 335, 337
Pahl, R. E., 16, 17–18
Parental care, inadequate, 64–5

Parents,
  death, 62–3, 68–9, 87, 89–90, 99,
    257
  employment, 112–13
  going out in evenings, 242–4
  health, 101–5, 232–4
  restrictions on, 183–5, 236–42
  subnormal living with, 91–5, 194
  support of and friendship with,
    285–7
  see also Attitude
Payne Report, 8
Petition for admission to institution,
    52
Pilot survey, 177
Police, 51, 53–4, 59, 61, 130–1
Poor Law, 52
Powell, Rt Hon. Enoch, 5
Practical aids, 322–5, 337
Precipitating factor, 57–69
Prevalence rates, 46–9
Prison authorities, 51
Problem families, *see* Family
Prostitution, 132
Proximity, *see* Nearness
Psychologist, educational, 335–7
Public Assistance Committee, 51–3,
    56
Public transport, 324

Quality of life, 165–6, 178–9, 230,
    236–61 *passim*

Rampton Hospital, 130
Refrigerator, 223
Regional Hospital Board, 20
Rehin, G. F. *et al.*, 387
Relationship(s),
  between mother and subnormal,
    202–4, 248, 306
  and residential care, 318–19, 327,
    337–9
  see also Family
Relatives of subnormal, 270–4
  aunt, 194
  grandparents, subnormal living
    with, 92
  sister, 194
  stepfather, 92, 194
  uncle, 194
  see also Father, Mother, Parents,
    Sib/Siblings
Relieving officer, 52

Residential care, 313–15, 317–22,
    325–41
  see also Hostel
Restrictions to which families of
    subnormals subjected, 183–4,
    236–40
Retarded, the profoundly, 317–19
    327
Rights of mentally handicapped
    people, 312
Robb, B., 7
Royal Commission on Mental
    Illness and Mental Deficiency,
    1954/7, 4
Running away, 131

Saenger, G. S., 31, 387
St Luke's Nursing Home, 338–9
Schizophrenia, 121
School
  ESN, 147–52, 157, 169–70
  ESN school-leavers, 37, 39, 161
  excluded from, 31, 147–52, 157
  ordinary, 147–52, 157
Seebohm Report, 8–10, 330, 342–3,
    391
Severely subnormal, age,
  those at home notified, 43, 54–6
  those in hospital admitted, 44–5
  those in hospital notified, 54–6
  structure, those at home, 43
  structure, those in hospital, 44–5
Sexual behaviour, promiscuous, 61
    132
Sexual offences, 131–2, 329
Shaw, C. H. *et al.*, 169
Sheffield Development Project, 159,
    312–15, 316–30, 342, 382–4
Sheffield Society for Mentally
    Handicapped Children, 165,
    261
Shopping, 221–4
Short-term care, 160–1, 197, 222,
    255–7, 304, 321–2
Sib/Sibling
  effect of older sibs on admission,
    100–1, 112
  help of, 112, 267–70, 281–3
  looking after subnormal, 96–7
  subnormality of, 106
  younger, effect of presence in
    household, 205
Skipper, J., 19, 340
Sleep, effect of subnormal on, 208–
    211

Social class, 341
  cross-tabulation with housing,
    73–4
  distribution of mongols, 76–7
  of families visited, 194–5
  father in manual and non-manual
    work, 73–80
  higher, mobility of, 74, 78–9
  large number of unknowns, 71, 80
  no association with admission,
    80–1
  relationship to socio-economic
    group, 31–2, 71, 388
Social contacts, 251–2
Social factors,
  in admission to hospital, 64–6
  in parents' outside activities, 240–2
  in planning hostels, 320
Social networks, *see* Networks
Social services, 9, 20–2, 310–11,
  315, 325–7, 342–4
Social workers, 3, 4, 5, 19, 22, 85,
  161–5, 204, 303–11, 325–6,
  328, 331–7, 391, 392
Social work help, 6–7, 317, 325
Special care unit, 147–8, 158–9, 176,
  227, 251, 304, 321
Stacey, M., 294
Stairs, negotiating, 213–15, 323
Stigma, stigmatized, 34, 206, 293
Stress on family, 126–7, 167–8,
  208–35 *passim*, 388
Structure
  for coping, 228–30, 293, 309,
    316–17, 320–1, 328
  of living, 248–52, 293, 316–17,
    320–1, 328
Subnormal
  abilities of, 135, 138
  boredom for, 226–7, 247
  going out alone, 224–6
  grimacing, 239
  living alone, 93
  naivity, 238–9, 247
  occupation for, 224–8
  over-activity, 226–7, 239
  physical condition of, 120, 143
  slavering, 239–40
  temperament of, 180–2
Subnormality, specialist in, **337**
Supervision
  needed by subnormal, 132–42,
    144, 175–7
  definitions, 132–4
  of mental defective, 3

Talk(ing)
  non-talkers, 289, 318
  sub-normal's ability to, 117–19,
    175, 195–200
Teachers, 335, 337
Telephone, 269, 287, 296, 324, 341
Tenants' associations, 331
Tizard, Professor Jack, 6–7, 9, 22,
  88–91, 115
Tolerance by neighbourhood, 263–4,
  284–5
Tönnies, F., 15
Townsend, Professor P., 32–3, 294,
  390
Training centres, 5, 11, 47, 113,
  145–59, 184–5, 212–13, 221,
  227, 229, 306–11, 313, 321, 335,
  389–90
Tranquillizers, 4
Transport, importance of punctual,
  229, 321

Unemployed Assistance Board, 51

Visit(ed)
  refusal to be, 162
  requirement to, 161
Visits for research,
  choice of families, 175–7
Voluntary associations, 3, 4
Volunteers, 8, 326, 392

Walker-Smith, Rt Hon. Derek, 4
Walking, 116–17, 140, 142–3, 175
Watkins Report, 7
Weekends, 246–8
Welfare services, basis on which
  they rest, 12–13
Wessex, developments in, 7, 8, 335–
  337
Whittingham Hospital, 8
Widow/Widowed Mother
  difficulties of, 222, 267
  going out, 245–6, 248
  holidays, 253, 254
  support by family, 270
Willmott, P., 16–17, 84
Wood Report, 3

Year of admission to hospital
  mildly subnormal, 42–3
  severely subnormal, 45–6
Young, M. *et al.*, 15, 390
Younger institution group,
  definition, 103

Routledge Social Science Series

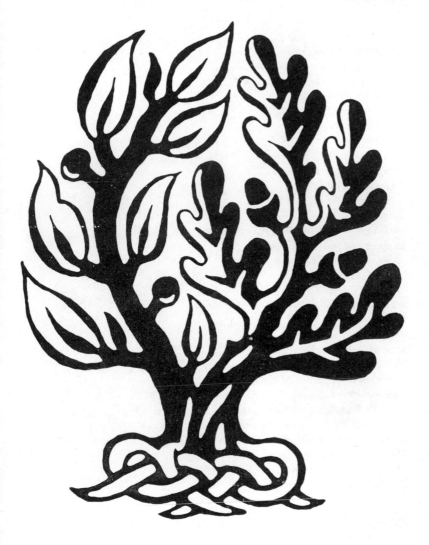

Routledge & Kegan Paul   London and Boston

68–74 Carter Lane   London EC4V 5EL
9 Park Street   Boston   Mass 02108

Contents

International Library of Sociology 3
General Sociology 3
Foreign Classics of Sociology 4
Social Structure 4
Sociology and Politics 4
Foreign Affairs 5
Criminology 5
Social Psychology 5
Sociology of the Family 6
Social Services 7
Sociology of Education 7
Sociology of Culture 8
Sociology of Religion 9
Sociology of Art and Literature 9
Sociology of Knowledge 9
Urban Sociology 9
Rural Sociology 10
Sociology of Industry and Distribution 10
Documentary 11
Anthropology 11
Sociology and Philosophy 12
International Library of Anthropology 12
International Library of Social Policy 12
International Library of Welfare and Philosophy 13
Primary Socialization, Language and Education 13
Reports of the Institute of Community Studies 13
Reports of the Institute for Social Studies in Medical Care 14
Medicine, Illness and Society 14
Monographs in Social Theory 14
Routledge Social Science Journals 15

*Authors wishing to submit manuscripts for any series in
this catalogue should send them to the Social Science Editor,
Routledge & Kegan Paul Ltd, 68–74 Carter Lane,
London EC4V 5EL*

● *Books so marked are available in paperback
All books are in Metric Demy 8vo format (216 × 138mm approx.)*

International Library of Sociology

General Editor John Rex

GENERAL SOCIOLOGY

Barnsley, J. H. The Social Reality of Ethics. *464 pp.*
Belshaw, Cyril. The Conditions of Social Performance. *An Exploratory Theory. 144 pp.*
Brown, Robert. Explanation in Social Science. *208 pp.*
● Rules and Laws in Sociology. *192 pp.*
Bruford, W. H. Chekhov and His Russia. *A Sociological Study. 244 pp.*
Cain, Maureen E. Society and the Policeman's Role. *326 pp.*
Gibson, Quentin. The Logic of Social Enquiry. *240 pp.*
Glucksmann, M. Structuralist Analysis in Contemporary Social Thought. *212 pp.*
Gurvitch, Georges. Sociology of Law. *Preface by Roscoe Pound. 264 pp.*
Hodge, H. A. Wilhelm Dilthey. *An Introduction. 184 pp.*
Homans, George C. Sentiments and Activities. *336 pp.*
Johnson, Harry M. Sociology: *a Systematic Introduction. Foreword by Robert K. Merton. 710 pp.*
Mannheim, Karl. Essays on Sociology and Social Psychology. *Edited by Paul Keckskemeti. With Editorial Note by Adolph Lowe. 344 pp.*
 Systematic Sociology: *An Introduction to the Study of Society. Edited by J. S. Erös and Professor W. A. C. Stewart. 220 pp.*
Martindale, Don. The Nature and Types of Sociological Theory. *292 pp.*
●**Maus, Heinz.** A Short History of Sociology. *234 pp.*
Mey, Harald. Field-Theory. *A Study of its Application in the Social Sciences. 352 pp.*
Myrdal, Gunnar. Value in Social Theory: *A Collection of Essays on Methodology. Edited by Paul Streeten. 332 pp.*
Ogburn, William F., and **Nimkoff, Meyer F.** A Handbook of Sociology. *Preface by Karl Mannheim. 656 pp. 46 figures. 35 tables.*
Parsons, Talcott, and **Smelser, Neil J.** Economy and Society: *A Study in the Integration of Economic and Social Theory. 362 pp.*
●**Rex, John.** Key Problems of Sociological Theory. *220 pp.*
 Discovering Sociology. *278 pp.*
 Sociology and the Demystification of the Modern World. *282 pp.*
●**Rex, John** (Ed.) Approaches to Sociology. *Contributions by Peter Abell, Frank Bechhofer, Basil Bernstein, Ronald Fletcher, David Frisby, Miriam Glucksmann, Peter Lassman, Herminio Martins, John Rex, Roland Robertson, John Westergaard and Jock Young. 302 pp.*
Rigby, A. Alternative Realities. *352 pp.*
Roche, M. Phenomenology, Language and the Social Sciences. *374 pp.*
Sahay, A. Sociological Analysis. *220 pp.*
Urry, John. Reference Groups and the Theory of Revolution. *244 pp.*
Weinberg, E. Development of Sociology in the Soviet Union. *173 pp.*

FOREIGN CLASSICS OF SOCIOLOGY

● **Durkheim, Emile.** Suicide. *A Study in Sociology. Edited and with an Introduction by George Simpson. 404 pp.*
Professional Ethics and Civic Morals. *Translated by Cornelia Brookfield. 288 pp.*

● **Gerth, H. H.,** and **Mills, C. Wright.** From Max Weber: *Essays in Sociology. 502 pp.*

● **Tönnies, Ferdinand.** Community and Association. (*Gemeinschaft und Gesellschaft.) Translated and Supplemented by Charles P. Loomis. Foreword by Pitirim A. Sorokin. 334 pp.*

SOCIAL STRUCTURE

Andreski, Stanislav. Military Organization and Society. *Foreword by Professor A. R. Radcliffe-Brown. 226 pp. 1 folder.*

Coontz, Sydney H. Population Theories and the Economic Interpretation. *202 pp.*

Coser, Lewis. The Functions of Social Conflict. *204 pp.*

Dickie-Clark, H. F. Marginal Situation: *A Sociological Study of a Coloured Group. 240 pp. 11 tables.*

Glaser, Barney, and **Strauss, Anselm L.** Status Passage. *A Formal Theory. 208 pp.*

Glass, D. V. (Ed.) Social Mobility in Britain. *Contributions by J. Berent, T. Bottomore, R. C. Chambers, J. Floud, D. V. Glass, J. R. Hall, H. T. Himmelweit, R. K. Kelsall, F. M. Martin, C. A. Moser, R. Mukherjee, and W. Ziegel. 420 pp.*

Jones, Garth N. Planned Organizational Change: *An Exploratory Study Using an Empirical Approach. 268 pp.*

Kelsall, R. K. Higher Civil Servants in Britain: *From 1870 to the Present Day. 268 pp. 31 tables.*

König, René. The Community. *232 pp. Illustrated.*

● **Lawton, Denis.** Social Class, Language and Education. *192 pp.*

McLeish, John. The Theory of Social Change: *Four Views Considered. 128 pp.*

Marsh, David C. The Changing Social Structure of England and Wales, *1871-1961. 288 pp.*

Mouzelis, Nicos. Organization and Bureaucracy. *An Analysis of Modern Theories. 240 pp.*

Mulkay, M. J. Functionalism, Exchange and Theoretical Strategy. *272 pp.*

Ossowski, Stanislaw. Class Structure in the Social Consciousness. *210 pp.*

Podgórecki, Adam. Law and Society. *About 300 pp.*

SOCIOLOGY AND POLITICS

Acton, T. A. Gypsy Politics and Social Change. *316 pp.*

Hechter, Michael. Internal Colonialism. *The Celtic Fringe in British National Development, 1536–1966. About 350 pp.*

Hertz, Frederick. Nationality in History and Politics: *A Psychology and Sociology of National Sentiment and Nationalism. 432 pp.*

Kornhauser, William. The Politics of Mass Society. *272 pp. 20 tables.*
Laidler, Harry W. History of Socialism. *Social-Economic Movements: An Historical and Comparative Survey of Socialism, Communism, Co-operation, Utopianism; and other Systems of Reform and Reconstruction. 992 pp.*
Lasswell, H. D. Analysis of Political Behaviour. *324 pp.*
Mannheim, Karl. Freedom, Power and Democratic Planning. *Edited by Hans Gerth and Ernest K. Bramstedt. 424 pp.*
Mansur, Fatma. Process of Independence. *Foreword by A. H. Hanson. 208 pp.*
Martin, David A. Pacifism: *an Historical and Sociological Study. 262 pp.*
Myrdal, Gunnar. The Political Element in the Development of Economic Theory. *Translated from the German by Paul Streeten. 282 pp.*
Wootton, Graham. Workers, Unions and the State. *188 pp.*

FOREIGN AFFAIRS: THEIR SOCIAL, POLITICAL AND ECONOMIC FOUNDATIONS

Mayer, J. P. Political Thought in France from the Revolution to the Fifth Republic. *164 pp.*

CRIMINOLOGY

Ancel, Marc. Social Defence: *A Modern Approach to Criminal Problems. Foreword by Leon Radzinowicz. 240 pp.*
Cain, Maureen E. Society and the Policeman's Role. *326 pp.*
Cloward, Richard A., and **Ohlin, Lloyd E.** Delinquency and Opportunity: *A Theory of Delinquent Gangs. 248 pp.*
Downes, David M. The Delinquent Solution. *A Study in Subcultural Theory. 296 pp.*
Dunlop, A. B., and **McCabe, S.** Young Men in Detention Centres. *192 pp.*
Friedlander, Kate. The Psycho-Analytical Approach to Juvenile Delinquency: *Theory, Case Studies, Treatment. 320 pp.*
Glueck, Sheldon, and **Eleanor.** Family Environment and Delinquency. *With the statistical assistance of Rose W. Kneznek. 340 pp.*
Lopez-Rey, Manuel. Crime. *An Analytical Appraisal. 288 pp.*
Mannheim, Hermann. Comparative Criminology: *a Text Book. Two volumes. 442 pp. and 380 pp.*
Morris, Terence. The Criminal Area: *A Study in Social Ecology. Foreword by Hermann Mannheim. 232 pp. 25 tables. 4 maps.*
Rock, Paul. Making People Pay. *338 pp.*
● **Taylor, Ian, Walton, Paul,** and **Young, Jock.** The New Criminology. *For a Social Theory of Deviance. 325 pp.*

SOCIAL PSYCHOLOGY

Bagley, Christopher. The Social Psychology of the Epileptic Child. *320 pp.*
Barbu, Zevedei. Problems of Historical Psychology. *248 pp.*
Blackburn, Julian. Psychology and the Social Pattern. *184 pp.*

●**Brittan, Arthur.** Meanings and Situations. *224 pp.*

Carroll, J. Break-Out from the Crystal Palace. *200 pp.*

●**Fleming, C. M.** Adolescence: Its Social Psychology. *With an Introduction to recent findings from the fields of Anthropology, Physiology, Medicine, Psychometrics and Sociometry. 288 pp.*

● The Social Psychology of Education: *An Introduction and Guide to Its Study. 136 pp.*

Homans, George C. The Human Group. *Foreword by Bernard DeVoto. Introduction by Robert K. Merton. 526 pp.*

● Social Behaviour: *its Elementary Forms. 416 pp.*

●**Klein, Josephine.** The Study of Groups. *226 pp. 31 figures. 5 tables.*

Linton, Ralph. The Cultural Background of Personality. *132 pp.*

●**Mayo, Elton.** The Social Problems of an Industrial Civilization. *With an appendix on the Political Problem. 180 pp.*

Ottaway, A. K. C. Learning Through Group Experience. *176 pp.*

Ridder, J. C. de. The Personality of the Urban African in South Africa. *A Thematic Apperception Test Study. 196 pp. 12 plates.*

●**Rose, Arnold M.** (Ed.) Human Behaviour and Social Processes: *an Interactionist Approach. Contributions by Arnold M. Rose, Ralph H. Turner, Anselm Strauss, Everett C. Hughes, E. Franklin Frazier, Howard S. Becker, et al. 696 pp.*

Smelser, Neil J. Theory of Collective Behaviour. *448 pp.*

Stephenson, Geoffrey M. The Development of Conscience. *128 pp.*

Young, Kimball. Handbook of Social Psychology. *658 pp. 16 figures. 10 tables.*

SOCIOLOGY OF THE FAMILY

Banks, J. A. Prosperity and Parenthood: *A Study of Family Planning among The Victorian Middle Classes. 262 pp.*

Bell, Colin R. Middle Class Families: *Social and Geographical Mobility. 224 pp.*

Burton, Lindy. Vulnerable Children. *272 pp.*

Gavron, Hannah. The Captive Wife: *Conflicts of Household Mothers. 190 pp.*

George, Victor, and **Wilding, Paul.** Motherless Families. *220 pp.*

Klein, Josephine. Samples from English Cultures.
 1. Three Preliminary Studies and Aspects of Adult Life in England. *447 pp.*
 2. Child-Rearing Practices and Index. *247 pp.*

Klein, Viola. Britain's Married Women Workers. *180 pp.*

 The Feminine Character. *History of an Ideology. 244 pp.*

McWhinnie, Alexina M. Adopted Children. *How They Grow Up. 304 pp.*

● **Myrdal, Alva,** and **Klein, Viola.** Women's Two Roles: *Home and Work. 238 pp. 27 tables.*

Parsons, Talcott, and **Bales, Robert F.** Family: Socialization and Interaction Process. *In collaboration with James Olds, Morris Zelditch and Philip E. Slater. 456 pp. 50 figures and tables.*

SOCIAL SERVICES

Bastide, Roger. The Sociology of Mental Disorder. *Translated from the French by Jean McNeil. 260 pp.*

Carlebach, Julius. Caring For Children in Trouble. *266 pp.*

Forder, R. A. (Ed.) Penelope Hall's Social Services of England and Wales. *352 pp.*

George, Victor. Foster Care. *Theory and Practice. 234 pp.*
Social Security: *Beveridge and After. 258 pp.*

George, V., and **Wilding, P.** Motherless Families. *248 pp.*

● **Goetschius, George W.** Working with Community Groups. *256 pp.*

Goetschius, George W., and **Tash, Joan.** Working with Unattached Youth. *416 pp.*

Hall, M. P., and **Howes, I. V.** The Church in Social Work. *A Study of Moral Welfare Work undertaken by the Church of England. 320 pp.*

Heywood, Jean S. Children in Care: *the Development of the Service for the Deprived Child. 264 pp.*

Hoenig, J., and **Hamilton, Marian W.** The De-Segregation of the Mentally Ill. *284 pp.*

Jones, Kathleen. Mental Health and Social Policy, 1845-1959. *264 pp.*

King, Roy D., Raynes, Norma V., and **Tizard, Jack.** Patterns of Residential Care. *356 pp.*

Leigh, John. Young People and Leisure. *256 pp.*

Morris, Mary. Voluntary Work and the Welfare State. *300 pp.*

Morris, Pauline. Put Away: *A Sociological Study of Institutions for the Mentally Retarded. 364 pp.*

Nokes, P. L. The Professional Task in Welfare Practice. *152 pp.*

Timms, Noel. Psychiatric Social Work in Great Britain (1939-1962). *280 pp.*

● Social Casework: *Principles and Practice. 256 pp.*

Young, A. F. Social Services in British Industry. *272 pp.*

Young, A. F., and **Ashton, E. T.** British Social Work in the Nineteenth Century. *288 pp.*

SOCIOLOGY OF EDUCATION

Banks, Olive. Parity and Prestige in English Secondary Education: a Study in Educational Sociology. *272 pp.*

Bentwich, Joseph. Education in Israel. *224 pp. 8 pp. plates.*

● **Blyth, W. A. L.** English Primary Education. *A Sociological Description.*
1. Schools. *232 pp.*
2. Background. *168 pp.*

Collier, K. G. The Social Purposes of Education: *Personal and Social Values in Education. 268 pp.*

Dale, R. R., and **Griffith, S.** Down Stream: *Failure in the Grammar School.*
108 pp.

Dore, R. P. Education in Tokugawa Japan. *356 pp. 9 pp. plates.*

Evans, K. M. Sociometry and Education. *158 pp.*

●**Ford, Julienne.** Social Class and the Comprehensive School. *192 pp.*

Foster, P. J. Education and Social Change in Ghana. *336 pp. 3 maps.*

Fraser, W. R. Education and Society in Modern France. *150 pp.*

Grace, Gerald R. Role Conflict and the Teacher. *About 200 pp.*

Hans, Nicholas. New Trends in Education in the Eighteenth Century.
278 pp. 19 tables.

● Comparative Education: *A Study of Educational Factors and Traditions.*
360 pp.

Hargreaves, David. Interpersonal Relations and Education. *432 pp.*

● Social Relations in a Secondary School. *240 pp.*

Holmes, Brian. Problems in Education. *A Comparative Approach. 336 pp.*

King, Ronald. Values and Involvement in a Grammar School. *164 pp.*

School Organization and Pupil Involvement. *A Study of Secondary Schools.*

●**Mannheim, Karl,** and **Stewart, W. A. C.** An Introduction to the Sociology
of Education. *206 pp.*

Morris, Raymond N. The Sixth Form and College Entrance. *231 pp.*

●**Musgrove, F.** Youth and the Social Order. *176 pp.*

●**Ottaway, A. K. C.** Education and Society: An Introduction to the Sociology
of Education. *With an Introduction by W. O. Lester Smith. 212 pp.*

Peers, Robert. Adult Education: *A Comparative Study. 398 pp.*

Pritchard, D. G. Education and the Handicapped: *1760 to 1960. 258 pp.*

Richardson, Helen. Adolescent Girls in Approved Schools. *308 pp.*

Stratta, Erica. The Education of Borstal Boys. *A Study of their Educational
Experiences prior to, and during, Borstal Training. 256 pp.*

Taylor, P. H., Reid, W. A., and **Holley, B. J.** The English Sixth Form.
A Case Study in Curriculum Research. 200 pp.

SOCIOLOGY OF CULTURE

Eppel, E. M., and **M.** Adolescents and Morality: *A Study of some Moral
Values and Dilemmas of Working Adolescents in the Context of a
changing Climate of Opinion. Foreword by W. J. H. Sprott. 268 pp.
39 tables.*

●**Fromm, Erich.** The Fear of Freedom. *286 pp.*

● The Sane Society. *400 pp.*

Mannheim, Karl. Essays on the Sociology of Culture. *Edited by Ernst
Mannheim in co-operation with Paul Kecskemeti. Editorial Note by
Adolph Lowe. 280 pp.*

Weber, Alfred. Farewell to European History: *or The Conquest of Nihilism.
Translated from the German by R. F. C. Hull. 224 pp.*

SOCIOLOGY OF RELIGION

Argyle, Michael and **Beit-Hallahmi, Benjamin.** The Social Psychology of
Religion. *About 256 pp.*
Nelson, G. K. Spiritualism and Society. *313 pp.*
Stark, Werner. The Sociology of Religion. *A Study of Christendom.*
  Volume I. *Established Religion. 248 pp.*
  Volume II. *Sectarian Religion. 368 pp.*
  Volume III. *The Universal Church. 464 pp.*
  Volume IV. *Types of Religious Man. 352 pp.*
  Volume V. *Types of Religious Culture. 464 pp.*
Turner, B. S. Weber and Islam. *216 pp.*
Watt, W. Montgomery. Islam and the Integration of Society. *320 pp.*

SOCIOLOGY OF ART AND LITERATURE

Jarvie, Ian C. Towards a Sociology of the Cinema. *A Comparative Essay
on the Structure and Functioning of a Major Entertainment Industry.
405 pp.*
Rust, Frances S. Dance in Society. *An Analysis of the Relationships between
the Social Dance and Society in England from the Middle Ages to the
Present Day. 256 pp. 8 pp. of plates.*
Schücking, L. L. The Sociology of Literary Taste. *112 pp.*
Wolff, Janet. Hermeneutic Philosophy and the Sociology of Art. *About
200 pp.*

SOCIOLOGY OF KNOWLEDGE

Diesing, P. Patterns of Discovery in the Social Sciences. *262 pp.*
●**Douglas, J. D.** (Ed.) Understanding Everyday Life. *370 pp.*
●**Hamilton, P.** Knowledge and Social Structure. *174 pp.*
Jarvie, I. C. Concepts and Society. *232 pp.*
Mannheim, Karl. Essays on the Sociology of Knowledge. *Edited by Paul
Kecskemeti. Editorial Note by Adolph Lowe. 353 pp.*
Remmling, Gunter W. (Ed.) Towards the Sociology of Knowledge. *Origin
and Development of a Sociological Thought Style. 463 pp.*
Stark, Werner. The Sociology of Knowledge: *An Essay in Aid of a Deeper
Understanding of the History of Ideas. 384 pp.*

URBAN SOCIOLOGY

Ashworth, William. The Genesis of Modern British Town Planning: *A
Study in Economic and Social History of the Nineteenth and Twentieth
Centuries. 288 pp.*
Cullingworth, J. B. Housing Needs and Planning Policy: *A Restatement of
the Problems of Housing Need and 'Overspill' in England and Wales.
232 pp. 44 tables. 8 maps.*

Dickinson, Robert E. City and Region: *A Geographical Interpretation* 608 pp. *125 figures.*
  The West European City: *A Geographical Interpretation. 600 pp. 129 maps. 29 plates.*
● The City Region in Western Europe. *320 pp. Maps.*
Humphreys, Alexander J. New Dubliners: *Urbanization and the Irish Family. Foreword by George C. Homans. 304 pp.*
Jackson, Brian. Working Class Community: *Some General Notions raised by a Series of Studies in Northern England. 192 pp.*
Jennings, Hilda. Societies in the Making: *a Study of Development and Redevelopment within a County Borough. Foreword by D. A. Clark. 286 pp.*
●**Mann, P. H.** An Approach to Urban Sociology. *240 pp.*
Morris, R. N., and **Mogey, J.** The Sociology of Housing. *Studies at Berinsfield. 232 pp. 4 pp. plates.*
Rosser, C., and **Harris, C.** The Family and Social Change. *A Study of Family and Kinship in a South Wales Town. 352 pp. 8 maps.*

RURAL SOCIOLOGY

Chambers, R. J. H. Settlement Schemes in Tropical Africa: *A Selective Study. 268 pp.*
Haswell, M. R. The Economics of Development in Village India. *120 pp.*
Littlejohn, James. Westrigg: *the Sociology of a Cheviot Parish. 172 pp. 5 figures.*
Mayer, Adrian C. Peasants in the Pacific. *A Study of Fiji Indian Rural Society. 248 pp. 20 plates.*
Williams, W. M. The Sociology of an English Village: *Gosforth. 272 pp. 12 figures. 13 tables.*

SOCIOLOGY OF INDUSTRY AND DISTRIBUTION

Anderson, Nels. Work and Leisure. *280 pp.*
●**Blau, Peter M.,** and **Scott, W. Richard.** Formal Organizations: *a Comparative approach. Introduction and Additional Bibliography by J. H. Smith. 326 pp.*
Eldridge, J. E. T. Industrial Disputes. *Essays in the Sociology of Industrial Relations. 288 pp.*
Hetzler, Stanley. Applied Measures for Promoting Technological Growth. *352 pp.*
  Technological Growth and Social Change. *Achieving Modernization. 269 pp.*
Hollowell, Peter G. The Lorry Driver. *272 pp.*
Jefferys, Margot, *with the assistance of Winifred Moss.* Mobility in the Labour Market: *Employment Changes in Battersea and Dagenham. Preface by Barbara Wootton. 186 pp. 51 tables.*

Millerson, Geoffrey. The Qualifying Associations: *a Study in Professionalization. 320 pp.*

Smelser, Neil J. Social Change in the Industrial Revolution: *An Application of Theory to the Lancashire Cotton Industry, 1770-1840. 468 pp. 12 figures. 14 tables.*

Williams, Gertrude. Recruitment to Skilled Trades. *240 pp.*

Young, A. F. Industrial Injuries Insurance: *an Examination of British Policy. 192 pp.*

DOCUMENTARY

Schlesinger, Rudolf (Ed.) Changing Attitudes in Soviet Russia.
  2. The Nationalities Problem and Soviet Administration. *Selected Readings on the Development of Soviet Nationalities Policies. Introduced by the editor. Translated by W. W. Gottlieb. 324 pp.*

ANTHROPOLOGY

Ammar, Hamed. Growing up in an Egyptian Village: *Silwa, Province of Aswan. 336 pp.*

Brandel-Syrier, Mia. Reeftown Elite. *A Study of Social Mobility in a Modern African Community on the Reef. 376 pp.*

Crook, David, and **Isabel.** Revolution in a Chinese Village: *Ten Mile Inn. 230 pp. 8 plates. 1 map.*

Dickie-Clark, H. F. The Marginal Situation. *A Sociological Study of a Coloured Group. 236 pp.*

Dube, S. C. Indian Village. *Foreword by Morris Edward Opler. 276 pp. 4 plates.*

  India's Changing Villages: *Human Factors in Community Development. 260 pp. 8 plates. 1 map.*

Firth, Raymond. Malay Fishermen. *Their Peasant Economy. 420 pp. 17 pp. plates.*

Firth, R., Hubert, J., and **Forge, A.** Families and their Relatives. *Kinship in a Middle-Class Sector of London: An Anthropological Study. 456 pp.*

Gulliver, P. H. Social Control in an African Society: a Study of the Arusha, Agricultural Masai of Northern Tanganyika. *320 pp. 8 plates. 10 figures.*

  Family Herds. *288 pp.*

Ishwaran, K. Shivapur. *A South Indian Village. 216 pp.*

  Tradition and Economy in Village India: *An Interactionist Approach. Foreword by Conrad Arensburg. 176 pp.*

Jarvie, Ian C. The Revolution in Anthropology. *268 pp.*

Jarvie, Ian C., and **Agassi, Joseph.** Hong Kong. *A Society in Transition. 396 pp. Illustrated with plates and maps.*

Little, Kenneth L. Mende of Sierra Leone. *308 pp. and folder.*

  Negroes in Britain. *With a New Introduction and Contemporary Study by Leonard Bloom. 320 pp.*

11

Lowie, Robert H. Social Organization. *494 pp.*

Mayer, Adrian, C. Caste and Kinship in Central India: *A Village and its Region. 328 pp. 16 plates. 15 figures. 16 tables.*

Peasants in the Pacific. *A Study of Fiji Indian Rural Society. 248 pp.*

Smith, Raymond T. The Negro Family in British Guiana: *Family Structure and Social Status in the Villages. With a Foreword by Meyer Fortes. 314 pp. 8 plates. 1 figure. 4 maps.*

SOCIOLOGY AND PHILOSOPHY

Barnsley, John H. The Social Reality of Ethics. *A Comparative Analysis of Moral Codes. 448 pp.*

Diesing, Paul. Patterns of Discovery in the Social Sciences. *362 pp.*

●**Douglas, Jack D.** (Ed.) Understanding Everyday Life. *Toward the Reconstruction of Sociological Knowledge. Contributions by Alan F. Blum. Aaron W. Cicourel, Norman K. Denzin, Jack D. Douglas, John Heeren, Peter McHugh, Peter K. Manning, Melvin Power, Matthew Speier, Roy Turner, D. Lawrence Wieder, Thomas P. Wilson and Don H. Zimmerman. 370 pp.*

Jarvie, Ian C. Concepts and Society. *216 pp.*

Pelz, Werner. The Scope of Understanding in Sociology. *Towards a more radical reorientation in the social humanistic sciences. 283 pp.*

Roche, Maurice. Phenomenology, Language and the Social Sciences. *371 pp.*

Sahay, Arun. Sociological Analysis. *212 pp.*

Sklair, Leslie. The Sociology of Progress. *320 pp.*

International Library of Anthropology

General Editor Adam Kuper

Brown, Paula. The Chimbu. *A Study of Change in the New Guinea Highlands. 151 pp.*

Lloyd, P. C. Power and Independence. *Urban Africans' Perception of Social Inequality. 264 pp.*

Pettigrew, Joyce. Robber Noblemen. *A Study of the Political System of the Sikh Jats. 284 pp.*

Van Den Berghe, Pierre L. Power and Privilege at an African University. *278 pp.*

International Library of Social Policy

General Editor Kathleen Jones

Bayley, M. Mental Handicap and Community Care. *426 pp.*

Butler, J. R. Family Doctors and Public Policy. *208 pp.*

Holman, Robert. Trading in Children. *A Study of Private Fostering. 355 pp.*

Jones, Kathleen. History of the Mental Health Service. *428 pp.*
Thomas, J. E. The English Prison Officer since 1850: *A Study in Conflict. 258 pp.*
Woodward, J. To Do the Sick No Harm. *A Study of the British Voluntary Hospital System to 1875. About 220 pp.*

International Library of Welfare and Philosophy

General Editors Noel Timms and David Watson

● **Plant, Raymond.** Community and Ideology. *104 pp.*

Primary Socialization, Language and Education

General Editor Basil Bernstein

Bernstein, Basil. Class, Codes and Control. *2 volumes.*
  1. *Theoretical Studies Towards a Sociology of Language. 254 pp.*
  2. *Applied Studies Towards a Sociology of Language. About 400 pp.*
Brandis, W., and **Bernstein, B.** Selection and Control. *176 pp.*
Brandis, Walter, and **Henderson, Dorothy.** Social Class, Language and Communication. *288 pp.*
Cook-Gumperz, Jenny. Social Control and Socialization. *A Study of Class Differences in the Language of Maternal Control. 290 pp.*
● **Gahagan, D. M.,** and **G. A.** Talk Reform. *Exploration in Language for Infant School Children. 160 pp.*
Robinson, W. P., and **Rackstraw, Susan D. A.** A Question of Answers. *2 volumes. 192 pp. and 180 pp.*
Turner, Geoffrey J., and **Mohan, Bernard A.** A Linguistic Description and Computer Programme for Children's Speech. *208 pp.*

Reports of the Institute of Community Studies

Cartwright, Ann. Human Relations and Hospital Care. *272 pp.*
● Parents and Family Planning Services. *306 pp.*
  Patients and their Doctors. *A Study of General Practice. 304 pp.*
● **Jackson, Brian.** Streaming: *an Education System in Miniature. 168 pp.*
Jackson, Brian, and **Marsden, Dennis.** Education and the Working Class: *Some General Themes raised by a Study of 88 Working-class Children in a Northern Industrial City. 268 pp. 2 folders.*
Marris, Peter. The Experience of Higher Education. *232 pp. 27 tables.*
  Loss and Change. *192 pp.*

Marris, Peter, and Rein, Martin. Dilemmas of Social Reform. *Poverty and Community Action in the United States. 256 pp.*

Marris, Peter, and Somerset, Anthony. African Businessmen. *A Study of Entrepreneurship and Development in Kenya. 256 pp.*

Mills, Richard. Young Outsiders: *a Study in Alternative Communities. 216 pp.*

Runciman, W. G. Relative Deprivation and Social Justice. *A Study of Attitudes to Social Inequality in Twentieth-Century England. 352 pp.*

Willmott, Peter. Adolescent Boys in East London. *230 pp.*

Willmott, Peter, and Young, Michael. Family and Class in a London Suburb. *202 pp. 47 tables.*

Young, Michael. Innovation and Research in Education. *192 pp.*

●Young, Michael, and McGeeney, Patrick. Learning Begins at Home. *A Study of a Junior School and its Parents. 128 pp.*

Young, Michael, and Willmott, Peter. Family and Kinship in East London. *Foreword by Richard M. Titmuss. 252 pp. 39 tables.*

The Symmetrical Family. *410 pp.*

Reports of the Institute for Social Studies in Medical Care

Cartwright, Ann, Hockey, Lisbeth, and Anderson, John L. Life Before Death. *310 pp.*

Dunnell, Karen, and Cartwright, Ann. Medicine Takers, Prescribers and Hoarders. *190 pp.*

Medicine, Illness and Society

General Editor W. M. Williams

Robinson, David. The Process of Becoming Ill. *142 pp.*

Stacey, Margaret, *et al.* Hospitals, Children and Their Families. *The Report of a Pilot Study. 202 pp.*

Monographs in Social Theory

General Editor Arthur Brittan

●Barnes, B. Scientific Knowledge and Sociological Theory. *About 200 pp.*

Bauman, Zygmunt. Culture as Praxis. *204 pp.*

● Dixon, Keith. Sociological Theory. *Pretence and Possibility. 142 pp.*

●Smith, Anthony D. The Concept of Social Change. *A Critique of the Functionalist Theory of Social Change. 208 pp.*

Routledge Social Science Journals

The British Journal of Sociology. *Edited by Terence P. Morris. Vol. 1, No. 1, March 1950 and Quarterly. Roy. 8vo. Back numbers available. An international journal with articles on all aspects of sociology.*

Economy and Society. *Vol. 1, No. 1. February 1972 and Quarterly. Metric Roy. 8vo. A journal for all social scientists covering sociology, philosophy, anthropology, economics and history. Back numbers available.*

Year Book of Social Policy in Britain, The. *Edited by Kathleen Jones. 1971. Published annually.*

Printed in Great Britain by Unwin Brothers Limited
The Gresham Press Old Woking Surrey
A member of the Staples Printing Group